The Complexity Paradox

The Complexity Paradox

The More Answers We Find,
the More Questions We Have

KENNETH L. MOSSMAN

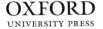

OXFORD
UNIVERSITY PRESS

Oxford University Press is a department of the University of
Oxford. It furthers the University's objective of excellence in research,
scholarship, and education by publishing worldwide.

Oxford   New York

Auckland   Cape Town   Dar es Salaam   Hong Kong   Karachi
Kuala Lumpur   Madrid   Melbourne   Mexico City   Nairobi
New Delhi   Shanghai   Taipei   Toronto

With offices in

Argentina   Austria   Brazil   Chile   Czech Republic   France   Greece
Guatemala   Hungary   Italy   Japan   Poland   Portugal   Singapore
South Korea   Switzerland   Thailand   Turkey   Ukraine   Vietnam

Oxford is a registered trademark of Oxford University Press
in the UK and certain other countries.

Published in the United States of America by
Oxford University Press
198 Madison Avenue, New York, NY 10016

Library of Congress Cataloging-in-Publication Data
Mossman, Kenneth L., 1946–2014.
The complexity paradox : the more answers we find, the more questions we have / Kenneth
Mossman.
pages cm
Includes glossary.
Includes bibliographical references and index.
ISBN 978–0–19–933034–8 (hardback)
1. Human biology—Philosophy.   2. Medicine—Philosophy.   3. Complexity
(Philosophy)   4. Biocomplexity.   I. Title.
QP34.5.M74 2014
612—dc23
2014005827

1 3 5 7 9 8 6 4 2
Printed in the United States of America
on acid-free paper

In memory of
Blaire V. Mossman

CONTENTS

Preface   xi
Acknowledgments   xvii
About the Author   xix

1. The Complexity Paradox   1

   WHAT IS LIFE?   7

      Information Storage and Retrieval   7

      Complex Structure and Organization   8

      Energy Use and Metabolism   9

      Responsiveness to Changes in the Environment   11

      Capacity for Growth and Development   12

   REDEFINING LIFE   13

   A ROADMAP TO THE BOOK   15

2. Laws to Live By   18

   NATURE HAS NO CHOICES   18

   THE MOTHER OF ALL LAWS   20

   LAWS ARE NOT ALWAYS RIGHT AND DO NOT PREDICT EVERYTHING   25

   LAWS OF PHYSICS AND REDUCTIONISM   28

   DETERMINISTIC LAWS AND LIFE   30

3. Forces of Nature   32

   MASS TRANSIT   33

   THE ELECTRIC SLIDE   38

   DRIVING FORCES   45

   ALL PUMPED UP   47

   MAY THE FORCE BE WITH YOU   49

4. Biological Complexity   51

  SYSTEM CONDITIONS AND STATES   52

  COMPLEXITY MADE SIMPLE   55

      Complex Biological Systems Have Many Components That Interact Nonlinearly
          and Are Interdependent   55
      Complex Systems Behave Unpredictably   56
      Complex Systems Show Fractal Geometry and Physiology   58
      Complex Systems Exhibit Emergent Properties   59

  COMPLEXITY IN ACTION   62

  COMPLEXITY IN HEALTH AND DISEASE   66

5. A Free and Independent Life   70

  THE IMPORTANCE OF BEING STABLE   71

  FEEDBACK CONTROL   78

  ACID-BASE BUFFERS   81

  RHYTHMS OF LIFE   82

  MORE THAN ENOUGH   83

  RANDOM WALKS   86

  THE WISDOM OF NATURE   89

6. Altered States   92

  SCHRÖDINGER'S CAT   93

  TOO MANY THINGS CAN GO WRONG   95

  SEARCH AND DESTROY   99

  IN THE EYE OF THE BEHOLDER   107

  MEDICINE WITHOUT BORDERS   109

  BEYOND THERAPY   111

  NOTHING IS SIMPLE   112

7. The Trinity   114

  THREE DISEASES   115

      Obesity   117
      Diabetes   119
      Heart Disease   120

  CAUSES AND RISKS   120

  WHERE'S WALDO?   126

  PUT THE GUN DOWN   131

8. The Mother of All Diseases   134

A BRIEF CANCER OVERVIEW   135

A COMPLEXITY PERSPECTIVE   141

   Disease Progression Is Unpredictable   142

   Complexity Is Evident at Multiple Scales   142

   Complex Systems Require Energy   142

   The Root Causes of Disease Are Masked by Complexity   143

   Complexity Offers Multiple Ways to Attack Disease   145

OTHER PERSPECTIVES   146

   Cancer Development Is a Multistage Process   146

   Cancer Is an Evolutionary and Ecological Process   147

   Cancer Is a Systems Biology Problem   148

A CONSOLIDATED VIEW   150

SEARCH AND DESTROY   152

COMPLEXITY AND PUBLIC HEALTH   154

   Screening   155

   Prevention   158

9. Brain Drain   163

UNIQUE COMPLEXITY   164

   The Brain as an Information Processor   165

   Brain States and Mental States   166

   Modularity and Plasticity   167

   Mind and Body   167

ROAD TO OBLIVION   168

10. Desperately Seeking Methuselah   177

SEEDS OF AGING   180

WORN-OUT BODIES   182

   Immune System Failure   182

   Slowed Metabolism   184

CHEATING DEATH   185

BUILDING BETTER HUMANS?   187

   Better Housekeeping   188

   Radical Solutions   189

   Inflammatory Control   189

   Making Sense of Aging   190

AGING AS COMPLEXITY   191

11. Emergence Medicine   193

    EMERGENCE   194

    DIMENSIONS OF COMPLEXITY   196

    EVOLUTION VERSUS FUNCTIONAL DYNAMICS   197

    BEYOND COMPREHENSION?   199

    A UNIFIED THEORY OF BIOLOGY   202

    PREDICTIONS   203

    FINAL THOUGHTS   206

Glossary   209
Notes   223
Selected Bibliography   249
Index   251

PREFACE

Recent discoveries and technological developments in the life sciences, especially in genomics, proteomics, informatics, and nanotechnology posit new challenges and possibilities for human medicine. Techno-optimists envision a bright future in which science and technology will remediate the miseries of the human condition. In the new age, people will live longer, healthier lives, and chronic degenerative diseases including Alzheimer's disease and cancer will become a thing of the past.

But is this realistic? Human biology and chronic human diseases are structurally and functionally complex. Complex systems behave unpredictably and cannot be reduced to simple quantitative or mathematical descriptions. Biological and physiologic complexity arises from the very large number of interacting network elements (molecules, cells, and so forth) and regulatory feedback loops over a wide range of spatial and temporal scales. Great strides have been made in medical diagnostics and therapy, and we have every reason to be optimistic about the future, but the inherent complexities of life limit what we can ultimately know and understand about the human body and disease.

Nonetheless, a complexity perspective promises to open new vistas to a better understanding of pathophysiologic processes. One of the key challenges in contemporary medicine and public health is early detection of chronic degenerative diseases. Finding and treating cancers and Alzheimer's disease at early stages saves lives and improves quality of life. A complexity perspective demands a multidisciplinary approach to solving these challenging diseases. Computational sciences, genomics, proteomics, and systems biology offer powerful ways to evaluate signaling networks and other features of complex systems to develop novel assays for drug effects and toxicities and to create new diagnostic and therapeutic tools for disease management.

This book is about complexity and its central role in human biology and medicine. "Complexity" means the whole is more than the sum of the parts. Behavior of many complex systems is inherently chaotic, which means it is impossible to predict and to describe fully in a quantitative way.[1] "Chaos" refers to nonlinear behaviors where small changes in one part of the system lead to disproportionate and unpredictable changes some time later in the entire system. This is often seen in drug therapies where unexpected complications are observed in parts of the body unrelated to the disease.

The unpredictable behavior that characterizes complexity arises from the sensitive dependence on initial conditions. What happens in the future is determined by what is happening now and has little to do with what happened in the past. Unless the system can be fully and accurately described at a particular time, any forecasting of system behavior is subject to large uncertainties. Even small inaccuracies in describing initial conditions mean that future behavior is unknowable. In complex biological systems, initial conditions cannot be fully described because the systems themselves are not fully understood.

Discovery in almost every field of science, including biology and medicine, has been based on the doctrine of reductionism, the idea that natural processes should be explainable by analyzing the component parts and that higher-level explanations cannot be fundamental. Reductionist explanations have been sought to explain higher brain cortical functions and economic and social phenomena. For example, the economic sciences and social dynamics, according to reductionists, should be explainable on the basis of human behavior. In turn, human behavior is explainable in terms of biological processes, which are further explained in terms of chemistry and physics.

But reductionist perspectives cannot explain complex phenomena. Language and other higher-order brain functions cannot be understood by examining individual neurons and their connections because language is an emergent property of the brain. Alzheimer's disease cannot be completely explained by examining aberrant proteins and neurofibrillary tangles. The disease and all its behavioral manifestations represent emergent properties of abnormal cortical functions.

In biology and medicine, ultimate explanations will come from systems-level perspectives. To be sure, our understanding of cancer has benefited considerably from a reductionist perspective—studies of cancerous cells and how they differ from normal ones. But cancer is a complex disease. As cancer progresses, it becomes more complex because the disease gradually becomes more than just a population of aberrant cells. Understanding cancer and other chronic degenerative diseases that ravage the body requires a holistic perspective that reveals disease-specific emergent properties.

Complexity demands we rethink our approach to medicine and disease. The cell theory of disease—a reductionist view proposed by Rudolf Virchow in the nineteenth century—argues that diseases like cancer can be completely understood at the cellular level. But the inherent uncertainties in complexity suggest otherwise. Biology and medicine are confronted by a complexity paradox—the more we learn about complex systems the more questions we ask. Our growing understanding of cancer is a good example. The discovery of cancer genes led to questions about how these genes regulate growth of cancer cells. The answers to those questions revealed that genes talk to one another through large, overlapping and complicated networks. Now many scientists are using network analysis and computational methods to explore how these networks function. What we learn from these studies will be important in addressing questions about how tumors grow and spread within the body.

Uncertainty means that we can never know everything there is to know about cancer and other chronic degenerative diseases. The specter of not knowing everything is the driving force behind research and the pursuit of knowledge to gradually chip away at our ignorance and learn enough about the disease to control it. The focus on complexity clearly distinguishes this book from the conventional approach taken in most general books on biology and medicine. The last half of the book addresses chronic degenerative human diseases as examples of complex phenomena emerging from the complexity of the human body itself. Alzheimer's disease, cancer, heart disease, obesity, and type 2 diabetes are discussed in detail because they represent key challenges in contemporary medicine and public health. Complexity is evident at every level of biological organization from subcellular organelles to organismal communities. A complexity perspective is a useful tool or framework in understanding the disease and controlling it. This book argues that the traditional medical approach of focusing on specific diseased tissues or organs should be supplemented with a holistic, system-wide approach that considers disease as a whole-body problem. Chronic diseases affect the entire person not just a specific tissue.

This book fills a critical niche in the world of biology, medicine, and public health. The human body and other complex systems cannot be easily unpacked and understood by examining component parts and their connections. Instead, interdisciplinary and system-level approaches are necessary to reveal characteristics of complexity and emergence in solving problems in health and management and prevention of disease.

The book makes significant predictions from complexity theory that lead to some surprising conclusions about health and disease.

- Chronic degenerative diseases arise as small perturbations in one part of the body but eventually have system-wide effects. To understand chronic disease is to understand the complexity of the human body.

- Complex diseases have no memory. Most chronic diseases take years if not decades to appear. Once the disease has developed, specific causes cannot be identified. Therapy is uncoupled from causality. Fortunately, treatment success is not contingent on knowing the cause. Doctors are trained to look for causes and why diseases happen. But once the disease is diagnosed, the cause(s), if any, don't matter. What matters is getting to the disease early enough that treatment can be effective.

- Diseases of complexity may occur spontaneously without any obvious cause. As a consequence, risks associated with small doses of disease-causing agents cannot be reliably measured because these small risks cannot be easily distinguished from spontaneous disease risks. Although disease probabilities can be assigned to a population, who in the population will get the disease is unknowable. The implications for public health policy are considerable because disease-causing agents, particularly carcinogens, are regulated to very low doses at enormous economic costs.

- The clinical course of disease and clinical response to therapy are unpredictable in the individual patient. However, certain tests are available to determine whether a patient is appropriately responsive to specific therapies.

- Chronic degenerative diseases like cancer and Alzheimer's disease cannot be eradicated, but early detection and therapy can delay progression and extend quality of life. Screening tests to detect disease in asymptomatic populations is not helpful for everyone. The effectiveness of screening tests is contingent on identifying high-risk groups.

In writing this book I have assumed an undergraduate knowledge of natural science primarily in biology and to a lesser extent in physics. The book introduces the phenomenon of complexity in human biology and medicine—an exciting and fast-moving field of science. Complexity demands we think about life processes in novel ways. Traditional scientific methods as presented in college science courses are often inadequate to explain emergence, chaos, and other characteristics of living complex systems. Reductionist approaches cannot fully explain system-level phenomena. What I am trying to accomplish here is to provide a new perspective on how we look at health and disease. The body is not simply a collection of independent physiological systems whose functions are coordinated by other integrating systems. Complexity argues everything is connected and changing one system may have consequences for other systems. In disease one or more tissues are directly affected by a pathological process, but that also means unrelated tissues feel the consequences because of the massive interconnectedness that is at the heart of complexity.

Complexity forces us to rethink how we do medicine and public health. What should a clinician do differently when considering a constellation of signs and symptoms within a complex system? How can complexity theory shape or guide public health programs when causal factors may be difficult if not impossible to identify? I discuss these and related questions as problems of complexity that require system-wide solutions rather than individual component analyses. For example, homeostasis is a concept used in medicine and physiology to refer to equilibrium or balance among various systems of the organism. Only through the framework of complexity theory can we understand how homeostasis is created and maintained in health and lost in disease.

The volume includes a select bibliography that will be useful to any reader who wishes to engage the issues further. The text is purely descriptive; no mathematical equations are included. Instead, figures are used to illustrate functional relationships. Some scientific language and medical terminology have been assumed. A glossary is included at the end of the book defining briefly many of the important terms used throughout.

The book may also serve as supplemental reading in the college classroom. This is not another textbook. Instead it is a collection of advanced topics focusing on complexity phenomena in human biology and medicine. The book is detailed and explores difficult subject material that is best suited to advanced study by students in graduate programs in biology, physiology, bioengineering, and related areas, and students studying medicine and veterinary medicine. The volume as a whole or as individual chapters could be offered as readings in college-level courses in basic medical sciences, biology, biochemistry, medical anthropology, physics, physiology, and public health.

A complexity perspective establishes a novel conceptual framework in biology. We usually think of Darwinian evolution, cell biology, and homeostasis as main theories of biology, and these are often taught as distinct and separate topics in the college science curriculum. Complexity science is rarely if ever discussed, yet it is the overarching theory that links traditional biological theories. A curriculum centered on complexity science as a unifying theme in biology provides for a comprehensive and inclusive exploration of the vast world of biology and medicine. The challenge in today's college classroom is building effective conceptual frameworks to allow students to organize and understand factual information. With Bing, Google, and other Internet search engines, students are able to gather facts about anything without ever leaving their dormitory rooms. Complexity theory provides the conceptual framework that allows students to make sense of all the biological data and concepts they run across.

The book is the product of my thinking about two very different challenges in biology and medicine—one research, the other teaching. The majority of my research career has been devoted to understanding the problem of cancer causation by low doses of ionizing radiation as encountered, for instance, in medical imaging. Measuring radiogenic cancer risks in populations has been very difficult, and estimates have large uncertainties. What we can say with a high level of confidence is that, if there is a risk from low-level radiation exposure, it is too small to measure reliably. We know quite a bit about the general behavior of cancers in the clinical setting, but information from epidemiologic studies to understand what causes cancer has been limited because radiogenic cancer leaves no unique signature and the number of nonradiogenic cancers overwhelms the number of radiogenic ones. This signal-to-noise problem is exacerbated at low doses of radiation. Cell and molecular studies have been very helpful in elucidating early events in carcinogenesis. What is missing is a complete understanding of the cancer process from the time cells become cancerous to the clinical presentation of disease, and this is where a complexity perspective is critically important: the notion that cancer is more than just a collection of bad cells and that the disease behaves as its own complex system nested in a larger complex system, the human body.

I have taught introductory college biology for many years and have always been troubled by the fragmented approach traditional college biology has taken. In many institutions, college biology is taught in two separate domains. One domain is "little" biology, focusing on the biology of cells or individual multicellular organisms. The second domain is "big" biology and looks at life on a population and global level, focusing on animal behavior, Darwinian evolution, ecology, population genetics, and such topics. What is missing is a coherent and comprehensive framework that ties together all of biology. That unifying principle is complexity.

The world is filled with phenomena that are exceedingly complex, including the function (and failure) of the biological processes that occur in our own bodies. Over the past few decades, researchers from a variety of disciplines, including physics, mathematics, computer science, social science, climatology, and biology, have attempted to understand the underlying forces that give rise to and shape complex phenomena. While there is a literature on complexity and human health, it is not a central part of either the college biology curriculum or the material that is taught to medical school students. This book fills that gap and has also been written to inspire researchers to incorporate principles of complexity theory into their research, and to give anyone interested in the complex nature of health and disease a sense of the power of complexity theory to explain disease-related phenomena.

Complexity is the biology and medicine of the twenty-first century. Contemporary problems in biology and medicine cannot be solved by the classical approaches of traditional scientific disciplines. Complexity-driven interdisciplinary organizations provide for novel strategies and creative out-of-the-box thinking to address contemporary problems in biology and medicine by consolidating computational sciences, neurobiology, systems biology, engineering, chemistry, and physics. Nothing in biology or medicine makes sense except in light of complexity.[2] Complexity is the unifying theory of life.

ACKNOWLEDGMENTS

During the six years I spent writing *The Complexity Paradox*, I had the good fortune to work with and be surrounded by many friends, colleagues, collaborators, and students without whose assistance I could not have completed the book.

My biggest challenge in writing this book was understanding normal and disease processes in living systems as problems of complexity. This meant thinking about biology and medicine in novel and unconventional ways. What was surprising to me was the extent to which features of complexity in a diverse set of natural systems inform the complexity of life. Lively discussions with Jerry Coursen, Peter Rez, and Tim Newman were very helpful in understanding chaos theory in complex systems and nonlinear dynamics that occur in many biological processes. Eli Fenichel was masterful in describing the complex nature of economic sciences. I thoroughly enjoyed conversations with Rob Page on the interesting complex behaviors observable in large social insect communities. Discussions with Jim Collins, Jim Elser, Manfred Laubichler, and John Nagy clarified what I thought about dynamic processes in ecological and evolutionary systems and how they contribute to complexity in cancer and other chronic human diseases. These discussions reinforced the importance of distinguishing evolutionary processes from functional dynamics in cancer and other diseases considered to have evolutionary origins. I had several highly informative discussions with Howard Kutchai on the central place of the macroscopic laws of physics in physiological processes from which complex behaviors emerge.

During my many years in the academy, I have had the good fortune of being surrounded by many talented and enthusiastic students. There are too many names to list here, but I call out Conley Kelley, Cassie Majestic, Taylor McGlone, and Dana Schulze in particular for their research and writing skills. Their work saved me many hours of searching for and assembling research materials.

I thank the medical records staffs at several hospitals and clinics in the Phoenix, Arizona, area for allowing me to review medical records of patients with diseases discussed in detail in the opening paragraphs of several chapters. Names of patients have been changed to protect patient and family privacy. An exception is the cholera case introducing chapter 3, "Forces of Nature." The death of Pyotr Ilyich Tchaikovsky from cholera is well known, and details of the case are in the public domain.

Mary Lou Bertucci copyedited the entire volume. Her magnificent writing skills and careful attention to detail turned my draft chapters into a readable tome. Sabine DeViche and James Baxter did a masterful job preparing a number of the figures. Miriam Gottlieb, Tim Jorgensen, and Virgil Renzulli made many helpful editorial comments.

Joan Bossert, my editor at Oxford University Press, has been a constant source of encouragement. From the beginning, Joan's keen sense of the importance of complexity science in neurobiology and other biomedical disciplines has guided me in structuring the book to reflect the diversity of applications of complexity in human biology and disease. I am grateful to Joan for believing in this book and shepherding my book proposal through the review process.

I take full responsibility for the contents of this book. I took great care to credit properly and reflect accurately the views and findings of others. Any errors, omissions, or misrepresentations are my fault and entirely unintentional.

Finally, I thank my late wife Blaire V. Mossman, who was a pillar of strength throughout the early research and manuscript-writing process. She served as a sounding board for many ideas, and her perspectives were particularly valuable to me in writing several chapters. This book is for you, sweetheart!

Kenneth L. Mossman
Scottsdale, Arizona
May 2013

ABOUT THE AUTHOR

Our brother Ken had a thirst for knowledge that drove him to excel in his academic pursuits. He was a scientist and a teacher. He could conceive of nothing better than life in academia. Over the course of his career he received many awards and much recognition for his achievements and contributions to the academic and scientific communities. He harboured no thought of retirement and entered his senior years with his interests and pursuits expanding. He was recently honoured to have been appointed by the President of the United States to serve on the bipartisan Defense Nuclear Facilities Safety Board and had temporarily moved from his longtime home in Scottsdale, Arizona, back to Washington, DC, where he had previously lived while in his first professorship at Georgetown University, with great anticipation for this new venture. Ken's appointment was confirmed in November 2013 and he was sworn in in early December. At the same time, he was anxiously awaiting the publication of this book. Ken, who had suffered the loss of his beloved wife Blaire to brain cancer in April 2011, suddenly and unexpectedly died of an apparent heart attack on January 8, 2014. He was 67 years old.

Samuel Mossman
Michael Mossman

1

The Complexity Paradox

There are two phenomenological domains in nature. The simple domain, which is neither exciting nor creative, is populated by events and processes characterized by linear dynamics and determinism; these linear systems are predictable and obedient to the laws of nature. For example, an apple falls from a tree; the sun rises in the East and sets in the West; we can accurately predict the trajectory of a baseball if we know its current position and velocity and then apply Newton's laws of motion with some adjustments. A system is defined as linear when the output is proportional to the input; if the system input is doubled, the system output is also doubled. Natural processes characterized by linear dynamics are at the heart of Newtonian mechanics and reflect the traditional Holy Grail of science—the use of objective, quantitative measurements to understand and predict the behavior of natural systems.

The French mathematician Pierre-Simon Laplace first articulated scientific determinism in 1814:

> We may regard the present state of the universe as the effect of its past and the cause of its future. An intellect which at a certain moment would know all forces that set nature in motion, and all positions of all items of which nature is composed, if this intellect were also vast enough to submit these data to analysis, it would embrace in a single formula the movements of the greatest bodies of the universe and those of the tiniest atom; for such an intellect nothing would be uncertain and the future just like the past would be present before its eyes.[1]

Implicit in Laplace's formalism is the notion that every event has a cause and the Universe is highly ordered and predictable. But not all natural systems are subject to complete quantitative descriptions and predictability. The principles of thermodynamics and quantum mechanics establish that some natural systems are indeterminate and express properties of uncertainty, entropy, and irreversibility—features that are incompatible with determinism. Instead, indeterminate systems behave in a nonlinear and unpredictable fashion. Unlike in a simple, linear system, in a nonlinear system, doubling the system input leads to something other than a doubling of the output. In nonlinear systems, initial conditions dictate system response; thus, without knowledge of initial conditions, system responses become unpredictable, and the future cannot be used to reconstruct the past. For example, current weather conditions are not helpful in reconstructing weather two weeks ago. In linear systems, the future is dictated by the past, and any future state of the system accurately recounts what happened in the past. Thus, nonlinear systems are endowed with an arrow of time that is absent in linear systems.

Nonlinear dynamics are at the heart of complex systems and represent the second domain of nature. Events and processes in the complexity domain are unpredictable and can be highly creative. As complexity processes progress, all sorts of surprises pop up along the way. The complexity domain encompasses a startling variety of natural phenomena, including complex weather patterns, cancer, cardiovascular physiology, Darwinian evolution, ecology, economic forecasting, and the shapes of snowflakes. In the context of complexity, Newtonian dynamics, the foundation of scientific prediction that has dominated science for over three hundred years, must be questioned and viewed as having limited application. Although much of the foundational work in nonlinear dynamics and complexity theory was initiated in the 1960s and 1970s, Henri Poincaré, arguably the most eminent scientist of his generation, first suggested that some phenomena in nature are too complex to reduce to simple mathematical treatment and escape understanding and prediction using classical approaches. His treatise on chance and sources of uncertainty foreshadowed developments of chaos theory almost a century later:

> Why have meteorologists such difficulty in predicting the weather with any certainty? Why is it that showers and even storms seem to come by chance, so that many people think it quite natural to pray for rain or fine weather, though they would consider it ridiculous to ask for an eclipse by prayer?. . . Small differences in the initial conditions produce very great ones in the final phenomenon. A small error in the former will produce an enormous error in the latter. Prediction becomes impossible, and we have the fortuitous phenomenon.[2]

Poincaré's idea of initial conditions showed that determinism and predictability are separate and distinct problems. If initial conditions are known exactly, then the behavior of complex systems can be predicted exactly. However, even the slightest error in describing initial conditions flips the system from deterministic to unpredictable. The evolution of such a system is often chaotic in the sense that a small perturbation in the initial state might lead to a radically different later state than would be produced by the unperturbed system. Chaos theory describes how deterministic systems can adopt behaviors that are impossible to predict.

It may be helpful to think about initial conditions and predictions in terms of a stock car race. The starting order should provide a fairly good prediction of the order of cars after the first few laps; although the prediction will not be perfect because of unforeseen events like crashes and engine failures, it will be a lot better than a random guess. Thereafter, the starting order becomes increasingly less predictive because cars pass one another, faster cars overlap the slower ones, tires are blown, and crashes occur. By the time the race is half over, the original order of cars is completely jumbled. Furthermore, knowing the order of the cars at the race's midpoint tells us nothing about the order of cars at the start of the race, or who the winner will be.

The uncoupling of the order of cars at the beginning and midpoint of the race occurs because of incomplete information about initial conditions. All we know is the starting order, but, to predict the order of cars at the midpoint, we would also need to know which cars will crash, which cars will overlap others, the speed of cars, the number of pit stops for any given car, and so forth. In other words, we need to do the impossible—predict the future. Only when initial conditions are fully known can the outcome of the race and the order of cars at any time during the race be predicted. However, initial conditions can never be known completely because human (driver) behavior and car performance are indeterminate factors influencing the race.[3]

Complexity forces us to think about natural phenomena in a holistic rather than elementalist way. Problems in complex systems are best resolved by looking at the whole picture rather than individual parts. Classical physics approaches do not apply to complex systems because these laws are valid only for linear dynamics.

Complexity also necessitates an inversion of Ockham's razor. Ockham's razor, or the principle of parsimony, attributed to William of Ockham, a fourteenth-century logician and Franciscan friar, asserts that, among competing explanations, the simplest one is preferred, all other things being equal. In science, it is used as a loosely guiding principle when evaluating competing scientific theories. By taking the simpler alternative (the one with the fewest parameters), the chance of compounding errors is reduced. But simplicity implies that understanding system components and their interactions is sufficient to explain system behavior. In complex systems, the assumptions of component independence and causality are invalid, requiring deeper explanations.

Reductionist explanations of complex systems do not account for emergent properties and nonlinear behaviors. Inherent uncertainties in complex systems due to incomplete knowledge of initial conditions mean we cannot fully understand complexity. Indeed, as complex systems become better defined, they are understood less: paradoxically, progress means more questions than answers. Even the act of measuring complexity introduces uncertainties in observations and explanations. However, while we cannot fully understand complexity, we can understand complexity better than we currently do. Consider meteorology: although exact weather predictions remain elusive, considerable progress has been made in forecasting. Thanks to better computer models, meteorologists are much better today at predicting weather conditions for the next week than they were twenty years ago. Still, even with improvement, the impact of complex systems like the weather far exceeds our knowledge of such systems.

Living systems are unique in nature because they are simultaneously simple and complex. Biological and physiologic complexity arises from the very large number of interacting network elements (molecules, cells, and so forth) and regulatory feedback loops over a wide range of spatial and temporal scales. Biological systems are complex as reflected by the presence of structural and functional features that repeat themselves at progressively lower spatial and temporal scales (called fractals). Fractal anatomy is seen in the tracheobronchial tree and in the His-Purkinje network that controls the heartbeat. Fractal processes like the fluctuations seen in the healthy heartbeat generate oscillatory behaviors that allow the body to adapt to changing environmental conditions including survival threats and stresses.

The coupling of simple, deterministic processes with complex structure and function is essential to survival. Although the fundamental engines of life are deterministic processes that obey the laws of physics, what truly define life are nonlinear and chaotic processes that occur as a result of relatively simple interactions within networks composed of large numbers of interconnected and interdependent elements. The result is that most biological processes, including the resting heart rate and blood sugar levels, exhibit dynamic behavior even though their outputs look stable. Not all complex systems in nature exhibit chaotic behaviors but, in general, living systems do as part of the adaptive response.

Networks appear at every level of biological organization—from gene regulatory networks at the subcellular level, to networks of cells in tissues, to social networks of individual multicellular organisms. Chaotic behavior manifests itself in a number of ways, most commonly as irregular fluctuations or oscillations in system outputs, which means that small changes in system inputs result in large, disproportionate changes in outputs. At the macroscopic level, nonlinear behaviors confer stability that allows for system adaptation. Heart rate looks predictable at the macroscopic level—at rest, the heart rate does not change very much when measured on an hourly basis. But when viewed at a microscopic level—measurements made every minute—heart rate fluctuates in a nonlinear and unpredictable way. These fluctuations allow for rapid changes in heart rate as physiological states demand.

Life is like riding a bicycle—stability is achieved when small, almost imperceptible steering adjustments are made by the rider to maintain balance. The human body uses feedback loops to maintain a stable state and physiological balance. Small variations occur constantly in heart rate, blood pressure, and other physiological parameters and serve as the agent of adaptation critical for survival. Without chaos, there is no life.

Deterministic processes are central to life because they follow well-known natural laws and are, therefore, predictable: outputs are always the same if conditions remain unchanged. Thus, the process of transporting molecular oxygen from the air sacs in the lungs to the blood for conveyance to the tissues is highly predictable and governed by the law of diffusion. On the other hand, large variations in the amount of oxygen delivered to tissues disrupt normal metabolism and physiological processes. Stability cannot be conserved if operating systems have highly variable operating characteristics.

Stability means the body's internal environment is relatively constant. In a healthy individual, body temperature is constant over time, so is the concentration of red blood cells in the circulating blood. Both are necessary for the body to operate efficiently. If body temperature and pH were allowed to vary, the functions of enzymes and other biologically important molecules would be compromised.

However, living systems also require an adaptive capacity; otherwise, changes in the external environment would threaten survival, just as the bicycle rider would topple over if he or she never adjusted steering. Although core body temperature is 37°C (98°F), the body can function quite well when external temperatures are much lower or higher than this. In Phoenix, Arizona, summer temperatures exceeding 43°C (110°F) are not uncommon. Although it is uncomfortable for some, everyone usually functions quite well because our core body temperature does not change much due to adaptive processes that increase cooling (like sweating) and decrease waste heat production. This reaction happens quickly and is facilitated by the nervous system and endocrine system—coordinating systems that exhibit nonlinear behavior.

Small changes in the environment often result in disproportionately large responses by the organism. A person threatening your life with a knife or a gun is a visual stimulus received by the brain. The human response is a cascade of quick reactions, characterized by accelerated heart rate, rapid breathing, and muscle contractions to escape the threat. All living systems are capable of toggling between a stable, vegetative state and a state of high arousal characterized by excitation and quick reactions to changing environmental conditions.

To move easily from a stable state to arousal requires the body to operate at the edge of chaos. Animals in nature clearly illustrate this situation. Animals in the wild continuously monitor the environment for both food and threats. They are constantly prepared to escape life-threatening situations and also to defend their territory from predators. We can never predict the precise behavior of humans or animals because initial conditions, including the presence of seemingly minor threats, can never be known exactly. We can never know precisely where Darwinian evolution might lead because the initial conditions that fully describe living systems, their environment and other determinants of evolution, cannot be known precisely. Evolution is a dimension of complexity that escapes prediction. The stock market is a byproduct of social interactions that is also complex; we can never predict future value of stocks exactly because initial conditions that govern future value cannot be known with certainty at the present time. To know the initial conditions of any complex system is to know the future.

The paradox of life, simultaneously simple and complex, simultaneously predictable and unpredictable, has been recognized for centuries. In the seventeenth century, René Descartes tried to explain some of the phenomena of the human body in mechanistic terms based on earlier studies by William Harvey on the structure of the heart and the flow of blood. Descartes's dualism doctrine, claiming a distinction between body and mind, allowed for the partitioning of "simple" mechanistic explanations about how the body worked and "complex," mysterious processes of the mind, including spirituality and consciousness.[4] Not until the twentieth century, however, did we realize that certain brain processes can be modeled mechanistically, but higher order neural processes such as language escape purely deterministic description.

Life is paradoxical because it exhibits apparently contradictory characteristics. How can relatively simple interneuron signaling explain language and other higher order brain functions? One would think that the nerve cells supporting language would have an equal level of complexity. The explanation is found in the concept of emergence—a phase-like transition occurring in systems made up of relatively simple but highly interconnected components that leads to complex system-level behavior. Communications between components may be very simple, yet the behavior of the system can be complex. The emergent behavior of the system can be explained in part by the components themselves, but the behavior of the components cannot explain the emergent properties of the system as a whole.

Complexity in living systems refers to their emergent properties and how system components relate to one another. Switching out certain components can have disastrous consequences because the massive interconnectedness among components might not be conserved, thus impacting the performance of the entire system. Replacing the auditory nerve tracts in a deaf person is not likely to restore normal hearing, because the complexities of neural networks supporting hearing cannot be fully reconstructed. We don't fully understand the architecture of the auditory cortex in the brain. Cochlear implants work because they enhance signaling in nerve tracts that are already there.

This is a book about human biology, human disease, and the physical laws and processes that govern life. The focus is on the simple and complex biological processes that operate at the same time and in parallel within living systems. Normal physiology requires the body to be stable in order to carry out functions efficiently but also have the capacity to respond rapidly and vigorously to changes in internal and external environmental inputs. Human disease may be viewed physiologically as a shift away from the delicate balance between stability and adaptability.

The uniformity of life is based on a broad spectrum of biochemical and physiological processes that humans share with lower life forms, including bacteria. Simple life processes are governed by the same suite of laws that explain many well-known phenomena in physics and chemistry. For example, one of the central laws in physics and chemistry and a key principle in sustaining life is the second law of thermodynamics. Although first formulated to describe heat flow, this law is a general description of the flow of energy in any system and is the underlying principle for almost every physiologic process. All life forms are based on the same set of chemical and physical processes. Thus, humans are a part of the continuum of life and occupy no special place in the biosphere.[5]

What distinguishes humans from other living species are complex processes, particularly those associated with the brain and neurobiological functions. What makes humans "human" and what it means to be "human" are questions that have been pondered by philosophers, scientists, and theologians for centuries and are well beyond the scope of this book.[6] Suffice it to say that the major competitive advantage of humans lies in the brain's unique ability to couple external social, informational, and technological systems in such a way as to evolve distributed cognitive networks. The two major distinctive features of humans are toolmaking and language. (Other species have these capabilities but to a lesser degree.) Human technological advancements have led to significant cultural and social changes. Today, exciting new developments are on the horizon in nanotechnology, biotechnology, information technology, and cognitive sciences (collectively referred to as NBIC technologies). One of the next great technological achievements for humankind will be the union of toolmaking and language—giving computers the ability to understand speech. Progress has been made in these areas of system complexity but is still far from "Hal," the conversational computer conceived in Stanley Kubrick's movie *2001: A Space Odyssey*.

What Is Life?

What distinguishes living systems from nonliving ones? What properties do humans and other life forms share that make them alive? To be sure, diversity and unity both describe the living world. Millions of species exist on Earth, including microscopic life forms and a wide variety of animal and plant species. Although species are distinctive, all living systems share five common and unifying characteristics.[7]

Information Storage and Retrieval

Living systems require a highly stable system of information storage and retrieval. A stable source of information is critical to directing the functions of the organism at the cellular level. Information storage also needs to be stable during growth and development of the body and maintenance of self-renewing tissues like the skin, small intestine, and bone marrow. The information needed for construction and operation of cells is coded in the DNA (deoxyribonucleic acid). The genetic information is stored in the linear arrangement of nitrogenous bases in the DNA. Because DNA contains the information for making proteins, it directs cell processes by determining which proteins are produced and when. Information transfer from DNA to protein is complex and involves important intermediary nucleic acids called messenger RNA (ribonucleic acid) that help regulate protein synthesis. Proteins carry out a number of critical functions, including catalyzing biochemical reactions and facilitating transport of select substances in and out of cells. These proteins are extraordinarily specific in their interactions. Genetic information storage and retrieval are essentially universal—all cells speak the same genetic language, have the same basic design, are made of the same construction materials, and operate using essentially the same processes.[8]

The complete sequence of bases in human DNA is now known. It is believed there are approximately 23,000 genes in the human genome. Genes vary in length from a few hundred bases to tens of thousands of bases. The normal functions of many of these genes are still not fully understood, however. DNA specimens from many individuals can now be examined to identify variants in the human genome. Today, DNA chip technology is capable of scanning tens of thousands of genetic variants. Recognizing and cataloging genetic variants will help identify specific genes that influence vulnerability to a wide spectrum of human diseases, including cancer.

Is DNA the molecule of life, the molecule that makes living systems "living"? In May 2010, J. C. Venter and Hamilton Smith of the J. Craig Venter Institute announced that they had successfully made a bacterium with an artificial genome capable of sustained proliferation.[9] Whether life has been created in a laboratory remains arguable, but there is no question a threshold has been crossed. It is now a bit easier to imagine Aldous Huxley's *Brave New World* in which life forms are designed by computer and then grown to specifications in assembly-line fashion.

If life is an emergent process of certain organic-based complex systems, is DNA a necessary and sufficient requirement for the emergence of complexity? It would seem that DNA is a necessary but not sufficient ingredient of life. Genetic determinism is clearly required to establish and maintain fundamental features of complex living systems from single cells to the complex organization of various human tissues and organs, and this genetic determinism is obvious over generations. The structure of the human body has not changed in any meaningful way over many millennia, but, in certain tissues like the brain, aspects of complexity and function develop beyond the influence of the DNA. Functioning neurons have limited capacity to divide and replace damaged ones. The development of this fixed neuron population in the brain is DNA directed and is necessary for establishing the fixed neural topology and architecture common in all humans. Early in life, humans have almost all the neurons they will ever have. However, what distinguishes the mature brain from the newborn brain are the number and complexity of synapses (connections between neurons) and the development of neural pathways that occurs as the result of aging and experiences. These postnatal synapse formations are not genetically determined and suggest that DNA has little influence on the development and control of higher-order cortical functioning.[10]

So, the secret of "life" is not in the DNA. Although DNA plays a critical role in information storage and retrieval, the molecule itself does nothing other than serve as a template for key cellular processes through RNA and protein synthesis. DNA does not code for emergent properties or, more generally, the remarkable capacity of living systems to self-assemble and maintain a high degree of order. The secret to life is the process of emergence in complex systems. To solve the riddle of life, we need to understand how emergence happens and how cooperativity occurs among independent cells. Is emergence like a phase transition, or is it another kind of change of state that occurs when a threshold of complexity is reached?

Complex Structure and Organization

Living systems are highly ordered and complex in both structure and function. This remarkable order is observable even in single cells. Cell functions are compartmentalized to improve efficiency. The separation of functions allows for many cellular processes to occur independently and in parallel. Even in bacteria, where there are few compartments, a high level of order is associated with metabolism and cellular reproduction. In multicellular organisms, higher-order processes in tissues and organs necessitate segregation of specific functions: gas exchange occurs in the lungs, and blood filtration occurs in the kidneys. In multicellular organisms, tissue specialization requires central orchestration to coordinate functions. In humans and other multicellular animals, coordination is endowed in an endocrine system, a nervous system, and an immune system.

How much complexity and organization is required to minimally sustain life? Life may be considered as the organization of energy processing above some, not yet understood, threshold of complexity. The simplest free-living organism known is *Mycoplasma genitalium*, a tiny parasitic bacterium that lives in the digestive and genital tracts of primates.[11] The bug's genome contains only 580,000 base pairs and 482 protein-coding genes. *M. genitalium* has a diameter of 200–300 nanometers, smaller than some large viruses. Whether some kind of cellular structure is a minimal requirement to sustain acquisition and processing of energy and some hereditary capabilities is not known. We do know that the simplest requirements for life include a genome set and matched environment. Life cannot be sustained unless there is a sufficiently complex yet stable system that can process energy in an environment that has the supporting characteristics for life.

Energy Use and Metabolism

Energy is used by living systems to build and maintain order. Order takes on many forms. At the molecular level, one type of order is concentration gradients that are maintained through steady-state processes. Concentration gradients allow for the movement of ions and molecules across cell membranes. Without gradients, net movement of critical nutrients such as oxygen and glucose into cells and carbon dioxide out of cells would not be possible. Controlled movement of ions and molecules is the basis for important physiologic functions such as the generation and propagation of nerve impulses, gas exchange in the lung, and blood filtration in the kidney. Living systems exist in a steady state, requiring the input of energy to maintain systems at an operating level that is essentially time invariant.

The key to maintaining concentration gradients across cells is the operation of molecular pumps that move molecules against their concentration gradient. Without such pumps, gradients run down until an equilibrium condition is reached, characterized by no net movement of molecules (Figure 1.1). This does not mean that molecules no longer can cross the cell membrane. They do, but as many molecules cross the membrane barrier in one direction as in the other. The gradient serves as the driving force for the net movement of molecules across the cell membrane.

When steady-state conditions cannot be maintained (for example, cells cannot power ion pumps because of lack of oxygenated blood), concentration gradients quickly decay to the equilibrium condition. In the absence of gradients, death occurs because of the lack of net movement of molecules that are necessary for key physiological processes. Without input of energy and maintenance of the steady-state biochemical and physiologic systems, decay to an equilibrium condition in which no energy flows through the system occurs. To sustain steady-state conditions, there must be a constant influx of energy.

The equilibrium state is a special case of the steady state. It represents the lowest energy state of the system. Equilibrium is attained only when there are no net fluxes through ion channels and no net fluxes through pumps. Equilibrium is, thus, achieved only when the cell is dead. The difference between steady-state and equilibrium conditions is the difference between life and death.[12]

Energy flow varies markedly among human organs. The distribution of energy flow densities shown in Figure 1.2 reflects resting conditions. When the body responds to stress or is engaged in heavy exercise, marked changes in the distribution occur. Energy flow to the heart and skeletal muscles increases strikingly but not at the expense of requirements for normal central nervous system and renal function that are critical to the support of homeostasis, which is the process of maintaining a constant internal environment. Homeostasis must be maintained whether the body is in a resting or highly active state. Physiologic adjustments must be made quickly, particularly when any organism is trying to avoid serious injury or death. The acute energy demands are met by mobilizing energy stores in skeletal muscle and in the

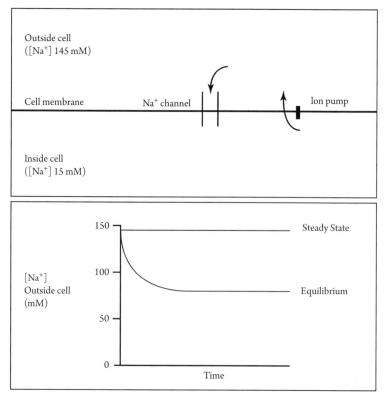

Figure 1.1 Steady-state processes are necessary to sustain life. The figure illustrates a simple steady-state system to maintain Na^+ concentration gradients across the cell membrane. Na^+ concentration is higher outside the cell than inside. When the sodium channel is open, Na^+ ions move into the cell by diffusion down the concentration gradient. This process will continue as long as a gradient is maintained. The Na^+ pump maintains the gradient by using energy to continue to pump Na^+ out of the cell. If the pump fails, steady-state conditions cannot be maintained, and the system quickly reaches equilibrium characterized by equal concentrations of Na^+ on either side of the membrane and zero net flow of Na^+.

liver (by converting glycogen, a storage form of glucose, to glucose). Further, the shift in energy flow to the heart and muscles is counterbalanced by reduced energy flow to the skin, intestines, and other organs that are less vital in the short term to maintaining homoeostasis. Usually, long-term energy demands (such as aerobic exercising) result in body weight loss if caloric intake remains constant.[13]

Energy flow density is a measure of metabolic activity. Oxygen consumption rate (a measure of metabolic rate) is very high in the brain, heart, and kidneys. The brain uses more oxygen than any other organ in the body, not surprising given the biological complexity and functions carried out by this organ. But on a per unit weight basis, the kidneys and heart have a higher energy flow density than the brain. The paired kidneys are only one-fourth as heavy as the brain yet consume about 20 percent of

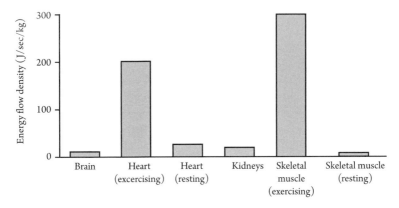

Figure 1.2 Energy flow density for selected metabolically active organs at rest and during exercise. Energy flow density is the energy flow rate (in joules per second) normalized to unit organ weight (in kilograms). Energy flow densities increase significantly in cardiac and skeletal muscle but do not change in the brain or kidneys during exercise.

the available oxygen in the body because of the energy demands for blood filtration and water and electrolyte balance.

Exercise does not cause an increase in functional requirements of the brain or kidneys. Blood flow to these organs does not change markedly during exercise, because these organs function optimally independent of the exercise state. The requirement for increased blood flow to muscle during exercise necessitates an increase in cardiac output. The increase in oxygen demand of the heart during exercise is met principally by augmenting coronary blood flow, because the resting heart extracts almost all the available oxygen. In skeletal muscle, both blood flow and oxygen extraction are increased significantly to meet physiologic demand.

Responsiveness to Changes in the Environment

Living systems can be thought of as complex organizational systems that are in a constant struggle to maintain their internal environments and respond appropriately to rapid changes in their external environments.

Because organisms reside in environments where abrupt changes can threaten survival, living systems must be able to respond to environmental changes (for example, toxins in the environment or threats from predators). Single-cell animals can respond by changing cell membrane characteristics to reduce or eliminate exposures to environmental threats. Some bacteria are even capable of physically moving away from a threatening environmental area. In multicellular organisms, the nervous system, endocrine system, and immune system coordinate responses to acute and chronic threats. Multicellular systems are linked to a sensory network (for vision, sound, touch, odor, and taste) that allows the organism to respond to ensure survival. Sensory networks are characterized by fast detection times so that organisms have sufficient time to respond to any perceived threats. The response to environmental changes occurs as a consequence of the requirement to maintain a constant internal environment for the maintenance and optimum operational efficiency of physiologic systems— namely, homeostasis.[14] Normal physiologic processes, including nerve impulse conduction, the heart beat, and blood filtration by the kidneys, lead to localized changes in homeostasis. The body expends considerable energy to return the systems to the steady-state condition and maintain homeostasis. If internal conditions are not stable, cellular metabolism and other important life processes could not operate in an optimal way. Disease diagnosis is based, in part, on observed deviations in specific physiologic parameters (for example, body temperature) from the homeostatic (normal) value.

Capacity for Growth and Development

Multicellular organisms must have extensive capacity to grow and to develop tissue specializations. Every multicellular organism starts out as a single cell. For humans, the usual nine-month gestation period requires that the fertilized egg undergo about forty divisions to reach a total cell population at birth of about one trillion cells. As the newborn further grows and develops, additional cell divisions take place, such that the adult has about ten trillion cells. Growth competence leads to a capacity for cell replacement. Damage or injury to tissues such as the skin or bone marrow can stimulate surviving cells to divide and replace damaged cells. Living systems enjoy dynamic steady states that are stable but not static. The human body changes continuously. Almost every cell in the body today was not there a few weeks or months ago (brain cells are an exception). Cells are continually replaced in cell renewal systems designed to supplant old functioning cells with new ones.[15]

Two divergent biological processes occur during growth and development. Cell proliferation through the process of mitosis results in the increase in cell numbers. One cell becomes two, two cells become four, and so on. In mitosis, the genetic information is conserved with a very high degree of fidelity, such that almost every cell in the adult contains the exact same genetic information as the fertilized egg from which it was derived.[16]

Differentiation is the process whereby cells acquire specialized functions. Multicellularity requires that the organism have specialized tissues to support different physiologic functions. Cells in the liver are different structurally and functionally from cells in the brain. Even though cells in different tissue have the same genetic makeup, specialization results by turning on or off certain genes in the genome. What distinguishes liver cells from brain cells are the genes activated or deactivated in one cell type but not in another. Deprogramming specialized cells so they acquire broader or different specializations necessitates control of gene regulation at the cellular level.

Cells that acquire specialization tend to lose their capacity to proliferate. Highly specialized cells such as brain cells, skeletal muscle cells, and red blood cells are not able to divide because they no longer have the proteins necessary to prepare for and to carry out mitosis. Cells that have a high proliferative capacity tend to be undifferentiated (that is, unspecialized) and lack the suite of proteins that confer specialized function, even though they retain the suite of proteins necessary for division. The reciprocal relationship between differentiation and proliferation is clearly illustrated in a rare form of bone marrow cancer called acute promyelocytic leukemia (APL).

Under normal conditions, promyelocytes do not divide and instead differentiate into mature white blood cells, but, in APL, the promyelocytes are transformed into cancer cells and do not differentiate. They seem to be stalled in an immature stage and retain the capacity to divide. The genetic defect for APL is a translocation involving chromosomes 15 and 17 that results in the activation of a cancer gene. The resulting fusion protein drives proliferation of promyelocytes and blocks differentiation.

The potential for differentiation and proliferation is a convergent property of stem cells. Stem cells share two important characteristics—self-renewal and differentiation. Whether a stem cell takes the path to self-renewal or the path to specialization depends on local environmental selection pressures. Stem cells exposed to certain growth factors may be stimulated to differentiate along a specific line of development. Stem cells are present in the early embryo and also to a limited extent in the adult. In the embryo, stem cells are pluripotent and have the capacity to differentiate into any tissue of the body. In the adult, stem cells reside in specific tissues and have a capacity to differentiate that is limited to the functions of that tissue. Bone marrow stem cells can make blood cells but not other types of cells. Because embryonic stem cells can become any tissue, in theory, they have enormous medical therapeutic potential for diseases such as Parkinson's and spinal cord injuries where the native tissue has little or no capacity to repair or replace damaged cells. The therapeutic value of adult stem cells has already been realized. Bone marrow stem cell transplantation is being successfully used for the treatment of multiple myeloma and other cancers.

Redefining Life

Characterizing living systems does not really help us understand what life is because it does not provide a deeper understanding of the essence of life. We do know that life would appear to be highly improbable in the context of the laws of physics. Indeed, life *appears* to defy the laws of nature. Life counters the natural tendency toward disorder by importing and channeling energy in the inexorable march toward complexity. Erwin Schrödinger in *What Is Life?* argues that life is distinct from other processes in nature.[17] But are these distinctive life processes governed by some heretofore unknown set of laws unrelated to the known laws of physics? Life's footprint on Earth is quite broad, not constrained to some narrow environmental requirements. We see life everywhere, from boiling hot springs in Yosemite to the dry valleys of Antarctica, from deep sea vents miles below the surface to willowy clouds miles above the ground. The discovery of life in extreme environments raises important questions about the possibility that life could arise through unknown processes and that extraterrestrial forms of life might exist. Clearly, the search for a definition of life is in its infancy. Some scientists are taking a reductionist approach by trying to build life from scratch. But life cannot be made in a test tube simply by mixing together various inorganic and organic substances. Although scientists at the J. Craig Venter Institute have been successful in getting a synthetic chromosome to function by inserting it into a living bacterium, it must be emphasized that this is not creation of life in a test tube. Life is not what Mary Shelley's *Frankenstein* would have us believe—something that can be created by simply assembling body parts.

The observation of a single type of life on Earth (carbon-based with a common genetic code and processes to make proteins) hampers any real effort to fully define life and set its boundaries because no comparisons are available. All life as we know it derives from a common set of processes evident in bacteria and human cells. Many species share the same metabolic processes to extract energy from the environment. Although other forms of life on Earth are possible in theory, they have yet to be observed and would appear unlikely because that would involve a new set of biological processes different from the one currently supporting millions of species and undetectable at the present time.

Our current definition of life is that it involves an emergent property of complex molecules (polymers) characterized by processes of self-assembly and the capacity to build and sustain order. All organisms are tightly coupled to their environments and require the constant exchange of matter and energy to sustain internal order. Complexity is hierarchical, and the degree of complexity in living organisms far exceeds that of any other known physical system. The capacity of proteins to self-assemble and build order and complexity is the essence of life. Although certain biological processes like diffusion and nerve impulse conduction can be adequately explained by physical laws, the phenomenon of "life" escapes physical interpretation.

Attempts to establish a purely mechanistic interpretation of life have uniformly failed. A mechanistic approach is reductionist and cannot account for the complexity and emergent properties of living systems. Reductionists take the position that, once the basic physical mechanisms operating a biological organism have been identified, life can be explained in terms of ordinary physics. But such reductionism fails to account for the hierarchy of complexity in biological systems. At each level of complexity, integration of system components leads to the emergence of new qualities that cannot be predicted at lower levels of complexity. Biology will never be reconciled with physics until hierarchal complexity and the properties of emergence are recognized and accounted for. The mystery of life is not in the forces that act on the individual macromolecules making up the organism but in how the collection of molecules operates in a coherent and cooperative way.[18]

A complete understanding of complex systems is beyond reach, and our understanding will always be incomplete. The more answers we get the more questions pop up. Complexity raises the interesting question of what is knowable and what is unknowable. The inherent uncertainties in complex systems means that not everything about the system can be known. But this shouldn't suggest that the system cannot be understood at some fundamental level. Human consciousness is likely never to be fully explained, but we are making considerable progress in understanding human awareness, sensory perception, and other cognitive processes. Complex human diseases are also subject to limits of understanding. Exact predictions about how tumors behave or how Alzheimer's disease progresses may be out of reach. However research advances and deeper understanding of the diseases themselves have led to a positivist perspective that we can conquer these diseases without fully understanding everything.

Astronomy provides the best-known example of scientific knowledge of phenomena that were once considered "unknowable." Planetary motion was considered by the ancient Greeks to be arbitrary and dictated by the gods. This entirely mysterious and theological interpretation eventually gave way to views by Ptolemy, Kepler, and others that planetary motion was predictable but in ill-defined ways. The mystery of planetary motion was removed by Newton and his laws of motion and by Einstein and others who contributed important modifications to Newtonian laws. There are other examples of phenomena once considered unknowable presented throughout this book.

Solving the complexity puzzle means developing unconventional approaches using conventional tools. There is no clear way forward because we are not sure what questions to ask. Complex systems are highly variable in nature and it is unlikely that a one-size-fits-all solution is realistic. Multidisciplinary approaches including biochemistry, chemistry, computational sciences, engineering sciences, neurobiology, and physiology will be needed to unravel the complexity of life. Perhaps the key is computational sciences. If the brain is any indication, complex systems and their emergent properties are a product of a very high degree of interconnectedness and interdependence among system components. This suggests that advanced network analyses and information processing will be key to understanding how complex systems function and emergent properties evolve. Whether advances in technology or computational techniques or other advances we have yet to imagine can answer some of the unanswered questions discussed in this book remains to be seen. It would be interesting to have some further perspective on how artificial intelligence, machine learning, and computational innovations might change the understanding of complex systems. In this regard, the points of view of data scientists, computer engineers, and network analysts who typically work in areas outside the life sciences will be important.

The ultimate goal of a multidisciplinary effort is to identify patterns and relationships in complex systems that lend themselves to quantitative expression. However, as discussed in the final chapter, a theory of complexity is not likely to lend itself to complete description by a set of mathematical equations. But we really don't know if that's the case. As we drill deeper and deeper into complexity phenomena certain fundamental principles might become evident. What is unknowable today might be knowable tomorrow.

A Roadmap to the Book

What is remarkable is that complex systems are driven by relatively simple physical processes. The processes are seen everywhere in nature and are not unique to life. A central feature of complex systems is the importing and processing of information from the environment. In life, information takes on two major forms—genetic information that is used to make proteins and energy that is used to power all life processes.

In chapters 2 and 3 the laws of physics driving biological processes are discussed. Life is concerned primarily with laws dealing with how energy flows and how it is processed. Chapter 2 discusses the second law of thermodynamics, perhaps the most important law in all of nature. It requires that energy always flows in a direction that increases disorder, and, under the second law, all natural systems tend toward disorder (increased entropy).

If the second law is true, how can life exist? Living systems are characterized by a high degree of internal order. Building order by importing energy from the environment does not violate the second law of thermodynamics because the cost of order building is increasing disorder exported back to the environment in the form of waste energy (body heat). Without an external source of energy, life would die out.

The body maintains internal order and physiologic functions by generating chemical, electrical, and mechanical forces. These forces of life are derived from chemical and electrical gradients across cell membranes. Chapter 3 explores simple, deterministic laws of physics that govern transport of molecules, production of electrical impulses, and generation of mechanical forces and pressures.

The rest of the book is devoted to the question of complexity in human biology and medicine. Chapter 4 explores complexity and nonlinear dynamics. Life is characterized by a variety of processes and organizational motifs over a wide range of scales. Biological systems have the capacity to replicate and evolve and to adapt or react to changing environmental conditions. The deterministic laws of physics discussed in chapters 2 and 3 are necessary but not sufficient to account for these cardinal features of life. Replication, evolution, and adaptability are consequences of biological complexity, characterized by physical and chemical processes operating far from thermodynamic equilibrium as nonlinear dynamical systems.

The human body runs efficiently because homeostasis is an inherent property of complexity and confers stability in biological systems. Chapter 5 discusses homeostasis—the maintenance of a stable internal environment—as a unifying principle of physiology and clinical medicine.

In chapter 6 disease is viewed as a spectrum of physiological states that are deviations from homeostasis. Cancer and other chronic degenerative diseases pose significant medical challenges because disease complexity makes medical management difficult. Unlike infectious diseases, where identifying and removing the causal agent (often a virus or a bacterium) usually returns the patient to health, there is usually no straightforward approach to prevention and management of complex diseases.

Chapters 7 through 9 explore biological complexity from the perspective of several important chronic, degenerative diseases. Chapter 7 discusses heart disease, obesity, and type 2 diabetes. Chapter 8 looks at cancer, actually a collection of more than one hundred separate diseases. Chapter 9 explores Alzheimer's disease as an example of neurodegenerative disease. These diseases are clinically distinct entities but share important characteristics coupled to complexity.

Age is the most powerful risk factor linking chronic degenerative diseases. Risk factors correlate with disease but are not themselves causal. How complexity theory informs the problem of aging is discussed in chapter 10. Although aging can be defined as progressive functional decline and increasing mortality over time, the process is not uniform and cannot be simply characterized. Can the processes of aging be retarded or stopped? If aging can be slowed can the onset of cancer and Alzheimer's disease be delayed? Can the human life span be increased indefinitely? By addressing design weaknesses, can we make a better human?

The final chapter explores principles of complexity to enrich our understanding of human biology and human disease. Complexity science offers interesting and somewhat surprising strategies to deal with Alzheimer's disease, cancer, and other challenging health issues. Complexity is the unifying theory that accounts for all biological principles—Darwinian evolution, cell theory, and homeostasis. Nothing makes sense in biology and medicine except in the light of complexity. A unified theory of biology needs to explain how dimensions of complexity, including homeostasis and evolution, relate to one another.

The secret to understanding biological complexity is the transition from elementalism to emergence, from simplicity to complexity. Before discussing complexity features in human biology and disease, let us step back and examine the nuts and bolts of life—deterministic processes that serve as the foundation of complexity. In the following chapter, we look at arguably the most important law in nature—the second law of thermodynamics—the law that makes life possible.

2

Laws to Live By

What is extraordinary about life is that the same cellular and subcellular processes are found in all the remarkably diverse forms of life. All living systems are complex, even down to simple bacterial cells. But "simple" bacterial cells use the same basic biological processes as the most specialized cells in the human. The structure of cell membranes that serve to separate the cell from its environment and control the movement of ions and molecules into and out of the cell are similar in bacterial cells and human cells. All living cells make proteins in essentially the same way, using a common genetic code. Cell metabolism and energy transformation in all living cells utilize the same chemical pathways. In fact, much of what we know about how human cells function comes in large part from the study of bacterial cells.

The uniformity of biochemical processes across all life reflects the cosmic imperative that physical laws are the same everywhere. Biological processes are invariant because they must obey the laws of physics. Diffusion, osmosis, and nerve impulse conduction can be understood and explained by the laws of physics. This chapter introduces major laws of physics that govern life processes. Human biology and disease can be understood in the context of compliance with these natural laws.

Nature Has No Choices

No one knows if there are "life laws," that is, unique laws that create and establish life. Although Erwin Schrödinger, the Nobel Prize–winning physicist, suggested there are laws that govern life, such laws have yet to be identified. Most scientists agree that, if such life laws exist, they are different from traditional laws of physics. Perhaps life is not the consequence of any new laws at all but instead is a remarkable emergent phenomenon of sustained order and complexity.

Life laws are different from *laws of life*. The laws of life describe the physical and chemical processes that support all life. These processes are identical in all life forms and obey the laws of physics. This is true at every level of biological complexity. The laws and equations that govern cellular events such as diffusion across cell membranes are the same laws and equations that describe physiologic processes in tissues, organs, and organ systems, at least to a first approximation.

However, the known laws of physics cannot account for or predict life. Life as we know it cannot be created from inert substances. Life comes from life; living cells come from other living cells. The laws of physics also cannot predict emergent properties of complex systems. For example, the human brain is the most complex system in the human body. Although laws of physics can explain how nerve impulses are generated and propagated, these laws cannot explain the phenomena of sensory perception that are emergent properties of the brain and involve the coordinated activities of billions of neurons and neuronal connections.

What do we mean by "laws?" Physical laws or laws of nature are scientific generalizations that represent a summary description of nature. Laws of nature can usually be expressed by simple mathematical equations. A law is a conceptual framework that facilitates organization of observations and other data in some meaningful way and also predicts future outcomes when system-dependent conditions are specified. Laws provide unexpected insights into observable phenomena. The ultimate goal of science and explanations of natural phenomena is the description of natural laws.[1]

Classical laws of physics include Newton's laws of motion and the laws of thermodynamics. By "classical laws," we mean those laws of physics that describe phenomena that are experienced on a daily basis, including gravitation, laws of motion, and electricity and magnetism. These laws were formulated in the seventeenth, eighteenth, and nineteenth centuries by such giants as Isaac Newton, Michael Faraday, and James Clerk Maxwell. Newton's laws have dominated theoretical physics since the eighteenth century.[2]

The laws of nature are universal; they operate in the same way everywhere in the Universe. A scientific law cannot be proven to be true but is considered to be true if tests of the law are always observed to be true. Thus, physical laws become established by accumulating scientific evidence that supports them.

Newtonian (classical) mechanics is the foundation on which our belief in a deterministic description of nature is based. "Determinism" means that predictions are invariant for a given set of inputs when the law is applied in appropriate circumstances. As discussed in chapter 1, deterministic laws predict past and future states if the state of the physical system is known at a particular time. The National Aeronautical and Space Administration (NASA) uses Newton's laws of motion in just this way to predict positions of spacecraft at any given time after a launch. In living systems, determinism applies at all levels of biological complexity from bacteria to complex multicellular organisms like humans. Single-cell and multicellular organisms must obey the laws of physics, but these laws are only incidental to biology.[3]

Newtonian determinism means that nature has no choices. Inherent in the Newtonian paradigm is the idea that systems can be described by a particular state at a given time. Changes in state can be understood and predicted in terms of the forces that act on the system in accordance with specific dynamical laws that are themselves state and system independent. The interaction between states and dynamical laws means that the state of the system at one moment determines its state at all previous and subsequent moments. Deterministic laws predict future states of systems.[4]

This is the value of classical laws of physics: the possibility of predictions. A change in a system parameter causes something else to change in the system in a predictable way, and the change is always to be expected when the law is properly applied. Clinical medicine depends on this deterministic quality of physical laws.

When a physician prescribes a drug to reduce blood pressure by causing the body to lose water, the physical law relating flow rate, flow resistance, and blood pressure comes into play. To maintain a constant blood flow rate, reducing flow resistance (by reducing blood volume through water loss) will result in reduced blood pressure because the heart does not have to work as hard to pump the blood.[5]

The Mother of All Laws

The physical laws governing life are concerned with processing energy. The body uses energy in many ways, and all processes are consistent with the known macroscopic laws of physics. The fundamental structure of these laws connects a flux to a driving force. A battery-powered flashlight provides a good example. As long as the battery is charged, a potential difference (driving force) exists, and electric current (flux) will power the light. When the battery is dead, there is no voltage and, therefore, no current to turn on the light. Biologically important processes like diffusion work the same way. Diffusion is the major transport process that moves molecules and ions into and out of cells. In diffusion, the flow of a substance across a biological membrane is determined principally by the driving force created by the concentration gradient or uneven distribution of the substance across the cell membrane. In the nervous system, the generation of electrical impulses depends on the flow of ions (electrically charged atoms) into and out of nerve cells. The uneven distribution of K^+ and Na^+ ions across the nerve axon membrane creates a potential difference and a concentration gradient that serves as the driving force for ionic flow across the membrane.

Living systems require a continuous external supply of energy to maintain the gradients necessary to power chemical, electrical, and mechanical processes. Cells store energy in phosphate bonds of adenosine triphosphate (ATP), the main energy source for most biological processes. The energy stored in ATP comes from the metabolism of carbohydrates and other energy-rich food sources. Organisms convert the energy stored in the chemical bonds in ATP molecules into mechanical energy, electrical energy, chemical energy, and heat. Multicellular organisms use available energy to build and sustain a high degree of order and to maintain a constant internal environment.

Most of the ATP energy is dissipated as waste heat. Waste heat is not useful in doing work, although some of it is used to maintain body temperature. The typical human body generates about 100 watts of power as waste heat, representing about 80 percent of the total power generated by the body. Thus, about 25 watts of power are actually used by the body to do work, including operating the most powerful computer we know of—the human brain. No man-made computer has the energy efficiency or computational power of the human brain.[6]

The primary laws governing energy processing are the laws of thermodynamics. These laws are deterministic and empirical in nature and cannot be derived mathematically from more basic principles. The laws of thermodynamics have been tested many times and never found to be invalid. The first and second laws of thermodynamics are central to our discussions of human biology and disease.[7] In Figure 2.1, compartments A and B represent the outside and inside of a human

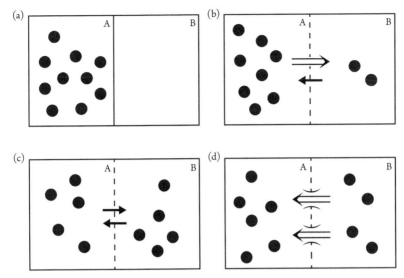

Figure 2.1 A simple closed system with two equal-sized compartments. In (a), sodium ions dissolved in water in compartment A cannot cross the membrane barrier into compartment B because all sodium channels are closed. In (b), sodium channels are open, and sodium molecules shown as dark circles move between compartments, but net flow (shown by the larger arrow) is from compartment A to compartment B because the concentration of Na^+ is higher in compartment A. In (c), net movement of sodium ions stops when the concentration gradient goes to zero, that is, the concentrations of Na^+ on either side of the membrane are equal. Sodium ions can still move from one compartment to the other, but, at equilibrium, movement in one direction is balanced by equal movement in the opposite direction. In (d), molecular pumps have been inserted in the membrane to pump sodium ions against the concentration gradient. Pumps sustain the gradient but require energy to operate.

cell, respectively. Compartment A contains water with sodium ions in solution, and Compartment B contains water only.[8] This is a thermodynamically closed system; the compartments are isolated from the environment so that no energy can enter or leave the system. The barrier between the two compartments is a membrane impermeable to the movement of sodium or water (Figure 2.1[a]). Sodium channels in the membrane, however, allow movement of sodium ions when open. When the channels are open, there is a net movement of sodium ions down its concentration gradient from compartment A into compartment B (Figure 2.1[b]). The sodium concentration gradient is the driving force for this to occur. Movement of sodium will continue until the concentration of sodium ions in both compartments is equal. At that point, the concentration gradient is zero, and an equilibrium condition has been reached (Figure 2.1[c]). Without a driving force, there can be no net movement of sodium. Prior to opening the channels, the energy state of the two-compartment system is the stored or potential energy established by the concentration gradient across the membrane. When the channels are open, the system proceeds to equilibrium, and the potential energy is converted to chemical kinetic energy as sodium ions move down its concentration gradient. The first law of thermodynamics says that the energy of the system prior to opening the membrane channels is equal to the energy of the system after it has reached equilibrium. Energy has neither been created nor destroyed; it has simply changed form.

Now suppose we start with the system in the equilibrium state as shown in Figure 2.1(c). Clearly, the system will not spontaneously proceed backward so that all the sodium ions return to compartment A, the initial condition as shown in Figure 2.1(a). But why should this not happen? If the reversal process did occur, the total energy of the system would still remain constant, so the first law would not be violated. There must be another principle independent of the first law that governs how energy flows in a system. The second law of thermodynamics dictates in what direction processes must proceed and is based on the "entropy" of the system. Entropy, a measure of the disorder of a system and also a measure of probability, is a characteristic of the state of the system and requires that processes move in a direction that results in an increase in disorder. The equilibrium condition is the most probable configuration of sodium ions when sodium ions can move between compartments. There are many ways in which the system can be in disorder but relatively few ways in which the system is ordered. An equal distribution of sodium ions across the two compartments is the most likely configuration of all possible configurations. The second law requires that a closed system can never proceed spontaneously in a direction that would increase its internal order. Entropy requires that the process be irreversible.

The equilibrium condition is reached when the system is at maximum disorder. Under the second law, sodium ions cannot spontaneously move in a net direction after equilibrium is reached because that would mean entropy is decreased and order increased. The only way that a nonequilibrium condition can be restored and the solute gradient sustained is to use molecular pumps that move the solute molecules against the concentration gradient, as illustrated in Figure 2.1(d). Pumps require an external source of energy to do this.

The second law of thermodynamics is arguably the most important law in biology. Sir Arthur Eddington called the second law the most important in nature. C. P. Snow said the second law is of such great depth and generality that it covers the Cosmos; he even went so far as to say not knowing the second law is equivalent to never having read Shakespeare. Paul Davies considers the second law the key fundamental physical law that governs life processes. It is a law that is not restricted to engineering or physics and is applicable to all of nature.[9]

The second law was formulated in the nineteenth century during the Industrial Revolution to understand the efficiency of heat engines. It describes the theoretical limits on the efficiency of engines but applies as well to living systems. According to the second law, only a portion of the available internal energy in a combustion engine can be used to power the engine; the remaining energy is dissipated as heat. In other words, although the first law holds that, even in irreversible processes, total energy is conserved, the second law says that not all the energy can be used to do useful work; some of the energy must be dissipated as waste. This waste energy contributes to entropy or disorder. The efficiency of a machine depends on how the machine is designed and works. The human body is a biochemical machine, and its efficiency depends on the source of energy and metabolism and other biological processes that convert chemical energy into other forms of energy to carry out vital processes.

Living systems are not heat engines but instead use isothermal processes to do work. Living systems do not depend on heat exchange or transport to do work but on other processes involving the change of energy from one form to another. For example, the chemical energy stored in glucose and other sugars is converted to electrical energy for nerve impulses. There are no heat gradients in the human body to do work. The operating temperature of the body is close to ambient temperature. Energy utilization is nonthermal because there are no thermal gradients in the body to channel energy flow. Nevertheless, living systems generate heat as waste energy that is required by the second law.

In the context of biology, the first law of thermodynamics says any biological process can occur as long as energy is conserved. The second law states that only those real processes that result in an increase in entropy in the Universe can occur spontaneously. For all other possible processes, energy needs to be added to the system for the process to go forward.

Erwin Schrödinger was one of the early physicists to ask how life can be explained in the light of the second law of thermodynamics. In his highly influential book *What Is Life?* he challenged the scientific community with two key questions: (1) What is the nature of the coded information in heritable material that explains heritable characteristics? (2) How can the spontaneous emergence of self-organized order in living systems be explained when the second law of thermodynamics requires systems to progress inexorably to states of increasing disorder?

Schrödinger's book was published in 1944, and within about twenty years we had the answer to his first question.[10] The answer to the second question has proven to be more challenging. Living systems are able to overcome the entropy requirements of the second law by constantly importing energy as open systems. What remains a mystery is how complex systems emerge through the process of self-assembly and organization. The work of Nobel laureate Ilya Prigogine in the 1960s and 1970s on dissipative structures and self-organizing systems has provided an important way forward in understanding life as complex systems.

Life processes require the second law of thermodynamics as a basis for powering diffusion, osmosis, and nerve impulse conduction. Living systems establish internal chemical and electrical gradients as driving forces by importing energy. Life is a remarkable phenomenon because of the way these gradients are sustained so that movement of ions and molecules always occurs. Structural and physiologic order is built and sustained by the conversion of energy from one form into another. Part of this energy conversion is used to do useful work, but some fraction of the energy must always be discarded as waste heat to increase entropy in the Universe. DNA-directed protein synthesis also builds order through the synthesis of complex structural and functional proteins. DNA is informational power in that highly ordered information, encoded in the linear sequence of bases in DNA, drives the synthesis of proteins that are critical in the structural and functional integrity of the cell and, by extension, multicellular system processes. DNA itself does not generate energy but is the information source that is necessary to build energy-dependent order. If DNA *defines* life, proteins *are* life! Order is a requirement of life because only highly ordered systems can replicate and because highly ordered systems can degrade energy gradients.

Biological processes balance changes in internal energy against changes in entropy. Only a fraction of the internal energy is free energy that can be used to do work. Consider protein folding. Proteins must be in the correct three-dimensional conformation to function properly. A protein is synthesized by the cell in the unfolded, nonfunctional state and has a low negative internal energy (that is, energy will tend to flow out of the molecular system and into the environment) and high entropy. The high entropy implies uncertainty in that many folded configurations of the protein are possible. Ultimately, protein folding occurs in such a way that the resulting conformation occupies the lowest energy state. The folded protein has low entropy and a large negative internal energy. The low entropy implies that only one conformational state is permitted. The decrease in entropy in the folding process suggests that the second law has been violated. But no violation occurs, because some of the energy transformation in the protein-folding process is waste energy that increases entropy. Although entropy is decreased in the cell, this is offset by an increase in entropy by dissipation of waste energy to the environment. It takes energy to create improbable, ordered configurations from disordered ones. As entropy (disorder) decreases, order must increase. Imported energy is used to create the spontaneous development of self-organized, emergent phenomena.

The second law is valid only for closed systems with no exchange of energy or entropy with the environment. All energy is internal to the system. The secret to life, then, is that it must be an open system that allows for environmental energy exchanges. In life, the second law is not violated, even though entropy may be decreased locally, as long as the total entropy of the environment is increased. Entropy in the form of body heat and other waste products is exported to the environment. This form of energy is not available to do work and contributes to the total entropy of the Universe. The only way to decrease entropy and increase order is to add energy to the system from an external source that requires the system to be open. By doing so, the system can be maintained in a nonequilibrium state and various kinds of work can be done since the nonequilibrium state serves as a driving force. If availability of external energy ceases, the system will inexorably go to equilibrium, and no work can be done. When that happens in living systems, death occurs.

Figure 2.1 assumes a closed system in which diffusion of solute molecules occurs in a system totally isolated from the environment. The system will ultimately reach equilibrium since there is no external source of energy to maintain gradients. In living cells, nonequilibrium conditions can be sustained by inserting molecular pumps into the cell membrane that continue to pump sodium ions against its concentration gradient (Figure 2.1[d]). The energy needed to run the molecular pumps comes from the external environment as energy-rich foods.

Overcoming the constraints of the second law of thermodynamics means that living systems operate far from equilibrium. The second law explains why there is degradation of energy available to do work, why nature seeks to break down gradients, and why order tends toward disorder. The second law also informs us that the process of emergence of internal order (negative entropy) within complex systems must be accompanied by export of even greater quantities of waste energy (entropy) to the environment, since the net change in entropy must be greater than zero.

The second law of thermodynamics also implies an arrow of time. The second law confines the direction in which processes can proceed. In a closed system, the state of the system always proceeds in the direction of increasing disorder. Such systems cannot spontaneously go backward and become more orderly. For living systems, disorder is death, and living systems cheat death by importing energy to maintain necessary order. The second law is consistent with the idea that, as complex systems evolve, they become more complex. Life forms have evolved from relatively simple cells like bacteria to complex multicellular forms like human beings.

In the history of physics, the second law represents a quantum leap forward in our understanding of nature. The Newtonian construct of reality has no arrow of time; Newton's time is reversible, whereby a particular state cannot be identified as being in the past or in the future. But this view is inconsistent with our everyday experiences. Time and direction are observed everywhere in nature. The formulation of the second law of thermodynamics was an important step in understanding the unavoidable connection between time and the natural world.[11] The second law means life is in a constant battle against death. We swim upstream against a great torrent of disorganization that tends to reduce everything to static equilibrium and sameness.[12] Living things constantly build order to overcome the tendency toward disorder. As the Red Queen said to Alice in Lewis Carroll's *Through the Looking-Glass*, "[I]t takes all the running you can do to keep in the same place."

Laws Are Not Always Right and Do Not Predict Everything

As mentioned previously, classical laws of physics can predict occurrences. The link to causal determinism in health and disease is obvious. Patients with asthma may be given a bronchodilator to ease breathing. Bronchodilators reduce resistance to air flow, causing a reduction in airway pressure, which eases breathing difficulties. The same relationship between flow, resistance, and pressure is seen in hemodynamics and derive from well-known laws of fluid dynamics.

The accuracy of predictions depends on whether characteristics or conditions of the system limit or invalidate the application of specific laws of physics. The behavior of real gases agrees to within 5 percent of the predictions of the ideal gas equation under conditions of standard temperatures and pressures. But at very low temperatures and very high pressures, predictions deviate significantly from observation. Ohm's law, as an example, is regularly used in electrical engineering to relate voltage and current, but its predictive value is diminished when dealing with semiconductor circuits. The predictive value of deterministic laws decreases with increasing

complexity of the system. Laws would be expected to be quite accurate in their predictions for simple physical systems such as a swinging pendulum, but physical laws
applied to living systems frequently fail or poorly predict outcomes because of the
inherent complexities of such systems.[13] This does not mean deterministic laws have
no utility in living systems, only that interpretation of predictions must be made
with caution. As long as assumptions and uncertainties are understood, use of deterministic equations can be of value in understanding the underlying basis of normal
and pathological functions.

All scientific laws or laws of nature are contingent, which means that certain
conditions must hold for the laws to be valid, to be applied properly, and to be
interpreted correctly. Conditions are specific characteristics of the system. When
these conditions are not met, the laws give incorrect predictions, but, when all
contingency requirements are satisfied, natural laws are considered universal
and always true. Newton's laws of motion are highly predictive when tracking the
motion of the planets or the position of a spacecraft, but these laws fail at the
atomic level, where quantum effects become important. The truth in the laws of
physics depends not on a strict logical analysis but on an accurate assessment of
the real world.

The accuracy of predictions depends on how well initial conditions are known.
If initial conditions can be completely specified, then all future states are knowable
regardless of the complexity of the system. However, since complete knowledge of
a system can never be achieved, certain assumptions must be made about the system, and these assumptions are important in determining the predictive value of
the applied law. Assumptions may be plausible, false, or unverifiable. A plausible
assumption is based on evidence from testing conditions of the system to see if it
is reasonable to believe the assumption is true. Assumptions may also be known to
be false but close enough to allow for reasonable interpretations of the law when an
assumption is not fully met. An assumption may also be unverifiable when it is not
possible to determine its validity. If unverifiable, the assumption may be accepted
as reasonable for the purposes of applying the law, but results must be interpreted
carefully because of the underlying uncertainties. In general, system conditions are
testable criteria that are used to support or override assumptions.

Take, for example, Newton's second law of motion. If an object is moving at constant velocity (that is, acceleration is zero), it will continue to remain in that state
of motion until an external force is applied to it. How well Newton's second law predicts the behavior of the object when a force is applied depends on the conditions of
the system. There are several assumptions that must be considered. The force acting
on the moving object must exist everywhere, the mass of the object must remain
unchanged, and any differences or inconsistencies between observations and predictions must be considered random statistical errors.[14]

In biological systems, complexity can compromise theory predictability. Complex
systems have characteristics including nonlinear dynamics and feedback loops that
are not accounted for by the classical laws of physics. When dealing with complex
systems like the human body, macroscopic laws of physics do not make very good
predictions. Application of a physical law to a part of a system does not necessarily take into account how the whole system might respond. For example, a child

with combined mitral valve stenosis (narrowing of the valve that directs blood flow from the left atrium to the left ventricle) and an atrial septal defect (a heart defect allowing blood to flow between the left atrium and the right atrium) has circulatory difficulties because the heart cannot pump oxygenated blood well. Repairing the septal defect will increase pressure across the mitral valve because blood is no longer shunted from the left atrium to the right atrium. But the increased pressure has a ripple effect and increases back pressure on the pulmonary veins, resulting in pulmonary hypertension and buildup of fluid in the lungs. The end result is the possibility of heart failure.[15]

Certain biological functions are so complex they cannot be understood at all in terms of physical laws. Human behavior, language, and other higher cortical functions of the brain cannot be predicted or understood on the basis of physical laws. Deterministic laws explain basic biological processes at the neuron and interneuron level. But at higher structural and functional levels of the brain, millions of neurons interconnect and interact in highly complex networks resulting in emergent properties. The exact condition of the complex system can never be fully described. To think otherwise reflects misunderstanding of how the laws of physics work and the complexity of biological systems.

Deterministic laws assume simple causal relations between system responses and system inputs. By "simple" is meant that a change in system inputs produces a proportional change in system response. The oscillatory motion of a mass attached to a spring can be fully understood and predicted when the oscillations are limited to the near-equilibrium condition and intrinsic forces, including the restoring force of the spring and the damping force and any external forces, are considered. In far-from-equilibrium conditions (large displacement of the mass from its resting position), the movement of the mass is not fully predictable because system dynamics become nonlinear and initial conditions of the system cannot be known exactly. In linear dynamics, the response of the system to a complex input is simply the sum of the responses to each of the simpler inputs making up the complex input. In nonlinear dynamics, a linear relation among simpler inputs does not exist.

In theory, the complex climate system is deterministic. Short-term and long-term changes in climate are knowable if initial conditions—the current state of the system—can be described exactly. If this situation holds, then the deterministic laws of physics will predict the state of the system at some time in the future. The difficulty is that we do not know or cannot account for all the factors that constitute the initial conditions. When we say that a system is completely known, we are really saying that the initial conditions of the system are completely describable. Climate forecasting, whether near-term or long-term, is made difficult by our lack of complete understanding of initial conditions.

Initial conditions codify the future and the past. Exact knowledge of the initial conditions means the future is already known. To predict the future is to know the future. Applying deterministic laws simply describes states of the system at some specific time in the past or in the future.

The problem of initial conditions may be incomprehensible and intractable when dealing with complex systems like the human body and climatology. In classical mechanics involving motions of a body in simple, well-described systems, initial conditions of the system are knowable. Knowledge of the mass, position, and velocity of the body and of the direction and magnitude of all forces acting on the body is all that is required to describe completely the initial conditions of the dynamic system. From there, application of Newton's laws of motion is all that is necessary to predict the position and velocity of the mass at any time in the future.

Laws of Physics and Reductionism

Reductionism has value by offering simplifying explanations. Indeed, it has had a powerful influence on scientific thinking for centuries. Although philosophers have argued the merits of a holistic versus a reductionist approach to the study of nature, the prevailing view has been that the atomist perspective would provide the route to understanding processes and mechanisms in otherwise complex systems. The assumption has always been that understanding the functioning of the parts is necessary to the understanding of the whole. Since the 1970s, this view has changed radically, as a growing understanding of complexities of natural systems clearly indicated that a solely reductionist approach was inadequate. What is missing is an understanding of system-level properties and behaviors that could not be explained or accounted for by studying only elemental components of the system.

The usefulness of the reductionist approach depends on the validity of assumptions underlying system characteristics. A reductionist approach assumes that (1) mechanisms are independent of level of organization (that is, mechanisms and behaviors at some higher level can be wholly explained by the behavior of the constituent parts) and (2) elemental constituents behave independently from one another and do not interact in a way that would result in a change in behavior at higher levels of system organization. In complex systems, these assumptions are not valid universally. Higher-order brain functions like language cannot be explained entirely on the basis of analysis of nerve cells and their connections. Emergent properties are a consequence of interdependence among tissue elements, a feature that is lost when examining the elements themselves.

Breaking down a complex system to its functional components provides partial knowledge about the behavior of that system; it clearly shows that the functions of the complex system are contingent on the interdependence, communication, and cooperativity of the components. Component properties are not necessarily transferred to the system level, and system-level properties are not necessarily found at the component level. Nevertheless, a reductionist approach has inherent value in understanding basic processes.

Deterministic laws of physics are valid only in limited circumstances in living systems. Living systems are complex, operate far from equilibrium, and exhibit nonlinear behaviors. The classical laws of physics predict behaviors for systems operating at or near equilibrium under linear dynamics. When living systems operate in a linear domain, they are predictable. Macroscopic laws of physics model basic biological processes such as diffusion, nerve signaling, and blood flow when these processes are isolated from the complex system. In this way, problems of contingency are reduced because nonlinear behavior and other characteristics of complex systems are eliminated or greatly reduced. The downside of reductionism is that complex behaviors cannot be accounted for in the isolated system.

Classic deterministic laws provide a first-order approximation of complex system behaviors. There is sufficient predictability in these laws to provide understanding of complex system behavior in the clinical setting. Blood pressure is a good example. Minute-by-minute measurements of blood pressure show fluctuations around a central value. While one cannot predict exactly the value of the next blood pressure reading, the average value from several sequential readings is a good first approximation of the status of the hemodynamic system. Physicians commonly compare the average blood pressure before and at appropriate times after administering antihypertensive medication to determine whether a blood-pressure drug works. If the drug is a diuretic, the laws of fluid dynamics predict that blood pressure will drop by reduction in total blood volume due to excretion of water. The exact change in blood pressure cannot be determined and is not clinically important. What matters is that blood pressure returns to or toward the normotensive range.

A reductionist approach provides for important insights about mechanisms and processes in complex biological systems. However, many features of biological systems are not amenable to a mechanistic analysis based on simple laws of physics. It is not possible to describe in mathematical terms the processes that govern higher cortical functions, including behavior, language, and consciousness. Reducing higher-order cortical functions to a set of mathematical equations may not be possible until the neurobiological correlates of mental functions and the causal connections between the brain and the mind are reasonably well understood. Whether mental functions can ever be described in this quantitative way is unknown, but it is unlikely.[16]

Reductionism is a simplification strategy that limits the number of parameters describing the system. A goal of the reductionist approach is to control complexity. Isolated systems can be manipulated so that processes are isolated in a linear domain. By isolating specific systems or subsystems under normal and disease conditions, the macroscopic laws of physics can be applied to investigate system behaviors in controlled environments and to evaluate key biological variables.

One of the central questions in systems biology is what minimal level of complexity leads to emergent behavior. It appears there is some level of complexity even in subcellular components.[17] Simplifying systems so complexity can be controlled seems to require that components themselves be nonliving. A great deal of useful work has been accomplished using isolated cell membranes, mitochondria, and other cell and tissue components. Computer and synthetic models also provide insightful knowledge about basic biological processes. Blood flow and diffusion of solute molecules from one biological compartment to another can be studied in this way (Figure 2.2).

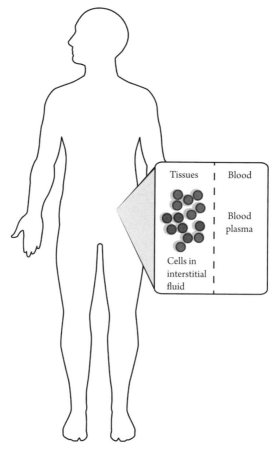

Figure 2.2 The goal of reductionism is to break down systems into component parts, assuming that studying the elements provides understanding of the system as a whole. The problem with complex systems is that the system is greater than the sum of the component parts. Accordingly, certain features of the system as a whole cannot be understood by studying the components.

Deterministic Laws and Life

The macroscopic laws of physics are at most approximate in the predictions they make. They do not describe normal or disease phenomena exactly because biological systems are complex and unpredictable. Although natural laws govern many fundamental life processes, life itself and what it means to be human are emergent properties that cannot be predicted or understood by these fundamental physical laws.

Every biological process necessary to sustain life may be understood in the context of the second law of thermodynamics and the flow of energy through open systems. Even in the brain the basic biological processes related to interneuron communications are fully explainable by laws of physics. The physical and chemical processes that support life are governed by thermodynamic-dependent macroscopic laws of classical mechanics and electromagnetism. Classical mechanics involves generation of forces in cells and tissues. Theories of electromagnetism are concerned with movement of charges and generation and propagation of electrical impulses.

Determinism is central to disease diagnosis. Clinical tests such as blood pressure measurements reflect the state of a system at a particular time. Blood pressure is a reflection of how hard the heart is working. As peripheral vascular resistance increases, the heart must pump harder and increase blood pressure. This is necessary to maintain adequate blood flow to tissues and organs. Hypertension or increased blood pressure is an important sign in many diseases. Disease diagnoses can be challenging because of the uncertain relationship among signs, symptoms, clinical test results, and specific pathologic states. This is particularly true for many neuropsychiatric disorders for which the underlying pathology and the related clinical signs are poorly understood. Deterministic laws can determine the physical states of a particular system, but the relationship between the physical states and disease is often unclear. In the next chapter, we look at specific physical laws and deterministic processes that are key to structural and functional complexity in human biology and disease.

3

Forces of Nature

On Wednesday, November 1, Pyotr, his brother Modest, and several friends went to the theater followed by a late dinner at a local restaurant. During the meal, Pyotr ordered a glass of water but was told that no boiled water was available. Because of an outbreak of cholera, the local health department had issued an advisory to boil all drinking water. Pyotr ignored the warnings and drank some cold, unboiled water anyway. The next day he complained of an upset stomach and diarrhea. The symptoms did not subside, and three days later, Pyotr was diagnosed with cholera. The signs and symptoms worsened; on Monday, November 6, just four days after initial symptoms, he died because of dehydration and kidney failure. The year was 1893. The place was Saint Petersburg, Russia. The cholera victim was Pyotr Ilyich Tchaikovsky, the famous Russian composer.[1]

Cholera is an acute diarrheal illness caused by a bacterial infection of the small intestine, *Vibrio cholerae*. The bug produces an intestinal toxin called an enterotoxin that promotes fluid and electrolyte secretion into the lumen of the small intestine, the space inside the intestines through which foods are transported and digested.

The severe diarrhea associated with cholera is a direct result of the action of the toxin on intestinal epithelial cells. The toxin causes chloride and bicarbonate ion channels to lock in the open position, and ions leak out of cells and into the intestinal lumen. Water follows the electrolytes, resulting in diarrhea characterized by massive water loss into the intestinal lumen. The movement of water out of cells is a consequence of osmosis, a fundamental transport process in living systems. As the cell becomes less concentrated because of the loss of chloride and bicarbonate ions, intracellular water moves out of the cell and into the more concentrated extracellular compartment (the intestinal lumen). In addition, because the intestinal cells contain toxin, any fluid that the body attempts to conserve is lost because of open channels in the cells and lack of absorptive ability. To exacerbate the fluid loss problem, cholera toxin also causes water channels, called aquaporins, to be inserted in intestinal cell membranes, facilitating movement of water into the intestinal lumen.[2]

Cholera is osmosis gone haywire. The uncontrolled loss of water and electrolytes from the body leads to reduced blood pressure and blood flow. Multiple organ failure and death occur unless replacement therapy is instituted quickly. Cholera reflects the central role of osmosis in normal human physiology. The movement of water from one physiologic compartment to another is the basis for many key biological processes. Osmosis is a deterministic, linear process; it meets the basic requirements of Newtonian physics. If the conductive properties of the exchange surface separating compartments (for example, the intracellular and extracellular fluid compartments) and the solute concentrations in the compartments are known, the osmotic behavior of water can be fully characterized and predicted.

As discussed in this chapter, living systems are complex, but at the heart of this complexity are elementary biological processes including diffusion, osmosis, and nerve impulse conduction that are governed by deterministic laws of physics.

Mass Transit

Movement of ions and molecules between biological compartments is the key to all biological processes; this movement is known as diffusion. In living systems, diffusion occurs when there is a difference in solute concentration inside and outside the cell and the solute can move across the cell membrane. The cell membrane has variable conductance properties allowing some solute molecules but not others to pass through. Membrane conductance is determined by which ion channels are open and closed. Solute molecules will move across the permeable membrane in the direction down the concentration gradient in accordance with the second law of thermodynamics. The gradient is the driving force for this movement. Energy is used to maintain concentration gradients so that diffusion can be sustained. Without constant replenishment of gradients, the system rapidly runs down to thermodynamic equilibrium, resulting in no net movement of solute molecules. Ionic gradients are keys to electrical impulses in the nervous system and in generating mechanical forces through contraction of skeletal and cardiac muscles.

Why is movement of ions and molecules critical to life? First, mass transport of molecules and ions is necessary to establish the internal environment. In higher animals, including humans, the chemical environment inside cells differs significantly from the cell's external environment within the body. This difference establishes the chemical gradients that drive transport processes. Feedback loops and other regulatory processes maintain this environmental difference. The fluid inside a cell (intracellular) consists of an aqueous solution containing relatively large amounts of potassium but small amounts of chloride, sodium, calcium, and magnesium. It also contains some organic anions (negatively charged ions) that cannot penetrate the membrane. Relative to intracellular fluid, extracellular fluid (that is, fluid outside the cell) is rich in sodium, chloride, calcium, and magnesium, but poor in potassium. Glucose, the main source of energy for the cell, is at higher concentrations outside the cell than inside.[3]

Second, the electrical activity foundational to all nervous system functions is based on diffusion of electrical charges across cell membranes. The nerve cell membrane is excitable; it can be stimulated to create small local electric currents. Potassium ions, sodium ions, and calcium ions are key electrolytes in this process. Each carries an electric charge. When charges move across the cell membrane, they induce a magnetic field that, in turn, establishes a local electric current and voltage within the membrane.[4]

Third, kinetic or mechanical forces generated by heart and skeletal muscle contraction derive from diffusion of calcium, potassium, sodium, and other electrolytes across cell membranes.

In living systems, diffusion usually refers to movement of solute molecules in a dilute aqueous solution. At equilibrium, solute molecules are uniformly distributed in the solvent, as we saw in Figure 2.1(c). Although individual solute molecules can move randomly from one compartment to another, there is no net movement of solute molecules, meaning that there are as many molecules moving in one direction as are moving in the opposite direction. Equilibrium represents maximum thermodynamic entropy.

Only small molecules that are not water soluble (known as nonpolar molecules) can easily transit the membrane because of the lipophilic nature of the membrane. Water molecules, water soluble ions or molecules, and large molecules like proteins either move through the membrane very slowly or cannot transit the membrane. The cell membrane serves to separate two aqueous fluids, the extracellular fluid and the intracellular fluid (cytoplasm). Permeability depends on lipid solubility properties, charge, chemistry, and molecular size. Semipermeable membranes provide selectivity in the environmental exchange of molecules.[5]

The rate of diffusion of specific solute molecules depends on the magnitude and direction of the concentration gradient, the permeability of the cell membrane, and the area and thickness of the membrane. In living systems, the area and thickness of the exchange surface is constant and rate of diffusion is determined primarily by the membrane conductance properties and the solute concentration gradient. If the membrane is permeable to the solute in question, the flow rate is directly proportional to the magnitude of the gradient. If the concentration difference is cut in half, the flow rate is also cut in half (Figure 3.1). Net movement of solute molecules tends to reduce the concentration gradient. The gradient will eventually run down to zero when thermodynamic equilibrium is reached, resulting in no net flow of solute molecules.[6]

Channel, carrier, and pump proteins mediate transport across biological membranes. Membranes are distinguishable by the nature of their protein content and arrangements. Semipermeable membranes contain channels that increase or decrease the membrane permeability to specific ions or molecules. Opening and closing channels (large transmembrane proteins inserted in the plasma membrane) alter membrane permeability and provide control over what can move into or out of cells. The rate of diffusion can also be increased by using carrier or chaperone proteins that bind to large or polar solute molecules and facilitate their movement through the cell membrane. Glucose uptake, for example, is a facilitated diffusion process. Glucose binds to the glucose transporter protein to get into the cell. The rate of diffusion under facilitated transport is limited by the availability of chaperone proteins and will reach a plateau when all carrier proteins are bound by solute molecules (Figure 3.1).

The cell uses two solute-specific strategies to sustain gradients. Ion pumps located in the cell membrane restore gradients by pumping electrolytes like sodium and potassium against their concentration gradients. This is an active transport process requiring energy, just like rowing a boat against a current. In the cardiac muscle cell (myocyte), contraction is contingent on the movement of calcium, potassium,

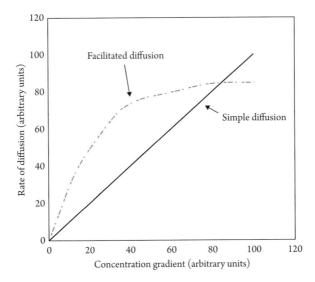

Figure 3.1 The rate of simple diffusion is a direct function of the concentration gradient. Over time, diffusion rates decrease unless the concentration gradient is maintained. The slope of the line is a measure of membrane permeability. In facilitated diffusion, the initial slope is steeper than in simple diffusion because facilitated diffusion increases permeability of specific solutes at low concentrations. However, the rate of facilitated diffusion levels off with increasing solute concentration because carrier proteins are saturated.

and sodium ions down their respective ion gradients. Gradients are sustained by continuously operating ion pumps. An intermembrane complex protein that pumps K^+ into the cell and Na^+ out, called the Na^+-K^+ ATPase pump, uses one molecule of adenosine triphosphate (ATP) to energize the transport of three Na^+ out of the cell for every two K^+ pumped into the cell. Other pumps move Na^+ and Ca^{++}.

Alternatively, solute gradients can be sustained by increasing consumption of solute molecules at the bottom of the gradient or increasing the supply of solute molecules at the top. In the lung, higher levels of oxygen are found in the alveolar air sacs than in blood plasma. This oxygen gradient is sustained by red blood cells that rapidly remove oxygen from the blood plasma. For glucose utilization, the gradient is established by sustaining higher levels of glucose in the fluid compartment outside the cell. This is accomplished primarily by the very high glucose use rate in the cell. Once glucose molecules enter the cell, they are immediately subject to glycolytic breakdown, keeping the concentration of glucose within the cell low.

Simple diffusion across the cell membrane is a passive process requiring no direct source of energy. But this is a bit misleading, since building and sustaining gradients that drive diffusion require energy. Reestablishing ion gradients necessitates that ions be moved against their concentration gradients via active transport. The ATP consumption rate to power pumps is tissue specific. Metabolically, active cells generate much of their ATP to run ion pumps.[7]

Tissues that have primary absorptive functions like the small intestine and the lungs feature large and very thin exchange surfaces. The larger the area of the exchange surface, the higher the rate of diffusion. The human small intestine is about six meters in length. If the intestine is considered a tube with a smooth luminal surface, the total absorptive area would be about 0.5 square meters. But, in actuality, the absorptive area is about 250 square meters—about the size of a tennis court. How can this be? The inner surface of the small intestine is not smooth but covered with microscopic finger-like projections, called villi. The villi protrude into the intestinal lumen, thus greatly increasing the absorptive surface area. The epithelial cells are thin and flat, providing minimal resistance to the diffusion of nutrients from the intestinal lumen to the blood plasma. The lung similarly offers a very large surface area to maximize oxygen movement from the alveolar air spaces into the blood plasma. Alveolar air sacs where diffusion occurs are organized into clusters like bunches of grapes, which increases surface area. The effective exchange surface area of the human lung is about 130 square meters. The alveoli are only one cell thick. When the thin, flat epithelial cells making up the walls of the alveoli thicken, as observed in certain chronic lung diseases, the diffusion of oxygen into the blood is severely compromised, requiring oxygen therapy. Osmosis is a special case of diffusion and provides the primary means by which water is transported into and out of cells. Osmosis occurs in biological systems because of the semipermeable nature of membranes. Cell membranes cannot be penetrated by large organic solutes such as polysaccharides and proteins such as albumin. Water molecules travel through the plasma membrane either by slowly diffusing across the phospholipid bilayer directly or via water channels (called aquaporins). These channels greatly increase the movement of water. Although water does the moving and not the solute molecules, it is the solute concentration gradient that serves as the driving force. If the solute concentration gradient goes to zero, osmosis will not occur.

The movement of water across the cell membrane during osmosis is consistent with the second law of thermodynamics. Osmosis occurs when there are two solutions of different concentrations separated by a semipermeable membrane; the system is said to be ordered and has negative entropy. When entropy is low, water moves from the area of low solute concentration to the area of higher solute concentration to balance solute concentrations. The second law of thermodynamics predicts the spontaneous net movement of water in a direction that increases the disorder of the system.

Only impermeable solute molecules have osmotic effects. The size, mass, or type of solute molecule (for example, a large protein molecule or a small ion) does not contribute to the osmotic effect. What matters is the concentration of impermeable solute molecules on each side of the semipermeable membrane.[8]

The flow of water across the semipermeable membrane exerts an osmotic pressure. The pressure is in the direction of the flow of water. For dilute solutions, osmotic pressure can be calculated using the ideal gas laws if the solute concentration, temperature, and membrane permeability characteristic are known. Under steady-state or homeostatic conditions where temperature, pH, and other physiological parameters are constant, the magnitude of the impermeable solute gradient is the principal determinant of osmotic pressure. Thus, osmotic pressure is a predictable quantity and can be calculated if the concentration gradient is known.[9]

A major function of the kidneys is osmoregulation, and they regulate water and electrolytes to within narrow limits. Osmoregulation balances intracellular and extracellular osmotic pressures and prevents net movement of water into or out of cells. Cell volume and hydration are critical to cell function. Too much or too little water compromises metabolism and other critical cellular processes. Plant cells generate turgor pressure by the osmotic movement of water into cells that allows certain plants to stand upright. Plant cells have a cell wall around the cell membrane that can withstand the internal osmotic pressure. Animal cells will burst if too much water enters the cells or will shrivel if too much water leaves the cell because of a lack of a cell wall.[10]

The regulation of water balance by the kidneys is controlled mainly by the antidiuretic hormone (ADH, also called vasopressin). In the presence of ADH, the body retains water. In the absence of ADH, the kidneys excrete water. ADH is produced by the hypothalamus and secreted by the posterior pituitary gland. The hypothalamus contains osmoreceptors that directly monitor the solute concentration (osmolality) of plasma and, when osmolality is high, signal the secretion of ADH. Retention of water by the kidney increases blood volume, thus reducing osmolality. ADH has the added effect of stimulating thirst. Water consumption also increases blood volume.

Water retention by the kidneys is facilitated by aquaporins (water channels) in the collecting ducts of the kidney. Water moves via osmosis from the collecting ducts into the kidney, where it is returned to the blood plasma. Any water remaining in the collecting ducts is excreted as urine. The kidney maintains an osmotic gradient in the renal medulla (inner portion of the kidney) to carefully regulate water content of the blood plasma. ADH acts on the collecting ducts to insert aquaporins into the membranes of cells lining the ducts. Since the solute (osmotic) concentration is higher outside the collecting ducts than in, water moves out of the collecting ducts by osmosis. In diabetes insipidus, ADH control is lost, leading to copious excretion of highly dilute urine because aquaporins are not available to return water to the blood plasma. Excessive urination is accompanied by excessive thirst, a physiological response to replace excreted water.[11]

Diffusion and osmosis are transport processes that operate over very short distances. Diffusion results from the random movements of atoms or small molecules (known as Brownian motion) as a result of their collisions with the molecules making up the surrounding medium. Large molecules like proteins might take as long as a hundred seconds or so to traverse a human cell (about 0.01 mm in diameter). Small solute molecules may take only about one-tenth of a second. Traversing a distance of 1 mm increases the diffusion time from the order of seconds to many minutes because the diffusion rate is proportional to the square of the distance traversed. This is the reason that tissues are highly vascularized, so all cells are close to oxygen and nutrients in the nearby capillary bed.[12] Individual cells could not survive if they depended on oxygen diffusion directly from the external environment. The respiratory and circulatory systems provide oxygen to cells through a process of long-distance blood transport. Once blood arrives in the capillary bed, oxygen and nutrients move out of the capillaries a short distance to the cells, and waste products move from the cells into the capillaries.

The Electric Slide

Movement of electrical charges (carried by ions) across cell membranes is used to generate electrical impulses that are key to nervous system function. The movements of ions across cell membranes induce electrical currents. Membrane voltages and currents can be calculated to a high degree of accuracy if conductance properties of the membrane and concentrations of ionic species across the membrane are known using established deterministic laws of physics (for example, Ohm's law and Coulomb's law).

Two key processes lead to electric currents in cell membranes. First, the cell maintains a constant concentration difference of ions across the cell membrane. Second, the cell membrane has variable conductance properties, which allows for the orchestrated movement of ions that is necessary in generating electrical impulses in the nervous system and elsewhere. Ions normally do not cross the cell membrane easily because of the nonpolar lipid bilayer in the inner portion of the membrane. Ion channels in the membrane facilitate ionic movement across the membrane. The conductance properties of the membrane can be regulated by opening and closing specific ion channels. Interestingly, classical laws of physics, when applied to voltage measurements in excited nerve cells, predicted membrane channels before laboratory methods were available to prove their existence.

Cells convert chemical energy into electrical energy by ions sliding down their electrochemical gradient. A voltage across the membrane is generated only when one or more ions are permeable and can move through the membrane. When there is no permeability to any ion, there is no membrane potential because, despite the presence of a chemical concentration gradient, there is no net charge imbalance across the membrane. The sodium-potassium pump is interesting in this regard. By pumping three sodium ions out of the cell for every two potassium ions pumped into the cell, the required charge imbalance across the membrane is established.

The cell membrane is like an electronic circuit with resistance and capacitance. The lipid bilayer is an insulator that separates charges (ions) located in the intracellular compartment from those in the extracellular compartment. Fluids both within and outside cells are good conductors of electric charge. The electric characteristics of cell membranes obey macroscopic laws of physics: Ohm's law (relating voltage with ion current and resistance), Fick's law (relating rate of diffusion with concentration gradient and membrane permeability), and the Goldman equation (determining the voltage, or equilibrium potential, across a cell's membrane based on the electrochemical gradient of all the ions that permeate the membrane).[13]

A resting membrane potential in most cells is generated by the relatively high permeability of potassium ions. Some potassium ion channels in the plasma membrane are "leaky," allowing for slow diffusion of the ion out of the cell. Potassium ions flow down their concentration gradient from the intracellular compartment (the cytoplasm) into the extracellular fluid space. The movement of potassium ions will continue unabated until the chemical gradient that drives potassium out of the cell is balanced by the electric gradient that tends to pull potassium ions back into the cell. The electric gradient results from the charge imbalance across the membrane created by the movement of potassium out of the cell. As potassium ions leave the cell, the inside of the cell becomes increasingly negative and has a tendency to pull positive charges back into the cell. The electric and chemical gradients work in opposing directions. When the forces driving potassium out of the cell and into the cell are balanced, potassium ions still enter and leave the cell, but they do so at the same rate; no net movement of potassium ions occurs. At this point, the membrane system is at equilibrium or balance, and the membrane potential is stable or "resting."[14] The total resting membrane potential is very close to the resting membrane potential for potassium only, because membrane permeability for potassium is much higher than it is for other ions. The value of the resting membrane potential is a deterministic quantity and can be calculated from Goldman's equation. Movement of potassium and other ions across the membrane depends on maintaining ion concentration gradients. This work is done by the ATP-powered ion pumps/transporters and/or exchangers such as the Na^+-K^+ ATPase pump. These pumps and exchangers work constantly to overcome the continuous degradation of gradients by movement of ions. The pumps get their energy from ATP produced primarily by the complete oxidation of glucose.

The resting membrane potential serves three main purposes. First, it provides a constant source of electrical energy because the membrane acts as a capacitor to store electric charge.[15] The membrane can be thought of as a battery that powers a number of biomolecular devices within the membrane. The membrane is an imperfect storage system or capacitor because potassium ions can slowly leak through the membrane. Ion pumps are critical to maintaining the electrical properties of the membrane. In the absence of these pumps, the membrane's capacitance would eventually go to zero.

Second, in excitable membranes, the electric potentials serve as cell signals. Excitable membranes are found in select cell types such as neurons, muscle cells, and certain secretory cells. In an excitable membrane, local changes in voltage in one part of the membrane lead to the opening or closing of ion channels that, in turn, produce a local current that travels rapidly to other parts of the cell membrane. Excitable membranes amplify changes in the membrane potential by triggering voltage oscillations and action potentials. Opening and closing ion channels change the resting potential. If the membrane potential is increased, it becomes less negative, and the membrane is said to be depolarized. If the membrane potential is decreased, it becomes more negative, and the membrane is said to be hyperpolarized.

Third, in sensory systems, including visual and auditory pathways, the resting membrane potential serves as a basis for environmental signal discrimination. Sensory cortices in the brain are endowed with a double coding capacity to interpret environmental signals. The resting membrane potential serves as a baseline whereby environmental signals can be compared and interpreted. In the absence of such a baseline, external signals would be difficult to distinguish from noise (that is, non-signal) in the system.

Nerve cells (neurons) have excitable membranes that carry a resting membrane potential of about -70 millivolts (mV). The voltage is negative because the interior of the cell is more negative than the outside of the cell due to leakage of potassium ions (positively charged) to the cell's exterior. Depolarization of the nerve cell membrane increases the membrane potential (for example, from -70 mV to -60 mV). Hyperpolarization decreases the membrane potential (for example, from -70 mV to

-80 mV). The cell can change its membrane potential by selectively altering membrane permeability to certain ions.

In nerve cells, a sufficiently large depolarization evokes an event called an action potential. The action potential is a sudden, very rapid change in the membrane potential going from a negative voltage to a positive one (Figure 3.2). The action potential is an all-or-nothing event and occurs only if the depolarization of the membrane potential exceeds some threshold value. If the threshold is exceeded, the action potential occurs every time; if not, there is no action potential. Action potentials are generated by special types of "voltage-gated" ion channels in the nerve cell membrane that allow sodium ions to enter the cell. (Voltage-gating is the opening or closing of the ion channel in response to a change in the membrane potential.) The sodium gradient is in the opposite direction of the potassium gradient because sodium concentration is higher outside the cell than inside.

Five functional types of proteins have been identified in neurons; these proteins support nerve signal generation and propagation: structural elements, enzymes, receptors, channels, and ion pumps. The nerve membrane is capable of storing, transmitting, and releasing electrical energy. The structural proteins hold cells together in junctions while stabilizing other proteins contained within the membrane to

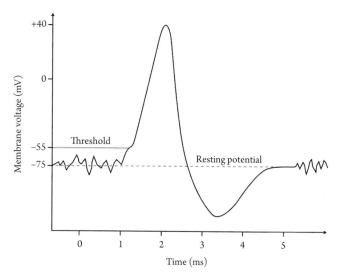

Figure 3.2 The action potential is a rapid membrane voltage transition. The all-or-none phenomenon occurs only when a voltage threshold is exceeded. If the threshold is exceeded, the membrane undergoes a rapid depolarization due to influx of sodium ions (the rising phase). The membrane voltage decreases as the membrane becomes repolarized due to sodium channels closing and potassium channels opening, allowing potassium to move into the cell. The membrane becomes hyperpolarized because of continued enhanced potassium conductance. Gradually, the membrane potential returns to the resting state. The duration of the action potential is about five milliseconds (ms). During that time interval, a second action potential cannot be generated because sodium channels cannot be opened.

maintain structure. Enzymes speed up chemical reactions for nerve and membrane function. Receptors recognize transmitter substances since the membrane of the cell must selectively recognize and bind to specific molecules. Pores or channels are specific regions where ions can enter or leave the cell based on their size and charge. The channels operate when the concentrations of ions differ inside and outside the cell. Thus, differing ion concentrations are a fundamental feature of neuron function, as pumps expend energy to expel certain ions from the cell and bring other ions into the cell.

The action potential is the language of communication between neurons. Nerves also send signals in the form of action potentials to control muscle movement and to stimulate secretions from certain types of glandular cells. The action potential and resting membrane potential are generated by membrane conductance properties primarily for potassium, sodium, and calcium. Whereas the resting membrane potential represents a relatively stable ground state, the action potential is a sudden, short-lived excited state.

The action potential in neurons results from a sudden influx of sodium ions into the cell (Figure 3.2). The spike is triggered by depolarization of the membrane leading to increased sodium conductance, inward current, and more depolarization. When the cell membrane is near its resting potential (about -70 mV), membrane permeability to sodium is low. If the membrane voltage is increased beyond a threshold (about -50 mV), voltage-gated sodium channels open, thus increasing membrane conductance for sodium. Sodium ions enter the cell, further increasing the membrane potential and opening more sodium channels in a positive feedback loop. Positive charge builds up on the interior membrane until the equilibrium potential for sodium is reached (about +40 mV). The rapid entry of sodium ions results in a reverse of voltage polarity in the membrane. When the sodium equilibrium potential is reached, net flow of sodium ceases because the inward flow due to the chemical concentration gradient is balanced by outward flow due to the electric charge gradient that pulls sodium ions out of the cell. When net flow of sodium is zero, the sodium channels close, and potassium channels open, allowing potassium ions to move out of the cell and causing repolarization of the membrane as the interior loses positive charge. The membrane eventually becomes hyperpolarized briefly because of excess potassium in the extracellular space. The membrane potential gradually returns to the resting membrane potential. The whole process of generating the action potential takes four to five milliseconds.

Distinct phase transitions with periods of depolarization, repolarization, and hyperpolarization characterize the action potential. The Na^+-K^+ ATPase pump operates continuously to restore the potassium gradient by pumping potassium into the cell and to restore the sodium gradient by pumping sodium out of the cell.[16]

Excitability requires the membrane to be at the resting potential when action potentials are not being generated. The typical negative resting potential is a result of selective ionic permeability to potassium and ion pumps that concentrate potassium inside the cell. Membrane potentials are sensitive to changes in the extracellular concentration of potassium. A ten-fold increase in extracellular potassium concentration is sufficient to abolish the resting potential. Excitable cells cannot generate action potentials in the absence of a negative resting potential because sodium channels cannot be opened. Sensitivity to changes in the extracellular potassium environment is tissue specific. Neurons are protected from large changes in potassium via the blood-brain barrier. But such protection is not available to cardiac tissue. Potassium chloride administered intravenously increases the extracellular potassium ion concentration, reducing its gradient, and the negative resting membrane potential is wiped out. Consequently, the cardiac ventricles can no longer contract and pump blood.[17]

Local anesthetics, including cocaine, lidocaine, and procaine, cause reversible local anesthesia by stabilizing the nerve cell membrane. Local anesthetic drugs act mainly by inhibiting sodium influx through sodium-specific ion channels in the neuronal cell membrane. When the influx of sodium is interrupted, an action potential cannot arise, and signal conduction is inhibited.[18]

The action potential is the same everywhere in the nervous system. The all-or-none character of the action potential and the shape of the action potential reflect biophysical determinism. Membrane conductance to specific ions and ion gradients determine the shape of the action potential. The shapes of the action potentials in cardiac pacemaker cells and neurons are different because of the role of calcium ions in the pacemaker spike.

Action potentials are generated in a special region of the neuron cell body called the axon hillock. The hillock is rich in sodium channels necessary to generate the action potential. The hillock is the region of the cell body that connects the axon to the neuron cell body. Action potentials generated in the hillock propagate down the axon and away from the neuron cell body (Figure 3.3). Action potentials propagate down the axon to either another neuron or a muscle cell or a secretory cell.

Nerve conduction velocities are limited by the need to regenerate the action potential along the axon because of energy losses and the time needed to generate the action potential. The nerve impulse dissipates energy as it moves down the axon. Action potentials must be regenerated at various points along the axon to refresh the signal. Action potentials are regenerated only when the resting membrane potential exceeds the voltage threshold. Regeneration of the action potential is constrained by the refractory periods caused by the process of sodium channel inactivation and the fact that sodium channels cannot reactivate until a short time after the membrane returns to its resting potential. Because of these delays, nerve signal velocities may only be one to two meters per second. In life-threatening situations or threat of serious injury, this may be too slow to achieve a timely neural response.

The nervous system is a fine-tuned detection and coordination system. Its primary role is to respond to environmental situations before they materialize fully. Once a "problem" is recognized, the solution becomes obvious. A nervous system does no good if the organism cannot respond in sufficient time to avoid injury or death.

Increased signal velocities provide a survival advantage. To increase speed, some axons are coated with myelin (called white matter), a lipoprotein insulator wrapped around the axon. Myelin increases electrical resistance across the cell membrane and decreases capacitance, thus preventing signal losses. When the nerve fiber is coated with myelin, signals literally hop down the axon in a process known as saltatory conduction. This increases the speed of conduction to about one hundred meters per second. Saltatory conduction is a consequence of the segmentation of myelin on the

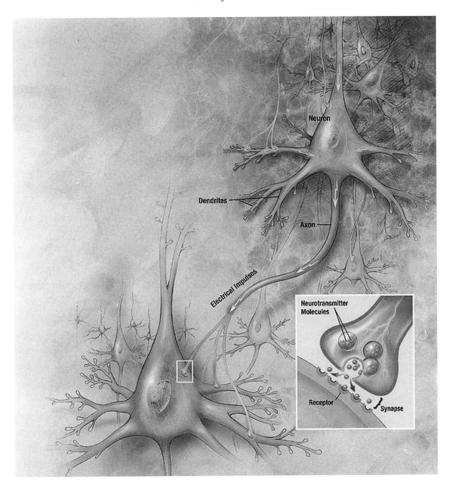

Figure 3.3 Anatomy of a neuron. The neuron consists of a cell body with numerous dendritic projections feeding into the cell. The axon is a specialized projection that carries action potentials away from the neuron to the next neuron. The axon terminus communicates with the dendrite of a neighboring neuron through a synapse. Synapses release neurotransmitters that depolarize or hyperpolarize the postsynaptic (dendritic) membrane. These voltages are summed by the neuron cell body; if the total voltage exceeds threshold, the neuron will fire an action potential down its axon. In the central nervous system, there are a thousand or more synaptic connections for each neuron. *Source:* National Institutes of Health, National Institute of Aging.

axon. Gaps of unmyelinated nerve fiber, called nodes of Ranvier, separate myelinated segments. The nodes are rich in sodium channels and are the loci for action potential regeneration. The action potential at one node passively depolarizes the adjacent node of Ranvier to threshold, triggering an action potential in this region that subsequently depolarizes the next node, and so forth. Myelin changes the

conduction properties of the axon. The electrical properties associated with myelina-
tion are deterministic and consistent with macroscopic laws of physics.[19]

Several important neurological diseases involve demyelination of the axon. The
destruction of the myelin sheath leads to slowed or blocked nerve conduction, and
this gives rise to numerous motor problems. Axon loss is the major cause of irreversible disability in patients with multiple sclerosis (MS), a chronic inflammatory
demyelinating disease of the central nervous system.[20]

The synapse is a second key component in neural communication. This is a specialized junction where a neuron communicates with a target cell or another nerve
cell. Neurons communicate by releasing neurotransmitters from the end of the axon
or by direct electrical connections called electrical synapses. When the axon releases
a chemical transmitter (a neurotransmitter), it diffuses across a small gap (the synaptic cleft) and activates specialized sites called receptors, situated on the target cell.
In neurons, the synaptic receptors are located in dendrites (Figure 3.3). The target
cell may also be a specialized region of a muscle cell or secretory cell.[21]

When neurotransmitters bind dendritic receptors, the membrane becomes
depolarized or hyperpolarized depending on whether the neurotransmitter is
excitatory or inhibitory (Figure 3.3). Receptors are usually binding sites located
on ion channels in the membrane. The channel opens when the neurotransmitter
is bound to the ion channel receptor site. Depolarization (increasing membrane
voltage) of the dendritic membrane occurs if the opened ion channel allows ions
to move into the cell. Acetylcholine is a very common excitatory neurotransmitter and opens sodium channels. The net movement of sodium ions across the dendritic membrane depolarizes the membrane. Gamma-aminobutyric acid (GABA)
is an inhibitory neurotransmitter and has the opposite effect. When it binds its
receptor, the membrane becomes hyperpolarized (that is, more negative membrane
voltage) because membrane conductance to potassium and chloride are increased.
Membrane voltages produced by local depolarizations and hyperpolarizations are
summed in the nerve cell body. If the integrated voltage is greater than threshold,
an action potential is generated at the axon hillock. Depolarization events in the
dendrites are more likely to lead to action potentials, whereas hyperpolarization
events are likely to be inhibitory. A single neuron in the brain may have a thousand
synaptic connections or more.[22]

Certain neurological and behavioral disorders have characteristic neurotransmitter signatures. Parkinson's disease, for example, is linked to low levels of dopamine in the brain and is characterized by spastic motion of the eyelids as well as
rhythmic tremors of the hands and other parts of the body. Thus, one approach to
treating Parkinson's disease is to increase the concentration of dopamine in the
brain. Some depression, anxiety disorders, and personality disorders are treated by a
class of drugs called SSRIs (selective serotonin reuptake inhibitors), including fluoxetine (Prozac), paroxetine (Paxil), and sertraline (Zoloft). Serotonin is an inhibitory
neurotransmitter associated with emotion and mood. Too little serotonin has been
linked to incidents of depression, problems with anger control, obsessive-compulsive
disorder, and suicide. SSRIs maintain adequate levels of serotonin by preventing the
reabsorption of serotonin from the synaptic cleft.[23] It is unclear how these drugs
actually alter mood and behavior because the relationship between changes in brain

chemistry and higher cortical functions governing behavior remains poorly understood and is clearly a problem of emergence in complex systems.

Driving Forces

The human body generates internal mechanical forces for movement, and these forces are the most obvious form of energy use in the human body. Walking, breathing, and eating all convert some of the chemical energy consumed in food into mechanical forces. The human body uses mechanical energy to carry out important physiological functions, including pumping blood, moving air into and out of the lungs, and transporting nutrients into tissues and waste products out of tissues.

Mechanical forces occur in two principal ways. Skeletal muscle contractions result from the cross-binding of specialized proteins called actin and myosin.[24] The cyclic coupling of actin and myosin in the muscle fibers results in muscular contraction and relaxation of skeletal muscle necessary for physical motion. The mechanical forces generated by muscular contraction can be modeled by Newton's laws of motion.[25] Skeletal muscles and joints act as a complicated system of levers that allow body movements.

Forces are also generated by changing pressures in body cavities. The heart uses pressure gradients as a driving force to move blood. Movement of blood through vessels and movement of air into and out of the lungs are based on the ideal gas laws. These laws describe forces generated in fluids and gases when pressures and volumes change. When the left ventricle of the heart contracts, the blood pressure inside the ventricle increases. Since the blood pressure is higher in the contracting ventricle than in the aorta (the main artery leaving the heart), blood moves down the pressure gradient and into the aorta.

Blood flow through the arterial system can be modeled in much the same way as water flow through pipes. Although blood is a complex fluid, certain reasonable, simplifying assumptions can be applied to predict blood flow as blood pressure or resistance to vascular flow changes. The basic job of the heart is to maintain blood flow through the various tissues and organs. If blood flow is reduced, the heart and circulatory system respond by increasing blood pressure. The heart pumps blood by rhythmically changing pressures in the pumping chambers. Blood flow through the arterial system is determined by the blood pressure and peripheral vascular resistance.

In physiology, pressure is measured instead of force. Pressure is force applied to a given surface area. To a first approximation, forces and pressures obey the classical laws of physics. Many physiological systems operate on the principle that normal function requires a balancing of pressures. Altering the pressure dynamics leads to physiologic dysfunction.

Forces and pressures act at every level of biological complexity. The balance of osmotic pressure and hydrostatic pressure in the capillary bed controls the direction of movement of nutrients and waste products to and from tissues. Osmotic pressure and hydrostatic pressure are functionally equivalent in their ability to drive water through a membrane but act in opposite directions in the capillary bed (Figure 3.4).

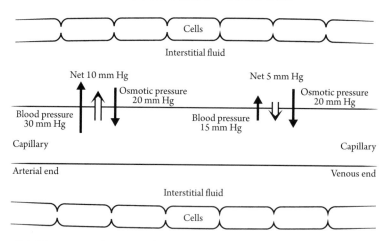

Figure 3.4 Movement of water and dissolved materials into and out of the capillary depends on the balance of hydrostatic and osmotic pressures. The longer dark arrow signifies direction of greater flow; the open arrow signifies direction of net flow. At the arterial end of the capillary bed, hydrostatic pressure exceeds osmotic pressure, resulting in a net flow of water and nutrients out of the capillary and into the interstitial spaces. At the venous end, hydrostatic pressure falls below the osmotic pressure, resulting in a net movement of water and solutes out of the interstitial space and into the capillary.

Capillaries are the smallest blood vessels in the body and bridge the arterial and venous circulations. The capillary wall separates the blood plasma compartment from the interstitial fluid compartment. Tissues and their constituent cells are bathed in the interstitial fluid from which they obtain nutrients and into which they excrete wastes. The blood plasma and interstitial fluid make up the extracellular fluid (ECF). Plasma constitutes 20 percent, while interstitial fluid makes up 80 percent of the ECF.[26] Capillaries are composed of a single layer of thin, flat epithelial cells. Most capillaries have pores (spaces) between the individual cells that make up the capillary wall.[27] Plasma fluid and small nutrient molecules can easily leave the capillary and enter the interstitial fluid through these pores, in a process called bulk flow. Blood cells and plasma proteins do not filter out of the capillaries by bulk flow because they are too large to fit through the pores.

Hydrostatic pressure is exerted by the blood plasma against capillary walls due to the blood pressure generated by the pumping action of the heart. Hydrostatic pressure is higher at the arterial end of the capillary bed and falls as the blood moves through the bed to the venous end because of frictional resistance of the capillaries and the increased cross-sectional area on the venous side of the bed. Hydrostatic pressure tends to force materials out of the capillaries and into the interstitial fluid space.

If the hydrostatic pressure was the only force present, there would be a continual loss of blood plasma (including water and solute molecules that can filter through the capillary walls). But under normal physiological conditions, little plasma volume is lost to the interstitial fluid compartment.

The reason for this is the osmotic pressure that counteracts the hydrostatic pressure and drives water from the interstitial fluid compartment back into the capillary and blood plasma. The composition of the interstitial fluid and the plasma is about the same, except that plasma also contains proteins not found in the interstitial fluid. These plasma proteins are too large to fit through capillary pores and cannot cross the capillary wall. Because of the presence of plasma proteins, the plasma has a higher solute concentration than does the interstitial fluid. Consequently, osmotic pressure causes interstitial fluid to be absorbed into the plasma compartment in the capillary.

Slight imbalances in the hydrostatic and osmotic pressures in the capillary bed allow for bulk movement of substances into or out of the capillaries. On the artery side of the bed, the hydrostatic pressure exceeds the osmotic pressure, and substances move out of the capillary into the interstitial space in a process called filtration. At the venous end, osmotic pressure exceeds the hydrostatic pressure and substances move into the capillary from the interstitial space in a process called reabsorption (Figure 3.4). There is normally slightly more filtration of fluid into the tissue spaces than is reabsorbed. About 90 percent of filtered fluid is reabsorbed; the remaining 10 percent flows into lymphatic vessels. The lymphatic system serves an important function by transporting proteins and other large molecules away from the interstitial spaces. These large molecules cannot be reabsorbed through capillary walls because they are too large. The lymphatic system is an auxiliary route by which fluids flow from the interstitial spaces to the blood plasma. Clearing proteins and other large molecules from the interstitial spaces is critical to maintaining the balance between filtration and absorption.

Perturbations in the delicate balance between hydrostatic and osmotic pressure affect the exchange of materials between the interstitial and plasma compartments. Tissue swelling (edema) is an important pathological process that occurs when this delicate balance is out of kilter. If excess fluid cannot be returned to the bloodstream, then interstitial fluid builds up, leading to swelling of the tissues. Edema can occur if there is a reduced concentration of plasma proteins. Kidney disease can result in the loss of blood proteins to the urine. A protein-deficient diet will also decrease plasma proteins. Edema also occurs if there is an increase in vascular permeability. In the generalized inflammatory response, tissue damage leads to the release of histamine from specialized cells of the immune system. Histamine increases the size of capillary pores. The rate of filtration increases because of the higher capillary permeability. Increased blood pressure in veins also causes edema. When blood flow slows at the vein end, blood can back up at the arterial end. The excess fluid increases the rate of filtration. Sitting for a long time (for example, on an airplane during a long transatlantic flight) leads to swelling in the lower legs because of a backup of blood in the veins. That is the reason it is important to stand up and stretch your legs to prevent the pooling of blood in the lower extremities.[28]

All Pumped Up

The cardiovascular system is composed of a complex network of vessels that provides nutrients to tissues and carries away waste products. Because diffusion distances are short (on the order of a few cell diameters), the vasculature is quite extensive such that any given cell is not far removed from the capillary bed. The extensive nature of the vascular network creates high peripheral vascular resistance that must be overcome by the heart to perfuse the tissues adequately. The heart pumps the entire blood volume about once every minute through sixty thousand miles of blood vessels—laid end to end they would circle the Earth two and a half times! As the heart beats, arterial blood pressure varies from a maximum during ventricular contraction to a minimum when the heart is resting and the ventricles are filling with blood. Large arteries have elastic walls that expand and contract to reduce variations in blood pressure as blood moves away from the heart.

Cardiac power (the amount of energy used by the heart per unit time) is the product of the blood pressure and blood flow. This is analogous to electric power based on Ohm's law, where power is the product of voltage and current. Assuming an average person at rest, the cardiac power is one to two watts (W). The heart generates about 5 percent of the useful work done by the body while at rest. During exercise or exertion, the heart increases its power output by increasing blood flow rate and blood pressure.[29]

The primary goal of the circulatory system is to maintain perfusion of the tissues by sustaining blood flow. The circulatory system adjusts blood flow by controlling arterial diameter to change vascular resistance. Mathematically, blood flow can be described by Poiseuille's law, which predicts flow characteristics for uniform liquids (called Newtonian fluids) where there is no appreciable turbulence. Poiseuille's equation identifies viscosity of the fluid (the thickness of a fluid or its fluidity) and the blood vessel radius as key determinants of peripheral vascular resistance. In the case of smooth flow (laminar flow), resistance depends linearly on the viscosity but on the fourth power of the radius of the blood vessel.[30]

The blood vessel radius is, therefore, a very powerful modifier of blood flow. If the blood vessel radius is decreased by one-half, resistance to blood flow increases sixteen times. Vasodilation (widening the vessel lumen) and vasoconstriction (narrowing the lumen) are key homeostatic controls of blood pressure. An important class of antihypertensive medications called beta blockers work by dilating blood vessels to reduce blood pressure.

Poiseuille's law is a good predictor of flow dynamics but only under certain conditions. These conditions are often not met in modeling flow of blood, particularly in the small arteries of the circulatory system. Blood is a heterogeneous fluid consisting primarily of red blood cells suspended in plasma.[31] Blood flow is compromised in diseased blood vessels. Atherosclerosis is a pathological process leading to the development of fatty deposits and plaques on arterial walls. The plaques cause blood flow to become turbulent. Eddies and vortices, the same kind as are commonly seen in streams as water passes around and over rocks, occur as the blood moves past the vascular wall abnormalities. Creation of these abnormal flow patterns causes blood flow to lose energy. The presence of arterial plaques also decreases the size of the blood vessel, further reducing blood flow.

The flow of crude oil through the Alaska oil pipeline is a good example of fluid mechanics and how flow can be optimized by adjustments of important flow properties. The Trans Alaska Pipeline System is eight hundred miles long and connects

Prudhoe Bay along the Alaska North Slope with the southern port city of Valdez, the northern-most year-around ice-free port in Alaska. Crude oil from the oil fields on Alaska's North Slope enters the pipeline at Prudhoe Bay and is heated to a temperature of about 150° F to decrease its viscosity and then pumped through a series of eleven pumping stations through a 48-inch diameter pipeline to Valdez at a flow rate approximating one to two million barrels per day. The movement of oil through the pipeline leaves a waxy deposit on the pipeline walls. Unless removed, wax buildup reduces the pipeline diameter and increases drag (flow resistance), thus reducing the flow rate. "Scraper pigs" are introduced into the pipeline on a regular basis to keep pipeline walls clean. Pumping heated oil and keeping the pipeline walls clean reduce flow resistance.[32]

May the Force Be with You

Physical forces act at the cellular level. These forces can change cell structure and function and, interestingly can directly affect when genes are expressed. Studies of bacteria grown in microgravity environments provide compelling evidence linking gravity and gene expression. Bacteria show unique changes in virulence, structure, and gene expression in the microgravity environment. The ability of a cell to sense its mechanical environment involves transmembrane proteins that act as tiny transducers to convert mechanical information in the environment to chemical information that trigger protein synthesis and other adaptive biochemical events in the cell. Environmental sensing is key to cell growth and differentiation in multicellular organisms. The firmness and cohesiveness of nearby tissue and the density of surrounding cells provide a physical environmental profile that dictates cell behavior. During human embryonic development, cells arrange themselves into tissues with interior cavities and multiple layers with distinct boundaries containing patterned arrangements of cell types. Cells in the embryo have the ability via contractile and protrusive activities to exert forces on one another and on the extracellular matrices they produce. These forces allow developing tissues to elongate, fold, segment, and form appendages.[33]

A wide range of important human diseases, including cancer, immune disorders, and cardiovascular and infectious diseases, are associated with abnormal physiological responses to mechanical forces. Little is known about the process of cellular biomechanics (how cells respond to mechanical force) especially the mechanism(s) of how this process affects both normal and diseased cells. The challenge is to understand how mechanical forces are integrated in cells and tissues and how this integration results in coordinated structural and functional changes at the cellular, tissue, organ, and organism level. Understanding how mechanical forces regulate cell and tissue function provides a valuable perspective on human biology and disease. There is enormous potential for advancing our understanding of systems biology and enhancing human health, including the development of new therapeutic modalities and novel tissue-engineering approaches to treat and prevent disease.

Cancer growth may be the consequence of balancing homeostatic or steady-state forces between the growing tumor and surrounding normal tissue. If the forces from the stroma (the tissue supporting structure) are greater than the forces from the growing tumor, the tumor will not grow and will die. Tumors grow and expand when tumor growth forces exceed opposing stromal forces. This is a particularly danger-ous and an acute problem when the volume for expansion is constrained. The brain is encased in a bony vault that allows little room for expansion. Primary brain tumors are often lethal because the growing tumor mass exerts pressure on healthy brain tissue that cannot be relieved by expansion.[34]

As discussed in this chapter, biological processes are, at an elementary level, deterministic. The fundamental processes underlying brain complexity—action potentials and membrane potentials—are deterministic and follow known laws of physics. When diseases like cholera are fully explainable at the deterministic level the disease course and outcomes are predictable. Signs and symptoms can be easily understood because they have all been seen before. Tchaikovsky's battle with chol-era followed a predictable course, and his death from severe diarrhea after drinking unboiled water was not unexpected.

But most diseases have an underlying complexity that cannot be explained by deterministic processes. Their clinical course is unpredictable. The complex char-acter of neurological and behavioral diseases derives from the complexity of the brain itself. Diffusion of ions across the cell membrane and generation of the mem-brane potential and action potential do not explain the emergent properties char-acteristic of brain complexity but are, nevertheless, necessary for observed complex behaviors. Thus, at higher orders of complexity, physiology transcends simple laws. Sensory tracking is a complex process involving the interplay of sensory structures (for example, the eye), nerve pathways to the cerebral cortex, and interpretation of neural information in the sensory cortex. When a baseball player tracks and catches a fly ball, the brain does not subconsciously solve Newton's equations of motion. Sensory tracking is much more complex and involves neural processing that is not fully understood. In fact, sensory tracking is not a higher-order cortical process reserved for humans or even primates. Anyone who has taken a dog out to play with a frisbee knows the dog probably uses the same brain functions as humans to snag the disc out of the air.

A major theme of this book is that processes underlying human biology and dis-ease are at a fundamental level predictable. At the heart of complexity is determin-ism and simplicity. The science of medicine depends on it. The macroscopic laws of physics discussed in this book are valid at equilibrium or near-equilibrium condi-tions. But life processes operate far from equilibrium and are nonlinear. Nonlinear dynamics can be unpredictable. As we will see in the next chapter, living systems are not predictable because of system complexity, nonlinear dynamics, and charac-teristics of chaos. Despite this, macroscopic laws of physics can be applied to living, complex systems: it is a question of knowing and appreciating the predictive and explanatory powers of these laws and their limitations. Even to a first approxima-tion, there is clear value in applying deterministic laws in clinical medicine. But how can the paradoxical characteristics of life—predictability good enough for medicine and unpredictability based on the complex, nonlinear properties of living systems—be reconciled?

4

Biological Complexity

Life is characterized by a variety of novel materials, processes, and organizational motifs over a wide range of biological scales—from the subcellular to social communities. Living systems have the capacity to replicate and evolve and to adapt or react to changing environmental conditions. Reproduction, evolution, and adaptability are consequences of biological complexity characterized by physical and chemical processes operating as nonlinear dynamical systems far from thermodynamic equilibrium.

Arguments have already been made that these cardinal features of life cannot be accounted for by the deterministic laws of physics. Complex systems, by virtue of their adaptive capacities, are endowed with an arrow of time whereby the future can be distinguished from the past. Dynamic memory erases itself. Old people look different from young people. Temporal asymmetry means that we can turn eggs into an omelet but cannot turn an omelet back into eggs.[1] As much as we would like to, we cannot turn the clock back. Anyone who has run a movie backward knows time cannot simply be reversed without encountering absurdities.[2]

The central challenge in unpacking biological complexity is figuring out how underlying deterministic processes operating in highly interconnected and interdependent environments lead to emergent properties. In sensory physiology, action potentials are generated at the sensory detector (eye, ear, taste buds). Information is coded as the spatial and temporal distributions of action potentials and interpreted by the brain to generate a sensory experience. Action potentials are deterministic and linear, but sensory perceptions are emergent and nonlinear. The generation of the action potential is well characterized, but we still have a long way to go to understand how neural signals are ultimately processed to drive higher cortical functions.

The taste stimulus-response function (Figure 4.1) illustrates higher cortical function complexity that cannot be completely understood on the basis of macroscopic laws of physics. The sigmoid-shaped curve bridges the biophysical events in taste buds with sensory events in the brain by relating magnitude of stimulus (as measured by concentration of tastant, that is, something that can stimulate the sense of taste) to perceived sweetness intensity (a measure of the central nervous system function). The dose-response curve is obtained using normal subjects given increasing concentrations of a tastant (sucrose) on the surface of the tongue and asked to grade the intensity of the sweetness response. The curve suggests that low concentrations of tastant elicit little or no response and that high tastant concentrations give rise to a saturation effect, whereby even higher concentrations do not further increase perceived intensity—the

taste sensation is as strong as it can get. The early sensory events, including the chemical binding of tastant to taste-cell membranes and the subsequent generation and
conduction of nerve impulses, are well characterized, but how the neural signal is translated into a sensory experience in the brain is not understood. Signal processing reflects
the complexities of the nervous system. Intensity responsiveness is more than just a
biophysical function of the taste-cell membrane receptors bound by tastant molecules.
We do not fully understand the biological processes that link triggering by the sensory
stimulus and the higher-level cortical response. Signal processing is so complex that it
can only be obtained in intact subjects. We can never understand fully how we experience taste by just examining the tongue. What is required is understanding the tongue,
the gustatory (taste) cortex in the brain, and everything in between that is involved in
making the taste experience. Studies of isolated sensory pathways provide incomplete
information about mechanisms of sensory perception. Complexity is a property of the
whole, not of specific components or groups of components.

In this chapter, we explore the characteristic features of complexity and what
properties of living systems make them complex. As we have seen, deterministic systems obey physical laws that serve as a prescription for a unique course of action. In
complex systems, however, there is no unique course of action. Instead, the system
may choose from a range of alternative paths. Complexity is a consequence of nonlinear dynamics and the capacity of systems to adapt. Complex systems have the capacity to transition to more elaborate and complex states through self-organization,
and this capacity leads to emergence, unpredictable behaviors, and other properties
of complexity.

There is now considerable interest in the search for definitive laws that explain
complexity, but it is unclear whether such laws even exist. Complexity, including emergence, is a property of nonlinear dynamic systems composed of highly integrated networks that, at their simplest level, obey the known laws of physics. If there are special
laws of complexity, they would not violate the classical laws of physics laws but would
complement them. In biology, identification of complexity laws would not necessarily
mean that we have discovered the secret of life, but such laws would go a long way to
explaining how the brain and other complex biological systems work. The search for
laws of complexity must be an interdisciplinary pursuit, and some of the most exciting advances are taking place at the nexus of biology, chemistry, physics, and computational sciences. Nevertheless, the uncertainty inherent in complex systems limits
what we can ultimately know about these systems. Complexity presents a challenging
but frustrating paradox—the more answers we get the more questions we ask.

System Conditions and States

Natural systems, including the human body, can occupy several possible conditions
that dictate system behavior. Conditions are determined by system energy content
and energy flow and are independent of system complexity. The conditions that
describe a simple system like a swinging pendulum also describe complex systems.[3]
System *conditions* are distinguished from system *states*. A system condition such as
equilibrium or nonequilibrium is a characteristic of the system as a whole. A state is

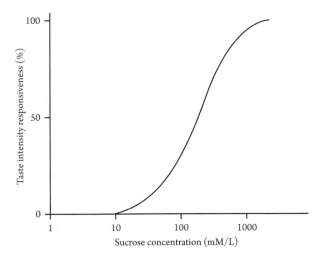

Figure 4.1 Sensory perception is a product of biological complexity and follows a nonlinear sigmoid response. At very low doses of a sensory stimulus (in this case, sucrose), response (perception of a sweet taste) is small. The intensity of sweetness increases as the concentration of sucrose is increased until a saturation point is reached. At that point, further increases in sucrose concentration do not elicit a greater response. The data couple concentration of sucrose against perception of sweetness but provide no information about mechanisms of sensory perception by the brain. *Source:* Figure redrawn from Mossman K, Shatzman A, Chencharick J. Long-term effects of radiotherapy on taste and salivary function in man. *International Journal of Radiation Oncology, Biology, Physics* 1982;8:991–997, with permission from Elsevier.

a specific description of the system at a particular time. For a swinging pendulum, the state is described completely by the position and momentum of the pendulum. System conditions dictate the dynamics of changes in system states over time.

When a system is in the equilibrium condition and in its lowest energy state, no further change can be expected within the system. In the thermodynamic sense, the system has zero entropy, meaning there is no net flow of energy through the system and that it is at maximum disorder. In our example, the swinging pendulum has come to rest. In living systems, equilibrium means death because there are no active gradient-driven processes. In the equilibrium condition, order associated with building and sustaining chemical and electrical gradients necessary for life is absent. Order has become disorder.

Systems can also exist in a stable near-equilibrium condition if an external source of energy can be continuously supplied. If no external energy source is available, the system will run down and eventually reach the equilibrium condition in accordance with the second law of thermodynamics. System stability is analogous to a battery that never goes dead because it is constantly being charged from an external energy source. Living systems are stable and avoid the equilibrium condition by importing high-quality energy and extracting the available energy through metabolism.

Systems in the near-equilibrium condition are linear. Small changes in the initial conditions produce proportional and predictable changes in system output. An example of a system in a near-equilibrium condition is a pendulum clock that uses a swinging pendulum as its time-keeping element.

A third condition is a system operating far from equilibrium. Here, behavior is no longer predictable because the system behaves in a nonlinear fashion. Unpredictability results from the capacity of the system to take on a number of surprising properties. Chaos, or small changes in one system variable that lead to unexpected changes in other system variables, cannot be modeled with simple mathematical equations. Chaos is a common property of nonlinear dynamical systems and demonstrates how the system can have complicated behavior that emerges as a consequence of nonlinear interactions.[4] The global climate system is an example of a complex, chaotic system. We cannot predict accurately long-term changes in the world's climate because we do not have a full understanding of all the variables in the system and how these variables interact to effect climate change.

Far-from-equilibrium conditions mean the system is subject to a large forcing agency that moves the system beyond regions of stability. In many cases, these systems will self-organize into more stable states called dissipative structures. As the system moves farther from equilibrium and becomes increasingly more unstable, a bifurcation or fork in the road is encountered, and the system can "choose" which fork to take. These bifurcations lead to more complex stable states. The system acquires complexity by internal differentiation. Internal differentiation can be thought of as the establishment of novel interaction networks among system components. Accordingly, reductionist approaches to understanding complex systems have limited utility because the system reflects coupled interactions among components that can be understood only by studying the whole rather than individual components. Everyday experiences, learning new skills, or learning a new language changes the brain through processes of internal differentiation that involve new synaptic connections among neurons and new neural networks.

The near-equilibrium and far-from-equilibrium conditions are not mutually exclusive. In fact, living systems require that these conditions coexist. Some biological processes such as diffusion across the cell membrane, which we saw in Figure 1.1, can be modeled as simple linear processes. Others such as heart contractions are nonlinear and demonstrate complex behaviors. Complexity confers both stability and adaptability. A strictly linear dynamical system is incapable of adaptation since a given input must produce a prescribed output. Complex adaptive systems exist at "the edge of chaos." Complex functions such as the heart rate are not constant over time but fluctuate unpredictably around a homeostatic or steady-state value. Complexity in living systems means that the system has the capacity to occupy simultaneously stable and unstable states. The system teeters at the edge of chaos, affording optimal adaptability. While something can go wrong at any time, the system can adapt in sometimes creative ways to adjust for the interruption in normal activity. That is the key to survival.

Complexity requires new ways of thinking about and understanding human biology and disease. A holistic or systems-level approach is nonreductive and considers both normal and disease states as consequences of multiple system interactions.

A systems approach requires that multiple variables be explored simultaneously to disentangle the dynamic structure that underlies system properties or behaviors of interest. The reductionist approach provides useful information about individual component behavior but cannot provide the insights critical to explaining system-level properties.

Complexity Made Simple

Complex systems are everywhere in nature. Complexity is not easily definable because it is so widespread in nature and takes on many forms and functions. It is evident in single cells, in multicellular organisms, in human social and behavioral networks, in ecology, and in climate systems. Murray Gell-Mann defines complexity as a quality that financial markets, complex immune systems, and ecological communities have in common. However complexity is defined, there are intriguing properties that all complex systems have in common. Complex systems consist of large networks of individual components, and complexity arises through the interactions and interdependence of components. The nature of interactions involves relatively simple signaling and information processing. To exist and function, complex systems use energy from the environment. Complexity endows the system with the capacity to adapt when the environment changes so the system can continue to exist and function.[5]

Complex Biological Systems Have Many Components That Interact Nonlinearly and Are Interdependent

Perhaps the key property of complex systems is the large number of parts that interact in a nonlinear fashion. Interactions are not predictable and often result in the creation of novel and creative structures. Life forms are the most complex systems in nature. Complexity is characterized by well-ordered multilevel organization, and multicomponent causal interactions.

A system is ordered when all components act or are arranged in a cooperative and systematic way. In biological systems, order is evident by the cooperation of diverse parts of an organism that perform a set of coherent and complementary functions. The brain and heart are highly ordered and perform specific functions in a coordinated fashion. Order may be discernible by the presence of spatial patterns. Orderliness is scalable in complex systems. In the human body, order is evident in individual cells, tissues, organs, and organ systems. The myriad forms of a living organism reflect the diversity and creativity inherent in complex systems.

Order can be quantified in terms of information content. If a system contains a hundred interconnected components, the information content of the system requires knowledge of each of the individual parts. But if the hundred parts are organized into ten identical groups of ten parts each, there are still a total of one hundred components but less information is required to explain the system because we now need to understand only ten parts. The latter case is less ordered and less complex than the former. The more highly ordered the system, the greater the amount of information necessary to describe the system. In contrast, disorder or entropy is the lack of information. In a thermodynamic sense, entropy describes the level of information. Living systems are highly ordered so have high negative entropy.[6] But quantity is not the only important information metric. The quality of information reflects the organization of the system. Organization refers to how well component parts interact and link together to achieve a unified functional purpose.

The quality of system information distinguishes complex systems from just complicated ones. Information quality reflects the richness of component interactions in complex systems. An automobile is highly ordered and has thousands of components, but it is not a complex system. The properties of the automobile are entirely predictable, explainable, and reducible to the properties of the component parts. Every component in an automobile can be switched out without compromising the automobile's operation. In a complex system, components interact in complicated ways, and replacing a component may have significant system consequences. We see this in transplantation medicine, where a new tissue or organ may fully restore a specific function, but system complexity leads to complications at the system level such as rejection of the transplanted tissue by the host immune system. Complexity is more about function than structure. The organized complexity of the eye is for the purpose of enabling the organism to see.[7] A system can be called complex if it can assume a large number of states or conformations (as determined by the number of components and connections) and if it can carry information.

Complex Systems Behave Unpredictably

The nonlinear dynamics inherent in complex systems leads to irregular and unpredictable behaviors. Small changes in one system parameter can lead to large changes in system responses. Nonlinear systems, unlike linear systems, do not exhibit properties of proportionality or independence. In nonlinear systems, the system output is not proportional to the system input. System components are also interdependent such that the combination of the effects of individual components is less than or more than the sum of the component effects. The result of the loss of the properties of linearity and independence is that the system can behave in an irregular and unpredictable way.

This disproportionate response is referred to as chaos. Chaos does not mean chaotic behavior and does not mean the system is operating wildly out of control. It means sensitivity to perturbations and unpredictability. In physiology, chaos is evident in a number of dynamical systems. The heart rate is not regular even during sleep; small unpredictable changes are always occurring. Although the heart rate may average seventy beats per minute over several hours, a careful analysis of heart rate on a minute-by-minute basis reveals a startlingly irregular pattern that cannot be predicted. Whether the heart rate "looks" stable or chaotic depends on the timescale of observation. Because of nonlinear dynamics, the heart rate at some time in the future can never be known exactly even though the average heart rate over a long time period may be stable (Figure 4.2).

Scientists began thinking about nonlinear dynamics (chaos) in physiologic systems in the 1960s and 1970s. Computational methods based on nonlinear dynamics are slowly working their way into clinical medicine and the analysis of physiological

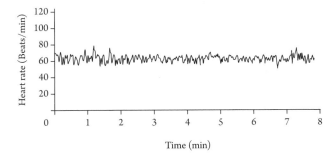

Figure 4.2 Heart rate time series in a healthy 22-year-old female subject. The mean heart rate is about sixty-five beats per minute. *Source:* Figure redrawn from Goldberger AL, et al. Fractal dynamics in physiology: alterations with disease and aging. *Proceedings of the National Academy of Sciences* 2002;99(Suppl. 1):2466–2472. Copyright 2002 National Academy of Sciences, U.S.A.

systems in health and disease. But the idea of nonlinear systems and the inherent unpredictable nature of such systems go back to the turn of the twentieth century and the work of the French mathematician Henri Poincaré.

As discussed in chapter 1, Poincaré championed a view that turned Newtonian physics and the notion of determinism on its head. The classical view as espoused by Pierre-Simon Laplace (1776) and others considered the Universe as entirely deterministic, meaning that knowledge of the current state of the system determined the past and the future. But Poincaré argued that, in complex systems, we can never know initial conditions exactly.

Living systems, thus, reflect deterministic chaos—simultaneously expressing deterministic and chaotic behaviors. Determinism holds true for all dynamic systems. However, the sensitive dependence on initial conditions makes predictions about system behavior impossible so that determinism no longer holds. For a chaotic system to be deterministic, initial conditions would need to be known completely and exactly. Uncertainty in complex systems takes two forms. First, complex systems exhibit chaotic behavior. Second, complex systems are indeterminant. There are many possible outcomes for a given input. Under nonlinear conditions, systems tend to bifurcate whereby the system "chooses" a particular state. Which fork is taken cannot be determined ahead of time unless initial conditions of the system are fully known.

Two common natural processes illustrate the point. Weather predictions beyond a week are inexact because of nonlinear dynamics in the complex weather system. The butterfly effect is a commonly used scientific metaphor that encapsulates the concept of sensitive dependence on initial conditions: a butterfly flaps its wings somewhere in Brazil and, at some time in the future, sets off a tornado in Texas. The creation of snowflakes is another example. No two snowflakes are identical; every snowflake pattern is unique and will always be so in the future. The structure of a snowflake is dependent on initial environmental conditions at the moment of creation and as the snowflake falls to earth. Very small changes in local temperature, pressure, and moisture content of the air influence snowflake structure. Snowflakes falling together show different structures because they experience different environmental influences that alter structure. Just the presence of a neighboring snowflake is enough to alter conditions and make predictions of snowflake structure impossible.[8]

Chaos may be difficult to distinguish from system noise. "Noise" is associated with random statistical fluctuations external to the system itself. Chaos is an intrinsic property of the system. A simple inspection of the heart rate tracing in Figure 4.2 cannot distinguish chaos from noise. Distinguishing the two requires statistical analysis to separate random external errors from inherent fluctuations in the system. Noise may be reduced but not entirely eliminated by measurement technique; chaos, however, cannot be reduced because it is an inherent property of the system. The distinction is important in medicine because chaos may reflect an underlying disease state. Noise tells us nothing about the underlying physiology and may interfere with interpretation of clinically relevant information.[9]

Complex Systems Show Fractal Geometry and Physiology

Fractal geometry and physiology are consequences of deterministic chaos. Fractals are random and irregular phenomena, most often associated with irregular geometric objects that display self-similarity. Fractal forms are composed of subunits (and sub-subunits, etc.) resembling the structure of the overall object (Figures 4.3 and 4.4). In theory, scale independence holds for all scales. But in reality, nature imposes upper and lower bounds over which scale invariant behavior applies. Fractals are found throughout the body. Fractal structures include bronchial branching, urinary collecting system, biliary duct structure in the liver, blood vessels in the heart, pulmonary blood flow, and arterial and venous trees.[10]

The branching pattern of the airway passages in the lungs is fractal. The lungs are a finely branching structure from the windpipe down to the terminal air sacs or alveoli where gas exchange occurs. Branching is uneven and occurs in unpredictable patterns (Figure 4.3). The human lung contains several hundred million alveoli. Although the lungs are compacted into a relatively small volume in the chest, the very high functional surface area derives from the fractal structure of the lungs. This fractal architecture facilitates gas exchange and pulmonary function by optimizing gas diffusion rates of oxygen and carbon dioxide in accordance with Fick's law of diffusion. Although biological complexity cannot be explained by classical laws of physics, the two are connected. The functional efficiency of the lung is dictated by its structural complexity and organization. In Fick's law of diffusion, the flow rate of oxygen from the alveoli into the blood plasma is directly proportional to the total area of the alveolar exchange surface.

The lung is an efficient organ of gas exchange because fractal architecture ensures components are properly connected in an integrated organ, airways and blood vessels are adequately correlated to allow well-matched ventilation, and blood flow and complex organization allow ventilation, blood perfusion, and gas exchange to function in a highly coordinated and efficient way. Physiological efficiency in gas exchange means the human lung has a high degree of complexity, correlativity, and connectivity. Meeting these design requirements introduces a number of problems, including how to design the gas exchanger so that all points can be efficiently

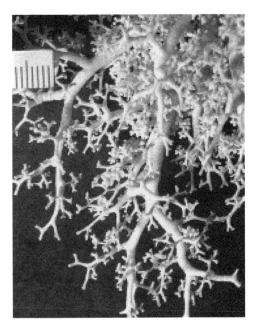

Figure 4.3 Lung cast showing fractal architecture. Fractal architecture facilitates gas exchange in the lung. Fractals are irregular shapes that are statistically similar to themselves on magnification over a range of length scales. *Source:* Reprinted with kind permission of Professor E. R. Weibel.

reached by air and blood and how to stabilize such a large exchange surface with so little tissue support. These difficulties are solved by use of fractal architecture.[11]

Fractal phenomena are also observed in physiologic processes. The patterns of variation in heart rate are repeated at smaller and smaller time scales (Figure 4.4). The underlying nonlinear dynamics leads to random and uncertain temporal patterns of heart rate. Nonlinear behavior allows for rapid alterations in heart rate as physiological requirements change.

Complex Systems Exhibit Emergent Properties

As systems increase in complexity, certain system-level properties emerge in a phase-like transition. Emergence is a consequence of complexity at multiple scales of organization. Living systems are thermodynamically open and multiscalar. A particular system behavior is considered emergent if it cannot be understood by studying the component parts at the finer scales of system organization. Emergence is unpredictable and represents larger-scale coherence. Interactions of components in the finer scales leads to structural or functional properties in the higher scales of the system that are absent in the components themselves. Emergence is identified with the capacity for self-assembly, such as inflammatory processes that involve cell aggregation. Cancer, for example, is a disease with emergent properties. Tumor growth and the acquisition

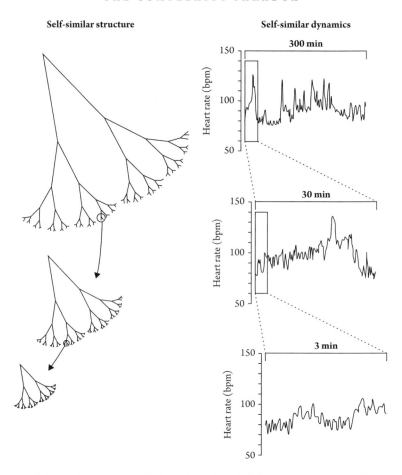

Figure 4.4 Fractal structure and physiology. On the left is a schematic of self-similarity observed in fractal structures. On the right is fractal-time series of heart rate. The structure at higher scales is repeated at lower scales. *Source:* Figure redrawn from Goldberger AL, et al. Fractal dynamics in physiology: alterations with disease and aging. *Proceedings of the National Academy of Sciences* 2002;99(Suppl. 1):2466–2472. Copyright 2002 National Academy of Sciences, U.S.A.

of metastatic potential are population-level properties that cannot be predicted very well by studying individual tumor cells.

In human biology, emergent properties at the tissue or organ level are contingent on a sufficient level of complexity at the cellular level. One of the great challenges in the new field of systems biology is the threshold level of complexity necessary for the appearance of emergent properties in the system. What system parameters and emergent properties dictate the threshold level? Once the threshold has been exceeded, what is the nature of the phase transitions that lead to the evolution of emergent behavior? Modeling emergence and complexity is difficult because these system properties appear abruptly and cannot be easily predicted.

Complex systems are composed of huge numbers of components and component interactions, and the nonlinear behavior of the system makes computational analyses exceedingly difficult.

The human body exhibits complexity over a broad range of scales. Complexity is evident from molecules to human social networks. Spatial (volume) dimensions in humans range up to twenty-seven orders of magnitude (Figure 4.5). Proteins range in size from a few amino acids in length to large macromolecules containing thousands of amino acids folded in complex three-dimensional configurations. Nonlinear dynamics is found in the simplest protein-mediated regulatory pathways, including negative feedback loops. Complex behavior can be seen in small populations of cells like the cardiac pacemaker cells that control heart rate.

The ten trillion (10^{13}) cells that make up the adult human body are organized into tissues and organs that carry out specific functions. Cardiovascular, endocrine, and nervous system functions all exhibit considerable complexity. Social complexity is well documented among insect societies such as ants and honeybees. In human populations, complexity is observed in stock market behavior and other social systems. Social complexity or "interconnections" among individuals in large populations is intergenerational and processes occur over time periods spanning years to decades. Nonlinear dynamical behavior in market economics leads to the unpredictability of future stock prices. Temporal processes are also scalable to about thirteen orders of magnitude. In general, biological processes are as fast or faster at lower scales because functions at higher scales such as in tissues and organs are contingent on lower-scale processes.

Emergent properties in complex systems result from chaos at lower scales that influences the behavior of the entire system by inducing self-organizational behavior at higher scales. At lower scales, interactions of components lead to negative and positive feedback processes that serve to stabilize the system. Emergence is a cooperative exercise among system scales. The interaction of components at lower scales

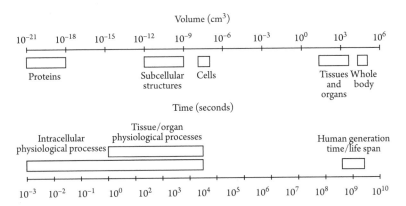

Figure 4.5 Human space-time. Both biological space (volume) and time occupy an extraordinary range of scales. Biological space is twenty-seven orders of magnitude. Biological time (excluding evolutionary processes) is up to thirteen orders of magnitude. Properties of complexity are evident at almost every spatial and temporal scale.

leads to novel and emergent properties at higher scales. In turn, the higher-level properties can influence the behavior of the lower-scale components. Nonlinear dynamical interactions among neurons in the brain lead to higher cortical functions. Neural plasticity or the capacity of the brain to modify itself in response to injury or disease is based on the capacity of neurons to establish new connections and create new neural networks. How the brain accomplishes this is poorly understood.

Complexity in Action

Living systems must be able to strike a balance between adaptability and stability. System complexity allows this to happen. Complex systems need to be stable to operate optimally. Most biological processes are enzyme mediated. Enzymes are large proteins that catalyze biochemical reactions and are sensitive to changes in their microenvironments, including pH (hydrogen ion concentration) and temperature. If the human internal environment is unstable and allowed to fluctuate, enzymatic activity cannot be maintained optimally. As a result, the body cannot operate efficiently.

But complex systems must also be adaptive and capable of responding to rapidly evolving environment conditions. If environmental conditions become life-threatening, the body must respond to ensure survival. The key to adaptability is systemwide endocrine and nervous systems that serve coordinating functions. Nonlinear dynamics permit these systems to initiate rapidly a cascade of events to reduce probability of harm and enhance survival. The response to environmental changes is a loss of stability and a move toward chaos. How the body *specifically* responds to a given threat is not predictable because initial conditions cannot be known exactly. No two people respond to identical threats in exactly the same way. Nonlinear dynamics returns the body to the stable state once the threat has dissipated.

Networks are the foundation of complexity. From a functional perspective, complex systems are organized into a very large community of interlocking networks. The nonlinear dynamical behavior characteristic of complex systems is endowed in network-level processes. Emergent properties in the brain are based on vast networks of neurons. Gene regulation in every cell in the body is contingent on the coordination of thousands of highly complex subnetworks of genes and proteins. Recent advances in network analysis provide exciting examples of the complex nature of neural networks and how these networks are disrupted in neurodevelopmental diseases. Bipolar disorder, depression, and schizophrenia are characterized by highly interconnected gene networks that may explain why some individuals express multiple disorders or are protected against some disorders but are predisposed to others. These fascinating studies also reveal some surprising results. Who could have foreseen that bipolar disorder and female breast cancer would be tightly negatively correlated in a disease co-occurrence network? The negative correlation may reflect a competition for genes regulating the cell cycle and cellular proliferation. One explanation is that genetic variations promote cell death in bipolar disorder but enhance cellular proliferation in breast cancer. The level of complexity in these networks is so high that we are unlikely to understand fully all of the complex interactions among the thousands of genes and environmental events underlying psychiatric disorders. The realistic challenge is identifying the common genes and processes in these diseases.[12]

Networks are critical to the reliable functioning of complex systems. Networks are patterns of interactions among biological elements (protein molecules, cells, and such) that carry out specific functions, including energy processing, synthesis of biologically important molecules, and feedback regulation of biological processes. Networks consist of nodes and edges. Nodes can be proteins, metabolites, genes, or cells. Edges are the interactions between nodes. The simple transcription regulatory network illustrated in Figure 4.6 is described by two nodes and one edge. The nodes are genes A and B, and the edge is the activation of a transcription factor, X_A. Regulatory networks are important in the cellular response to many environmental and regulatory signals. In more complex networks, thousands of nodes each with multiple edges may be present. Single transcription factors may regulate transcription rates for several genes.

Networks function at all levels of biological complexity and include transcription regulatory networks, signal transduction networks, and neural networks. Cancer at the molecular level may be thought of a disease of networks where networks regulating control of cell proliferation and genome integrity have been corrupted.[13]

Cancer arises because of mutations in genes that control cell growth and proliferation. *MYC* is an important cancer gene that serves as a transcription factor regulating the expression of about 15 percent of all genes. The *MYC* subnetwork (Figure 4.7) is highly complex. Because of interacting regulatory functions, mutations in *MYC* have significant consequences downstream for other nodes (genes) in the network. These nodal alterations in turn can cause changes in other nodes in other networks. The end result is a loss of significant regulatory control of cell growth and division leading to cancer. Changes in *MYC* have potentially serious consequences because of the scope of its regulatory influence. In the central part of the network, edges or interactive opportunities greatly exceed the number of

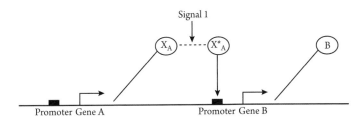

Figure 4.6 A simple transcription regulatory network. Transcriptional regulation is the process by which genes regulate the transcription of other genes. Gene A directly regulates gene B because X_A, the protein encoded by A, is a transcription factor for gene B, that is, it binds to DNA on a specific site near the sequence coding for B, called a promoter region of B, and activates or inhibits its rate of transcription. In the presence of a signal (shown as signal 1 for example, a hormone), X_A is activated and regulates the rate of transcription of B. When the signal is terminated, X_A is inactivated, and no regulation of gene B transcription occurs.

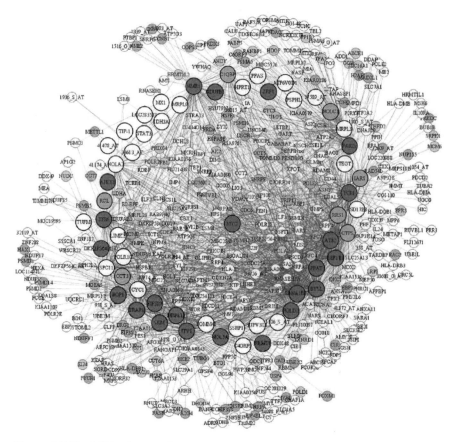

Figure 4.7 The *MYC* subnetwork. The *MYC* proto-oncogene is a transcription factor that regulates expression of 15 percent of all genes. When it is mutated, cancer results. *Source:* Basso K, et al. Reverse engineering of regulatory networks in human B cells. *Nature Genetics* 2005;37:382–390. Figure reproduced with the permission of Nature Publishing Group.

nodes, leading to a high degree of complexity. Changes in a small part of the network can have significant effects on the entire network and beyond. The *MYC* cancer gene is associated with many common cancers such as breast cancer and lung cancer.[14]

Gene function is controlled by an elaborate network of functional elements and switches arranged in a complex and redundant hierarchy. Networks regulate how cells, tissues, and organs develop and function. These regulatory networks determine whether a cell becomes part of the liver or the brain. Scientists are just beginning to map and explore these networks. Understanding network malfunction may hold keys to managing human disease and developing new drugs and treatments. The Encyclopedia of DNA Elements (ENCODE) project first reported in 2012 the nature of the functional elements in the human genome. ENCODE is a multinational effort to map regions of transcription, transcription factor association, chromatin structure, and histone modification. ENCODE documents for the first time that regions of DNA often referred to as "junk DNA" are not "junk" at all but are active in controlling genetic activity.

The Human Genome Project determined the entire base sequence of DNA. The ENCODE project goes a giant step further by exploring the functional dynamics of the genome. The genetic blueprint is not simply the information coded in the linear arrangement of nitrogenous bases. Instead, the genome is a dynamic entity in which the synthesis of gene products is tightly regulated by functional elements organized in complex interactive networks. Depending on how they are organized, functional elements constitute the information needed to build all the types of cells, body organs, and, ultimately, an entire person from a single genome. Functional dynamics in the human genome will force us to rethink what is meant by a gene. The finding that gene regulation can be influenced by remote functional elements upends the long-held belief that gene transcription is dominated by nearby regulatory elements.[15]

Networks are the functional units of complex biological systems. The human brain is the ultimate information-processing network. No current human-made computer can even approach this level of computing power. In biological networks, feedback loops confer stability (called steady states). The steady state is not a point estimate but represents a range of values because feedback results in oscillatory behavior. Steady-state body temperature is not exactly 37°C but varies between about 36°C and 38°C in normal individuals. Biological oscillations are important to allow for rapid adaptation of the system to environmental changes. Oscillatory behavior is evident in a wide range of biological systems, including the cardiac cycle, intestinal smooth-muscle contraction during digestion, insulin release from the pancreas, and the dilation-constriction cycle of the iris of the eye. Oscillations occur only in non-linear dynamical systems.

Negative feedback operates to minimize deviations in the state variable from the steady-state value. Thermostatic control of room temperature is a good example of oscillatory behavior in network control. Typically, a thermostat is located some distance away from a heating unit. The heater is either on or off depending on whether the room temperature is above or below the set-point (steady-state) temperature. The heater is turned on if the room temperature falls below the set point but is turned off when the room temperature exceeds or is at the set point. The time it takes for the room temperature to begin to fall after the heater is turned off is a measure of the lag time in the system. Generally, it takes time for the heat at the source to dissipate after it turns off. This results in an overshoot in the temperature at the thermostat. Clearly, the temperature will cycle or oscillate, with the period of oscillation increasing as the time lag (related to the distance between the heat source and thermostat) increases. This same sort of feedback loop is essential to the control of many biological processes.[16]

Systems biology is a relatively new field of study in the life sciences that focuses on networks and the complex interactions of elements within biological systems. Systems biology provides a holistic approach to the study of biology, as opposed to the traditional reductionist or elementalist approach that focuses on individual components as a way of understanding complex systems. Biological networks are poorly understood even in single-celled organisms. There are few network systems for which complete node-and-edge descriptions are fully characterized. Very little is known about how individual networks behave over time and how networks interact with one another at the system level. If the subnetwork in Figure 4.7 is representative, total understanding of network behavior from a computational perspective is an almost impossible problem.

The grand goal in systems biology is a complete synthesis of life processes in a systems context. In the second decade of the twenty-first century, achieving the goal looks impossible. Moreover, solving all the unknown number of differential equations that describe network behaviors is beyond the computational power of even the most powerful computers available today. Further, it is inconceivable that we can view and understand the entirety of complexity of the human body. Because of complexity, studying a part of one network influences the behavior of other networks. The networks that are of interest will generally be determined not by the system being evaluated but by the particular questions that are asked about it. Complex systems carry a type of irreducible or deep uncertainty. The human body itself will always remain more complex than can be captured at any one time, and what is observed when one looks at any part of the system is determined by the purposes of the inquiry. So, for example, fully investigating the behavior of the *MYC* subnetwork in Figure 4.7 includes exploring what happens to a single component or group of components in the network when another component is modified in some way. But because of the high degree of interconnectedness in the network, manipulating one part of the system leads to unintended changes elsewhere in the system. If you try to avoid this problem by isolating the components of interest, then the importance of interconnectedness at the system level is lost. The *MYC* subnetwork is a small, complex system within each cell. The problem becomes enormously more complex when scaling up to the whole body where trillions of cells interact in complex ways. The nature of the question being asked is what is important. The query identifies the particular networks of the system that are relevant, and they, in turn, define the boundaries of the system for the purpose of the inquiry.[17]

Complexity in Health and Disease

A complexity perspective puts a whole new spin on human biology and disease. Complexity requires a multidimensional and multisystems approach. Physiology is not isolated to specific tissues and organs. Although we go to medical specialists for diseases of specific tissues or organs, effective disease management often involves a multisystem and multidisciplinary approach. How the kidneys control blood pressure and water and electrolyte balance requires an understanding of how the kidneys, endocrine system, nervous system, and cardiovascular system interact. Physiologic controls are system-wide. A complex system perspective provides important insights into how subsystems in the human body interrelate and coordinate multiple functions in a coherent fashion.

The practice of medicine illustrates this clearly. Drugs can produce complications in unrelated body systems. Statin-class drugs are commonly used to treat elevated blood lipids and have proved successful in doing so; but these drugs can cause constipation and other effects in the digestive system. The medical profession has recognized for many decades that there is "no free lunch." Almost every diagnostic test and medical treatment is associated with some complication. Cancer patients, perhaps more than others, experience this firsthand. In some cases, patients claim the treatment to be worse than the disease. The challenge in medicine has always been to do as much good as possible without harming the patient, but the problem seems magnified in a disease like cancer that often requires aggressive and toxic therapies. Understanding biological complexity is key to optimizing the ratio of benefits to risks.

Disease causation and development also reflect system complexity. Complex diseases result from component failure (for example, cell damage) that may occur spontaneously. Stuff just happens. Many cancers appear for no apparent reason. For diseases linked to environmental factors like lung cancer, agent exposure increases the risk of disease over and above the spontaneous disease rate in a dose-dependent fashion. The issue is further complicated by the fact that complex diseases have no causal signatures. Spontaneous lung cancer and smoking-induced lung cancer are not clinically distinguishable. Knowledge of causation plays no role in diagnosis or treatment. This implies that environmental causal agents act by increasing the spontaneous rate of disease rather than initiating novel mechanisms of disease.[18] The implications for public health are significant. Spontaneity of disease means complex disease cannot be eradicated. The disease process is natural and cannot be avoided. All that public health measures can do is to reduce the disease burden related to environmental causation. Completely eradicating cigarette smoking will reduce but will not entirely eliminate lung cancer.

Even for diseases like whooping cough, for which a single causal agent has been identified, elements of multifactorial causation are evident. Not everyone who is exposed to the causal agent for whooping cough, *Bordetella pertussis*, gets the disease, but everyone who has the disease is infected with *B. pertussis*. The bacterium is a necessary and sufficient cause of whooping cough, but constitutional factors such as immune response explain why some people who are infected do not get the disease. For some diseases, including many cancers, causal factors and pathogenesis are not fully understood. Known causal factors interact synergistically to produce effects that cannot be predicted by evaluating each possible causal factor individually. Lack of knowledge of causality and pathogenesis might not impact treatment, but effective strategies for disease prevention are compromised.

Some diseases appear to be associated with a change in system complexity. Normal oscillatory patterns may be altered in disease states. One of the most thoroughly studied oscillatory systems is the heart pacemaker. These are specialized cells located in the right atrium of the heart that emit electrical impulses to control the heartbeat. Certain arrhythmias are associated with regularity in the oscillatory pattern of the heart rate. Normally, the heart rate displays chaos and an irregular pattern (Figure 4.2). Ironically, the disease state looks as if order came out of disorder. Whether changes in complexity are a root cause of disease or a manifestation of disease is not clear. The relationship is itself complex and disease specific.[19]

The theory of complexity loss suggests that aging and disease are associated with a breakdown of complexity in normal structure and function that reduces the adaptive capacity of the individual. However, the relationship of complexity with aging and disease may not be that straightforward. Some diseases like cancer suggest complexity may actually increase—disease progression is associated with increased complexity (as measured by degree of tumor heterogeneity), unpredictable disease behavior, and reduced efficacy of therapy. Measuring complexity is difficult and involves fractal analysis and nonlinear dynamics. How tests of complexity should be used and analyzed remains uncertain, but what seems clear is that no single measure is adequate for sufficient characterization of the complexity of a physiologic system.[20]

Chaos theory is earning increased attention in medicine. Analysis of clinical data by specialists in nonlinear dynamics is of particular interest in understanding normal and pathological functions of the brain, heart, and immune systems. More generally, complexity is forcing us to rethink the concept of homeostasis in physiology and medicine. Homeostasis is generally defined as the maintenance of a constant internal environment characterized as a single stable state. The concept of homeostasis is central to the practice of medicine, and most diseases are defined quantitatively as deviations from homeostasis. A patient may be diagnosed as anemic because the red blood cell count is well below normal, homeostatic levels.

Complexity suggests homeostasis consists of an array of stable states. Homeostatic values are not constant but fluctuate over time. The implications are clear for the diagnosis and treatment of many diseases. The temporal pattern of the disease-related physiologic parameter may be more important than a snapshot single-value estimate. The prostate specific antigen (PSA) test as a screening tool for prostate cancer is problematic because single readings tell us little about the status of the prostate. The PSA test is nonspecific since levels may be elevated for various reasons, including the presence of cancer. The diagnostic value of the test lies in temporal trend analysis rather than evaluation of point estimates.[21]

A complexity perspective demands a multidisciplinary approach to solving contemporary challenges in medicine and public health—solving cancer, neurodegenerative disease (for example, Alzheimer's disease), and cardiovascular diseases. Computational sciences, genomics, proteomics, and systems biology offer powerful ways to evaluate signaling networks and other features of complex systems to develop biomarkers of disease and new diagnostic and therapeutic methods for disease management.

Complexity implies that there are multiple ways to attack a disease. Cancers and hypertension are diseases usually treated by drug combinations. Each drug attacks a particular system component or process or has a different toxicity. Complexity theory can inform therapeutic approaches to optimize the efficacy of multidrug combinations. A complexity analysis would include drug-drug interactions and analysis of toxicities. Do drugs interact synergistically? Are there overlapping drug toxicities?

Complexity forces us to confront the notion of asymptotic limits of knowledge and to realize that a full and complete understanding of health and disease is likely out of reach. A complexity lens is a powerful way of looking at life. It promises to open new vistas to a better understanding of pathophysiologic processes. The application of complexity to diagnostic and therapeutic medicine is still in its infancy, but clearer definitions of what is meant by complexity and reliable methods to measure complexity hold considerable promise for a better understanding of pathophysiology and how complexity-dependent physiologic processes change with age and disease.

In the next chapter, we take a closer look at complex system stability and the concept of homeostasis as a quantitative and objective way of defining what is normal and what is disease. Homeostasis has usually been thought of as reflecting steady-state conditions, which represent constant levels of a biological parameter over time. But that view is changing with the recognition that the human body is a complex entity of interacting subsystems. The body is not in a steady state, defined, for example, as constant body temperature, but is, nevertheless, stable. Heart rate, hormone levels in the blood, body temperature, and other physiological parameters fluctuate over time but over a limited range. What do these fluctuations and associated unpredictability mean for health and disease?

5

A Free and Independent Life

Alison Taylor is a forty-three-year-old Caucasian female who leads an active lifestyle. She does not smoke or drink. She is married with a daughter and son. At age fourteen, she was diagnosed with type 1 diabetes (insulin-dependent diabetes) and has been taking insulin ever since to control her blood sugar. Recently, her insulin pump began to malfunction; because of that, her blood glucose levels became difficult to manage. She visited a local hospital emergency room, complaining of headaches, nausea, sensations of dehydration, frequent urination, and overwhelming thirst. A physical examination revealed dry mucous membranes and wheezing and crackling in her lungs. Laboratory tests showed her blood glucose level was 495 milligrams per deciliter (one milligram, or mg, is 1/1000 of a gram; a deciliter, or dL, is 100 milliliters). Normal blood glucose values are within the range of 70–110 mg/dL. When asked about her uncontrolled blood sugar, Alison said she had not changed her insulin-treatment regimen but admitted that her blood sugars had been "out of control" the previous week and that her insulin pump had not been working properly. Alison was admitted to the medical-surgical floor of the hospital and immediately put on insulin therapy to control her blood sugar. By the next day, Alison's blood glucose level was 135 mg per deciliter, but she still had severe headaches. While in the hospital, she was put on a low-carbohydrate diet. By the second day, Alison was eating well and was well hydrated; her blood sugar was also under control. She was discharged the evening of the second day and advised to replace her insulin pump and maintain her regular insulin regimen. Since her abnormal sugars might also be due to diet, she was also advised to maintain a diet of 1,800 kilocalories per day. The usual American diet is about 2,200 kilocalories per day. She was also instructed to have a close follow-up with her primary care doctor.

Type 1 diabetes is a classic example of system stability run amok. Blood glucose levels are normally under tight regulatory control by the endocrine system. If levels of blood glucose get too high (usually after a meal), the pancreas secretes insulin to lower blood glucose by increasing glucose utilization by skeletal muscle and other tissues and by converting glucose to glycogen (a storage form of glucose) in the liver. If glucose levels are too low, the pancreas secretes another hormone, called glucagon, that converts liver glycogen back into glucose. Sustained low levels of blood glucose can lead to loss of consciousness and compromised physiological function in other tissues and organs. Coma is a serious risk in type 1 diabetic patients with poorly managed blood glucose levels. Sustained high levels of glucose can have serious clinical repercussions by affecting the integrity of blood vessels, leading to long-term neurological, kidney, cardiovascular, and eye problems. Alison Taylor is at risk for these chronic diseases if she cannot get control of her blood glucose over the long term.

The Importance of Being Stable

This chapter explores stability in complex biological systems. Claude Bernard claimed that higher organisms, including humans, have a "free and independent life" because they sustain a constant internal environment separate from the external environment. The organism continuously strives to maintain constancy of the internal environment by making adjustments to physiological parameters like body temperature in response to small external perturbations.[1] Maintaining an internal environment that is significantly different from the external environment requires energy and complex coordination among regulatory systems, including the cardiovascular system, endocrine system, immune system, and nervous system.

Stability means that system states do not vary over time. But how do living systems maintain stability in the face of constantly changing external environments? Everyday activities lead to changes in the internal environment that constantly require readjustment. Digestion generates internal heat that must be dissipated to keep the body's core temperature at or near 37°C. Physical activity and exercise raise the body's temperature by generating heat in muscles. Sweating after a good workout is one way the body returns to normal temperature. Mental activities and other functions of the nervous system continuously degrade ion gradients that require recharging. The ion gradients are part of the internal environment and serve as a driving force for electrical impulses much as a rechargeable battery powers a mobile phone. The body also maintains tight control over an array of biologically important molecules, including electrolytes and cells like red blood cells that have a limited life span and must be replaced constantly.

Threats of injury or death initiate adaptive responses that wreak havoc on the internal environment. The nature of the response reflects the magnitude of the stress or threat and involves physiological processes that perturb the internal environment often in significant ways. Success in countering threats requires that the body detect the threat (usually through sight or sound) in sufficient time to elicit an effective response. When survival is threatened, an acute adaptation response, sometimes referred to as the "flight-or-fight" response, leads to enhanced cardiopulmonary function, shunting blood to the heart and muscles and away from the skin and digestive organs (Figure 5.1). The immune system and inflammatory response are suppressed in favor of redirecting sources of energy toward support for cardiopulmonary and skeletal muscle function. A threatened organism needs to escape the threat and can do so in the short term without an optimally functioning immune system or digestive system. The common phrase "white as a ghost" refers to the blanching of skin when blood flow destined for the skin is redirected to the heart and muscles in response to a frightening or sudden threat situation. Once the threat has dissipated, the body restores the constant internal environment by reversing the threat-initiated adaptive changes.

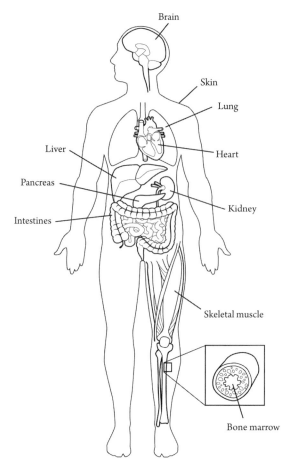

Figure 5.1 Threats to survival or of serious harm trigger a complex stress response that involves a number of tissues and organs. The brain processes sensory inputs (primarily auditory and visual) that lead to the release of hormones and electrical impulses directed at specific target organs. The cardiovascular system responds by shunting blood to the skeletal muscles and heart and away from the skin and intestines. The liver converts glycogen back into glucose and accelerates glucose use by tissues in response to pancreatic hormones. Other tissue functions are either suppressed (for example, the inflammatory response) or enhanced (for example, lung function).

What triggers the body's reaction to environmental signals? Whether a defense like fever, stress, and anxiety or other response is expressed depends on its costs of expression and whether it can be induced quickly. Certain defenses like the flight-or-fight response are very costly and responding to false alarms is inefficient and expensive in terms of energy expenditures. Signal discrimination is used to distinguish between a true signal and noise. Signals—the sound of a rattlesnake or the sight of a scorpion—are interpreted in terms of the probability of harm and the severity of the consequences. Threats can usually be safely ignored if the signal represents a low-probability, low-consequence event (the snake is in a covered glass tank) but a signal signifying a high-consequence event (serious harm or death) likely will elicit a response whether the event is high probability or low probability.

Sensitivity is a measure of how well the system detects a signal when one is really there—the ability to distinguish signal from noise. However to achieve high sensitivity the detector may also be biased and express a high number of false alarms. If everything is interpreted as signal then sensitivity is one hundred percent but at a cost of a high frequency of false alarms (what is interpreted as signal is really noise). Detection efficiency is achieved by tuning the system—dampening detector sensitivity enough to reduce excessive false alarms. Efficiency is achieved to a large degree through learning and experience. These same principles apply to signal detection theory in diagnostic medicine. Distinguishing between disease (the signal) and pseudodisease (the noise) in cancer screening tests centers on the problem of false positives and is discussed in some detail in chapter 8.

Stabilization of the internal system environment allows for resistance to functional changes due to small perturbations in the external environment. In living systems, stabilization of the internal environment is called homoeostasis and represents an outgrowth of self-organization of complex systems. Coherence of structure and function is a striking feature of biological complexity, but how morphology leads to specialized tissue and organ functions remains one of the central problems in all of biology. A complex system perspective posits design as the product of emergence of complexity from self-organized systems of interacting components. Thus, sophisticated structures and functions emerge from interactions among elements and networks at lower levels of organization. The neo-Darwinist perspective argues that good design is a product of natural selection whereby desirable function/structure genes are favored over less desirable genes. But only the complexity perspective can adequately account for stability, an important inherent property of biological systems.[2]

System stability is important for two reasons. First, building and maintaining order in complex systems requires a stable internal environment. Complexity and order are natural consequences of spontaneous self-organization and self-assembly. In multicellular organisms like humans, order comes in two forms. Order is established in metabolically active tissues that require constituent cells to proliferate and maintain structure in support of tissue functions. A good example is the bone marrow. The bone marrow is constantly making new blood cells because these cells have a finite life span. The number of circulating blood cells is under tight regulatory control and, in the healthy individual, does not vary much with time. However, when control is lost as in leukemia, blood cell counts can run wild. A second type of order is seen in the establishment and maintenance of chemical and electrical gradients across cell membranes. Second, constituent cells in multicellular organisms are highly specialized and operate optimally only within a narrow range of environmental conditions. Since the body is an ensemble of functionally and spatially distinct compartments, homeostasis enables the body to survive in diverse external environments by maintaining a constant internal environment. Loss of control of the internal environment results in death or disease because of the narrow range of environmental parameters that cells require to function. Cells in the human body are different from bacteria and other single-celled organisms that live and function as individual units. Single-celled creatures are unspecialized and perform all the necessary functions to survive in an ever-changing environment, within a tolerable range. Single-celled organisms in general can tolerate wide swings in environmental conditions, but there are still limits. Bacteria that grow in fresh water grow poorly or die in brackish or sea water. Single-cell organisms that grow at ambient temperatures cannot grow in very cold or very hot environments. Cells of multicellular organisms, on the other hand, are highly specialized and perform a narrow range of functions. Their environment must be carefully controlled in order to survive because they do not have the capacity or the complete toolkit necessary to adapt to the wider range of environmental conditions that single-celled organisms can. The cost of cell and tissue specialization necessary for multicellular organisms to grow and survive is the loss of the capacity of individual cells to adapt to changing environments.

The body's response to changes in its internal environment is a useful model of health and disease. What is particularly important and revealing is the kinetics of recovery of system states from physiologic challenges. How rapidly an individual's blood glucose level returns to normal after a glucose challenge reveals important information about glucose regulation. The kinetics of recovery is usually determined by serial measurements. Single measurements provide incomplete information about the "health" of the system or presence of a pathophysiologic condition. Diagnosis of diabetes type 1 includes a glucose tolerance test. The body is challenged with a single oral dose of glucose, and blood levels are then measured serially over three hours to determine to what extent and how rapidly blood glucose returns to normal levels. Prediabetic or diabetic conditions are diagnosed based on peak values of blood glucose and how rapidly blood glucose levels decrease after the test dose is given.

The most revealing information is obtained when the system is observed under controlled perturbations. The resting electrocardiogram provides incomplete information about the electrical conductivity of the heart. Serious cardiac pathologies may be missed under such measurement conditions. However, when the electrocardiogram is obtained under controlled exercise, as on a treadmill, changes in electrical patterns may become evident as cardiac demand increases. Dynamical tests reflect the tendency of complex systems to return to stable configurations when perturbed.

A key approach to disease diagnosis in Western medicine is comparison of a patient's clinical profile (including blood pressure, red blood cell count, and heart rate) against established normal values that represent homeostasis. At your next visit, ask your doctor for a copy of a clinical laboratory report. In it, you will see a list of the ordered blood tests, your results, and the ranges of normal for the tests (Table 5.1). Any results out of the range of normal are usually tagged for the doctor's attention.[3] Deviations from normal values may reflect disease but are not unique determinants of disease. Many diseases share the same signs, and further clinical evaluation is needed to make a definitive diagnosis. The success of disease therapy also relies on notions of normal values. Return of clinical test results to the range of normal is a primary goal of therapeutic medicine. Most prostate cancer patients have prostate specific antigen (PSA) levels that exceed the normal range of 0–4 nanograms per milliliter of blood. Diminution in PSA levels reflects responses to therapy. In theory, total surgical removal of the prostate gland reduces the PSA level to zero because therapy removes all viable prostate tissue.[4]

Table 5.1 **Some Normal Clinical Laboratory Values**

Test	Normal Range	Test	Normal Range
Arterial blood gases		Serum proteins	
Carbon dioxide (pCO$_2$)	33–44 mm Hg	Total	6.0–7.8 g/dL
Oxygen (pO$_2$)	75–105 mm Hg	Albumin	3.5–5.5. g/dL
Blood acidity (pH)	7.35–7.45	Globulin	2.3–3.5 g/dL
Serum electrolytes		Other serum constituents	
Sodium ion (Na$^+$)	135–147 mEq/L	Creatinine	0.6–1.2 mg/dL
Chloride (Cl$^-$)	95–105 mEq/L	Glucose (fasting)	70–110 mg/dL
Potassium ion (K$^+$)	3.5–5.0 mEq/L	Urea nitrogen (BUN)	7–18 mg/dL
Bicarbonate ion (HCO$_3$)	22–28 mEq/L		
Calcium (Ca^{++})	8.4–10.0 mg/dL		
Inorganic P (P$_i$)	3.0–4.5 mg/dL		

Source: Koeppen BM, Stantop BA. *Renal Physiology* 4th ed. Philadelphia: Elsevier; 2007. Selected data taken from Appendix B, 183.

The idea that multicellular organisms have the capacity to control their internal environment was first realized in the 1850s by Claude Bernard, a celebrated French scientist frequently credited with founding the fields of experimental medicine and physiology. Bernard developed the concept of the *milieu interieur* based primarily on three lines of investigation: studies of the glycogenic function of the liver, regulation of temperature by vasomotor nerves, and the role of the pancreas in digestion. These investigations suggested that the temperature of the blood and the glucose level in the blood are actively regulated and, under normal conditions, remain at constant levels over time. Constancy of the internal environment was entirely consistent with Bernard's belief that living systems obey the known laws of physics and chemistry. He rejected the early views of vitalism that posited the existence of "life forces" separate from the laws of nature.

A constant internal environment is a unifying principle of physiology and has served as a major focus of physiology research for over a hundred years. Interestingly, the idea of a *milieu interieur* never took hold during Bernard's lifetime. At about the time Bernard introduced his constancy theory, Charles Darwin announced his theory of evolution by natural selection. Bernard's theory initially could not be resolved with Darwinism. How could the diversity of species in the same local environment be explained if the internal environment was constant? What clarified the idea of the *milieu interieur* were studies comparing ionic concentrations of body fluids with the external environment. The internal fluids of marine animals, such as ocean crabs and lobsters, were as salty as sea water. Animals in fresh water, however, had internal fluids that were much less salty. The internal environment appeared to be increasingly independent of the external environment as one proceeded up the evolutionary ladder. This provides the basis for the "free life" of higher organisms. The uncoupling of the internal and external environments in higher organisms led to reconciliation with Darwin's theory of evolution and launched Bernard's *milieu interieur* as an important central theme in organismal physiology.

The Darwinian hurdle and the lack of laboratory methods to measure accurately the chemical composition of the internal and external environment delayed acceptance of Bernard's constancy hypothesis by more than fifty years. Walter Cannon, a Harvard physiologist, was a principal architect in its resurrection. In the years between the world wars, Cannon explored mechanisms of stability and coined the term *homeostasis* to describe the *milieu interieur*. But Cannon went beyond a simple revival of Bernard's theory by proposing that management of a stable environment is based on self-regulating homeostatic "agencies" within the body. The parasympathetic and sympathetic divisions of the autonomic nervous system were keys to homeostatic control. The autonomic nervous system regulates the heart, glands, visceral organs, and smooth muscle; this system is further broken down into the parasympathetic and sympathetic divisions that counterbalance each other in the regulation of many tissues and organs. Cannon's discussion of homeostasis in his *Wisdom of the Body* argues that internal stability requires management of necessary supplies, including water, electrolytes, and sugars, and the capacity of the body to maintain adequate reserves. Cannon saw homeostasis as key to the evolutionary emergence of higher organisms, specifically the brain and the progression of intelligence in higher organisms such as humans.

Cannon considered "homeostasis" in a Hippocratic context of the healing power of nature. Homeostasis is a quantitative definition of health and normality. Cannon was an early proponent of quantitative and objective medicine and viewed modern medicine as the art and science of facilitating homeostatic control and self-regulating adjustments of the body. Cannon's Hippocratic interpretation differs from Bernard's view, which stressed the technical control of nature. Bernard supported the notion of a therapeutic determinism in physiology and nature. Human domination of nature was an important theme in Bernard's work.[5]

The classical view of homeostasis as developed by Bernard and Cannon is consistent with steady-state dynamics in which key biological parameters like heart rate, blood pressure, and blood sugar are constant over time. Changes in physiologic parameters because of environmental stresses, disease, or injury initiate an adaptive response that tends to return the system state toward normal. Normal values have ranges reflecting interindividual variability. Bernard and Cannon also considered homeostasis as a localized rather than system-wide control process; physiological adjustments are made in specific tissues and organs.

Bernard's constancy hypothesis had broad appeal beyond biology and medicine. The concept of *milieu interieur* led Norbert Wiener, a mathematician and philosopher, to the development of cybernetics and feedback loops as central principles underlying system-control engineering. Simple control systems are used to maintain temperature in the face of fluctuating environmental conditions or to maintain constant output from an electronic device receiving variable inputs. Wiener also viewed human diseases, particularly in the nervous system, as aberrations of control systems.[6]

As we have learned more about homeostasis, the steady-state view has evolved into a more complex concept. Allostasis is a physiological concept introduced by Bruce McEwen in 2002 to describe the capacity of animals with hormonal and autonomic nervous systems to respond in such a way as to survive stressful changes.[7] It differs from homeostatic mechanisms, which are feedback systems that preserve the internal status quo. Allostasis is accomplished through evolved complex physiological systems that alter homeostatic parameters in response to chronic stress and in preparation for response to a perceived future threat.

Allostasis suggests that living systems do not have constant internal environments. Instead, the internal environment fluctuates around some normal, homeostatic, or set-point value. Most people have a resting heart rate about seventy beats per minute; but, at any moment, heart rate is highly irregular, and the instantaneous heart rate cannot be predicted (see Figure 4.2 in previous chapter). A steady-state perspective has given way to an understanding based on complexity in which biological parameters are seen as fluctuating around a central value. Whereas steady state is a product of linear dynamics with predictable outcomes, a nonlinear approach reflects complexity and the inability to predict future system states accurately. Over long time intervals, homeostatic parameters look constant and essentially invariant, but a closer look at system fluctuations over finer timescales reveals extraordinary details and variations that appear random and unpredictable.

Concentrations of substances in blood plasma, saliva, and other bodily fluids are also not constant. Instead, they fluctuate in an oscillatory pattern around a central value that approximates substance-specific steady states. The observed oscillatory patterns derive from nonlinear dynamics associated with the changing rates of production and elimination of the substance (for example, a hormone). Concentrations at any point in time are unpredictable because rates of production and elimination are dependent on prior conditions of the system that can never be known exactly. Levels of prostate specific antigen (PSA) in the blood and control of cell production in cell-renewal tissues like bone marrow are examples of this type of chaotic behavior. Average values can be calculated and are often useful to measure the state of the system, but central estimates by themselves provide no information about dynamic behavior.

The continuous fluctuations actually observed in physiological systems are necessary for the system to be adaptable. Small changes in environmental conditions necessitate physiological responses to maintain a constant internal environment. Homeostasis in Bernard's and Cannon's view does not adequately reflect the complexity of physiological systems. A thermodynamic perspective addresses the central role of energy processing in fluctuating systems. Organisms utilize external sources of energy to maintain a highly organized internal environment that fluctuates within tolerable limits. Fluctuations reflect life at the edge of chaos, where physiological systems flip-flop between stability and nonlinear adaptive behavior.

Life exists as open thermodynamic systems operating between near- and far-from-equilibrium states. As such, living systems are perched at the edge of chaos. How does life balance the need for stability yet maintain the capacity to adapt as environmental conditions require for survival? The remainder of this chapter explores three key strategies. First, even the simplest organisms have feedback control and buffering systems that tend to minimize fluctuations in the internal environment. Second, living systems have a multitude of oscillatory systems that facilitate adaptation to environmental change. Third, living systems are robust and have a reserve capacity and redundancy of systems allowing for sustained homeostasis when resources are limited or injury has occurred.[8]

Feedback Control

Homeostatic control systems can be quite simple relative to the complex systems they control. Regulating the level of a protein in a cell is achieved by using the protein product as its own regulator. In addition to its intended functions, the protein serves as a transcription factor. When excess amounts of protein are produced, production is shut down because the protein binds the DNA promoter region, thus preventing a reading of the DNA that is necessary to produce the protein. When too little protein is made, the promoter region is not bound by the protein product, allowing for transcription. The probability the promoter region is bound depends on the amount of protein available. Excess amounts of protein increase the probability the promoter region will be bound.

Most life-sustaining control systems, including control of blood sugar and body temperature, use negative feedback. A negative feedback loop tends to stabilize the output of the system. Negative feedback is triggered when the system output (for example, level of blood glucose or body temperature) deviates from the system set point. If the output is *higher* than the set point, negative feedback lowers the output toward the set-point value. If the output is *lower* than the set point, the system responds by raising the output in the direction toward the set point. So, negative feedback, in effect, sets the system back on track by reversing any deviations of output. Over time, the system output is stabilized and approximates the set-point value. Thus, negative feedback is a self-correcting system: if the system goes too far in one direction, a correction is made in the opposite direction.

Negative feedback loops are contingent on informational feedback within the system. In the protein example, the concentration of protein is the information used by the system to regulate further production of the protein. The behavior of the feedback system is governed by the system set point and response rate. In biological systems, the system set point is the homeostatic value. The set point for body temperature is 37°C. Thermal regulation, such as sweating during exercise, seeks to return core body temperature to the set point.

System response dictates how quickly homeostasis is reestablished following perturbations. Not all perturbations are serious or life threatening, but, for those that are, response must be rapid, else serious damage or death may occur. For example, a sudden, significant loss of blood requires a rapid cardiovascular response to maintain blood pressure and organ perfusion. Sustained high fever can irreversibly damage the brain, so immediate measures must be taken to restore the body to its core temperature.

Negative feedback systems have three features in common. First, they have some sort of sensor that can compare the current state of the system to a desired set point. Second, there is a mechanism that can respond when there is a difference between the current state and the desired set point. Third, the direction of the response is always opposite the direction of the deviation with respect to the set point. Control of room temperature is a good example of negative feedback in action (Figure 5.2).

In living systems, the delay between sensing a signal and responding to it is tissue-function specific. It usually takes tens of minutes for blood sugar levels to return to normal levels after eating a carbohydrate meal or for the heart rate to return to resting levels after a brief workout. But threats to survival or serious injury elicit responses in less than one second. The speed of response is dictated by whether electrical or chemical signals link signal detection and physiologic response. Responses to survival or injury threats are mediated by the nervous system. Nerve impulses can travel about one hundred meters per second along insulated nerve fibers. Hormones such as insulin to control blood sugar are chemical signals that act at a much slower rate.

Feedback systems in humans are complex because they are usually interlocking. Multiple sensory systems are used to detect and characterize environmental signals. Sensory-dependent coding facilitates signal characterization. Auditory and visual signals provide different but complementary information about the nature of the source of the signal. Sensing the environmental signal must occur faster than the physiological response to the signal; otherwise, the sensor can never get an accurate enough reading to stabilize the system.

The challenge is that different sensory signals like hearing and vision move through different neural networks and are processed at different speeds. A gun is used to start sprinters, instead of a flash, because reaction time is faster for a bang than it is for a flash. The cells in the auditory cortex can change their firing rate more quickly in response to a bang than the visual cortex cells can in response to a flash. The brain must account for speed disparities between and within its various sensory channels if it is to determine the timing relationships of features in the world. As long as incoming sensory data are acquired not too far

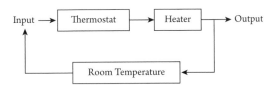

Figure 5.2 Control of room temperature is a common negative-feedback system. The thermostat compares the temperature of the air in the room to some ideal, predetermined setting. If the room is too cool, the system responds by starting the heater to raise the temperature. If the room is too warm, the sensor sends a signal to turn off the heater. The cycle repeats indefinitely, as information (temperature) about the system's status is constantly fed back into the system. Because of their cyclical nature, feedback systems are often referred to as feedback loops. Eventually, the room temperature stabilizes at the set-point temperature.

apart in time, the brain has the capacity to resynchronize the signals that were synchronized in the real world.

The human brain has quite good resolution when making temporal judgments. Two visual stimuli can be accurately deemed simultaneous down to five milliseconds, and their order can be assessed down to twenty-millisecond resolutions. The time interval may be different for hearing or touch. If the visual brain wants to get events correct in a temporal context, it may have to wait about a tenth of a second, the time needed for the slowest information to arrive. Accumulating as much data as possible has the advantage of more fully characterizing the environment.

But the brief waiting period also has the disadvantage of pushing perception into the past. Living too far in the past compromises the capacity to respond to threats quickly. The tenth-of-a-second window may be the smallest delay that allows higher areas of the brain to account for sensory-processing delays while still operating near the boundary of present time.[9]

Physiological responses to environmental signals are also multidimensional. Interlocking physiological systems controlled by the hypothalamus increase or decrease core body temperature. Shivering or sweating, decreasing or increasing blood flow through the skin, and speeding or slowing the metabolic rate can be adjusted depending on the thermal gradient between the environment and the body.

A small number of important biological processes are controlled by positive feedback loops. In positive feedback, an increase in the output feeds back to cause a further increase in the output. Everyone has experienced the screeching noise associated with positive feedback in a public address system. When the microphone picks up sound from its own loudspeakers and these sounds are reamplified enough, the effect can be loud squealing or howling noises from the loudspeakers. Nerve signals are generated by localized positive feedback loops in the membrane of the nerve axon. The generation of the nerve signal occurs when a change in the membrane potential causes a slight leakage of sodium ions through sodium channels, resulting in a further change in the membrane potential, which, in turn, causes more sodium channels to open, and so on. The slight initial sodium leakage results in an explosion of sodium across the axonal membrane, creating the nerve action potential.

Uterine contractions during labor in pregnancy are controlled by a positive feedback loop. Labor contraction stimulates secretion of oxytocin, a hormone secreted by the posterior pituitary gland that acts on uterine smooth muscle. Increases in frequency and intensity of contractions cause more oxytocin to be released. Another example is the process of blood clotting. Positive feedback is initiated when injured tissue releases chemical signals that activate platelets in the blood. The activated platelets release chemicals to activate more platelets, causing a rapid cascade and formation of a blood clot.

A positive feedback loop is inherently unstable and will become uncontrollable unless constrained by some limiting process. In the case of the nerve action potential, the process terminates when the sodium electrochemical gradient reaches zero. In the case of pregnancy, the birth of the child causes uterine contractions to stop.

Understanding response to a physiological stimulus is a systems-level problem requiring approaches that can elucidate the connectivity among signaling networks. To maintain homeostasis within the tissue/organ environment, an intricate signaling network system responds to specific signals. Homeostatic signaling networks are generally organized into functional modules regulated by negative and positive feedback control loops.

Acid-Base Buffers

The interstitial fluid compartment and blood plasma (collectively the extracellular fluid compartment) are under homeostatic control to maintain constant pH, temperature, and protein and electrolyte concentrations. All cells are bathed in interstitial fluids, and a stable chemical and physical environment is necessary for physiologic efficiency. The pH of the cell environment is particularly important because of its effects on biochemical reactions and molecular transport. Significant fluctuations in pH disrupt normal biochemical reactions catalyzed by pH-dependent enzymes. Membrane physiology is altered if the pH deviates significantly from physiologic levels, thus affecting transport of ions and molecules into and out of cells.[10]

Under normal physiological conditions, blood pH is maintained within a narrow range (pH = 7.35–7.45). The principal way blood pH is kept constant is by acid-base buffers dissolved in the blood. These buffers confer resistance to a change in the pH when hydrogen ions (protons) or hydroxyl ions are added or removed. Such buffers typically consist of a weak acid and its salt.

The carbonic-acid-bicarbonate buffer is the key buffer for maintaining acid-base balance in the blood. In dilute aqueous solution, carbon dioxide and water (the end products of the complete oxidation of glucose) combine to form carbonic acid (H_2CO_3). Carbonic acid readily dissociates into the bicarbonate ion (HCO_3^-) and a hydrogen ion (H^+) in aqueous solution.[11]

Buffering works because the concentrations of carbonic acid (the weak acid) and bicarbonate ion (the salt) are large compared to the quantity of hydrogen ions added or removed. When pH is lowered by adding hydrogen ions, some of the bicarbonate ions in the buffer are converted to carbonic acid by using up most of the hydrogen ions added; when hydrogen ions are removed from solution, some carbonic acid molecules are dissociated, freeing up hydrogen ions to replenish what was lost. The effect on the pH of the solution will be small, as long as the amount of hydrogen ions added or removed is not too great.

Control of pH is an integrative physiologic exercise. In addition to buffers, the kidneys and lungs also help control blood pH. Processes that tend to decrease pH, such as strenuous exercise, may be too great for the buffer alone to control blood pH effectively. The lungs and kidneys serve as excretory organs and help control the amounts of CO_2 and HCO_3^- in the blood. The lungs remove excess CO_2 from the blood. The kidneys remove excess HCO_3^-.

Rhythms of Life

Homeostasis depends on the oscillatory behavior of physiological control systems. A static system is not adaptable. Oscillatory behavior facilitates rapid response to environmental conditions. Oscillators do not appear in static systems (that is, systems at thermodynamic equilibrium) because there is no energy exchange. Biological oscillators require that the system be open thermodynamically and exchange mass and energy with the environment. Oscillators occur in nonequilibrium thermodynamic systems.

Oscillators make complex systems work but are not necessarily complex themselves. In actuality, oscillatory behavior is highly system specific. Oscillators are subject to external forces that keep the system oscillating and change the amplitude and frequency of oscillations. Damping occurs when forces reduce amplitude. Nonlinear relationships exist between forces and fluxes in oscillatory systems.[12] Oscillatory behavior is evident at every level of biological complexity, including intracellular biochemical pathways, resting membrane potential in the nerve axon, hormone receptors and hormone production in the endocrine system, and cell production in self-renewal tissues like bone marrow. Oscillatory behavior of protein levels and many other substances in the blood occurs when rates of production and elimination are not constant but depend on prior concentrations of the protein. Other types of oscillations are generated by temporal changes in cell membrane electrical-conductance properties.[13]

One of the simplest types of oscillators occurs in cardiac pacemaker cells and can operate with only four molecular channels, two ions, two ion pumps, and an ATP (adenosine triphosphate) to energize the process. Membrane potential oscillates with time, and changes are a result of potassium ions crossing membranes (Figure 5.3). Rhythmic oscillations in the membrane potential control the heart beat. The membrane oscillator is represented by a control loop in which membrane potential changes evoke conductance changes and vice versa. At the beginning of the oscillation, the membrane potential diminishes as a result of the opening of the voltage-sensitive calcium channel. Calcium enters the cell because the calcium concentration in the compartment outside the cell is much higher than it is within. The increasing levels of calcium inside the cell cause the opening of the potassium channel. Potassium moves out of the cell because the concentration of potassium inside the cell is higher than it is outside. The net movement of potassium out of the cell causes an increase in the membrane potential. The process begins over again. Underlying the transmembrane movement of calcium and potassium are the continuous ATP-powered pumps that sustain the ion gradients necessary for the oscillator to function. Potassium is recovered by the cell through the Na^+-K^+ ATPase pump, and calcium is pumped out of the cell by a separate enzyme-mediated pump.

If the amplitude of the oscillations is sufficiently high to exceed the membrane threshold for an action potential (about -50 millivolts), a burst will form at the crest of the slow oscillation. The formation of the nerve action potential occurs in milliseconds, much faster than the pacemaker cells' oscillation frequency of about one hundred per minute. The pacemaker cells act as a random impulse generator. Although the normal heart beats on average at the rate of seventy beats per minute, the heart rate is quite random over shorter time intervals.

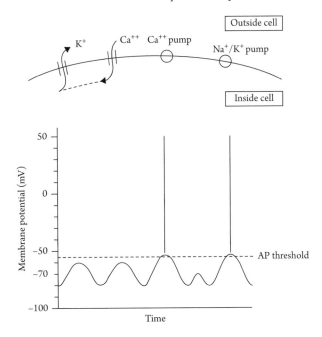

Figure 5.3 Heart pacemaker cells use a simple oscillator system to regulate the heartbeat. Cell membrane potential due to movement of potassium ions across the membrane oscillates about an average value of -70 mV (millivolts). If the membrane potential exceeds -55 mV, an action potential (shown as vertical lines) is generated, leading to heart muscle contraction.

The spontaneous oscillations occurring in sensory nerve fibers (for example, hearing and vision) facilitate signal characterization by providing additional coding information. Background system noise facilitates signal recognition. Without spontaneous background oscillations, small true signals might not be recognizable since the brain has nothing to compare them to. Spontaneous oscillations allow discrimination of signals that have a more regular pattern.[14]

More Than Enough

In the United States, the human life span is about seventy-five to eighty years. To operate efficiently for a lifetime, the body must be engineered for reliability. Reliability occurs when the system is robust and has adequate reserve capacity in vital systems to withstand sudden, life-threatening changes and has the capacity to adapt to gradual changes occurring in the internal environment as a result of exertion, stress, and organic diseases.

Robustness is the capacity of the system to respond flexibly. It is a property of complexity that allows a system to maintain function despite external and internal changes. Redundancy is a form of robustness that occurs when a duplicate component in the system is activated. If a gene is inactivated or knocked out, redundancy ensures the gene network still functions by activating duplicates of the gene. Degeneracy defines a different organizational complexity contributing to robustness. Within biological systems, degeneracy refers to circumstances where structurally dissimilar components or modules or pathways can perform similar functions. Degeneracy is, thus, a relational property that requires comparing the behavior of two or more components. In particular, if degeneracy is present in a pair of components, there will exist conditions where the pair will appear functionally redundant but other conditions where they will appear functionally distinct.

Robustness is a scalable characteristic of biological complexity. Evidence of degeneracy appears at every level of biology from subcellular to organismal physiological processes. Homeostasis cannot be sustained unless the system is robust. Maintenance of the core body temperature involves degenerative processes that include different activities such as shivering and sweating.

Perhaps the best example of robustness in living systems is the redundancy in the genetic code. Many different nucleotide sequences encode the same protein. In cell metabolism, multiple, parallel biosynthetic and catabolic pathways exist. A large array of food sources and end products provide for an enormous variety of diets that are nutritionally equivalent. In the immune system, populations of antibodies and other antigen-recognition molecules are degenerate. Networks in the nervous system have enormous degeneracy in local circuitry, long-range connections, and neural dynamics. Many body movements are degenerate because they involve different patterns of muscle contraction and relaxation that yield equivalent outcomes. Sensory signaling involves multiple modalities that are degenerate because information obtained by any one modality often overlaps that obtained by others.

The capacity for robustness appears to be both ubiquitous and significant for biological systems. Robustness provides for the ability to survive in an environment with changing internal and external conditions. Robustness characterizes mechanisms that produce flexible behavior as well as mechanisms that support homeostasis by keeping physiologic properties stable.[15]

Reserve capacity is also a key reliability function in living systems. Tissues reserve is not the same as degeneracy. Reserve refers to excess capacity to carry out physiological functions. The human body has two kidneys but only one is needed to maintain water and electrolyte balance and filter toxic products. This reserve capacity allows individuals to donate one kidney to another in kidney failure.

The observation that, when paired organs like the kidney fail, they tend to do so in tandem is a consequence of reserve capacity. Renal function appears normal until almost all the renal mass is rendered nonfunctional by diseases like diabetes and hypertension. Paired organs often sustain damage simultaneously, not sequentially.

Not every tissue is endowed with a reserve capacity. But those that are either have excess tissue or the capacity to repair and replace healthy tissue. The liver is capable of regenerating itself if a threshold amount of normal tissue remains. Other tissues such as the skin, bone marrow, and small intestine have a self-renewal capacity that continually produces new, functional cells to replace old cells. Self-renewal requires tissue-specific stem cells as a source of functional cells. The nervous tissue has little or no capacity to regenerate. However, brain plasticity allows for healthy areas of the brain to take over functions lost by damage to other brain areas. The brain has the remarkable capacity to "relearn" certain motor and sensory functions when specific areas of the brain sustain injury.[16]

Engineers use safety margins to describe reserve capacity and overall stability in systems. Building codes, safety regulations, and design manuals lay out clear standards for factors of safety. The higher the safety factor, the more secure a structure is from external forces and inherent flaws in the system that creep in during design, construction, and aging. Large safety margins mean that normal functioning occurs in spite of large variations in system outputs. Depending on the system, safety margins may be as high as ten or more to ensure adequate protection under extreme conditions. Interestingly, the system of levees in New Orleans was constructed with a safety margin of only 1.3, clearly not adequate enough to withstand the natural forces generated by Hurricane Katrina in 2005.[17]

In human biology, safety margins are tissue specific (Table 5.2). Safety margins allow for adequate protection of homoeostasis, except under the most severe, life-threatening conditions.[18] Reserve capacity ensures that vital organ systems and tissues are reliable and can sustain homoeostasis and continue to function. Even if a part of the tissue is destroyed or fails to function, homoeostasis can be maintained. The body can function fully with one kidney and one lung. There are a sufficient number of nephrons in one kidney and alveoli in one lung to maintain homeostasis. The kidneys and lungs have high margins of safety because of their central role in homeostasis. These tissues regulate the fluid compartment outside the cell by controlling water retention, electrolyte balance, and concentrations of respiratory gases.

There is a delicate balance between robustness and fragility in biological systems. The human body has its weak points. The brain and heart are "critical" organs because damage can lead to total system failure. The ability of critical tissues to respond to acute damage or loss of blood flow is limited because reserve capacities

Table 5.2 **Reserve Capacity in Selected Physiologic Systems**

Physiologic Parameter	*Normal level*	*Functional Threshold Level*
Blood glucose	100 mg/dL	50 mg/dL
Blood calcium	10 mg/dL	6 mg/dL
Blood filtration rate in kidneys	85–125 mL/min	60 mL/min
Blood pressure (systolic)	110–120 mm Hg	70–80 mm Hg
Diffusion capacity of lungs	20–30 mL/min/mm Hg O_2	<15 mL/min/mm Hg O_2

Sources: The data for blood glucose, blood calcium, blood filtration, and blood pressure are from Cannon WB. *The Wisdom of the Body*, New York: Norton; 1932. Data for lung diffusion capacity are from Weibel ER. What makes a good lung? *Swiss Medical Weekly* 2009;139:375–386.

and the time necessary for tissue repair, replacement, or remodeling is not fast and complete enough to sustain homeostasis. A sudden obstruction of a coronary artery leads to severe heart damage and possibly death because the body is not engineered to circumvent the sudden loss of critical tissue function.

Random Walks

Life processes are random or stochastic in nature. A stochastic process evolves in time or space subject to the laws of probability. The simplest type of stochastic process is the random walk, a process consisting of a sequence of changes each of whose characteristics (including magnitude and direction) is determined by chance. Stochastic processes are used to describe diffusion and other important biological processes in which a particle or molecule moves in straight-line steps but random direction. Random behavior is a consequence of the second law of thermodynamics and the requirement of natural systems to maximize entropy.

Events in complex systems occur because of chance interactions among elements. Biochemical reactions occur by chance interactions of molecules. Reaction probabilities increase with the concentration of the reactants. Enzymes, the largest class of proteins in cells, act as catalysts and increase the probability of preferred reactions occurring by lowering the activation energy of the reaction. The Mendelian laws of genetics follow simple laws of probability and describe how genetic traits in parents are randomly distributed among offspring. Stochastic processes in complex systems are consistent with the macroscopic laws of physics but cannot be derived from them.

Why does random behavior occur in complex systems? All molecules have kinetic energy that fuels random movement. Drug molecules injected into a vein are immediately subjected to small currents and other hemodynamic effects in the blood. Very little is known about the nature of these *local* events except that their occurrence and behavior are very complicated and not subject to the simple laws of physics. After some time, molecules will be distributed according to chance, that is, randomly. Uniform distribution does not depend on macroscopic blood flow throughout the body, although blood flow facilitates mixing. A small quantity of solute will still distribute evenly over time because of random motion. The ultimate consequence is that we cannot know how any individual molecule will behave and where in the complex system it will be located at any given time.[19]

Although individual events or states in a stochastic or random process are probabilistic, the outcomes in a large population of identical events or states are deterministic or predictable. Determinism is a population-level characteristic. The sex of a particular child cannot be predicted before fertilization. In theory, the chances of being male are 50 percent and of being female are 50 percent. In a large population of newborns subject to no external forces determining sex, the number of males and females is equal. Radioactive decay is also a stochastic process. In a population of radioactive atoms, which atoms decay in the next defined time interval cannot be predicted, but the behavior of a large population of radioactive atoms is predictable and defined by the radioactive decay half-life, a constant for each species of radionuclide. The behavior of the population is predictable, but that of individual members is not. The minimum population size needed to characterize a stochastic process depends on the probability of occurrence of the event or state. Determining the probability of being male requires observations in a small population because the probability is high. Only a small number of coin tosses is needed to establish the probability of heads for a fair coin.

Physiology is based on stochastic processes. Diffusion occurs because of random movement of molecules. Thermal motion shows no preferred direction. A molecule in a cell is just as likely to move in one direction as in any other. Two consequences of continuous random movement are keys to diffusion. First, molecules tend to disperse from areas of high concentration in accordance with the thermodynamic imperative that systems inexorably move toward greater disorder. Second, molecules of different types tend to intermix.

Randomness is also evident at higher levels of biological organization. The flow of blood through any tissue or organ is a random process. When a blood cell encounters a fork in a blood vessel, which fork is taken is probabilistic and determined by the resistive characteristics of the branch. A cell is more likely to enter a larger branch because resistance is lower there. With branches of equal size and resistance, there is an equal chance the blood cell will go to the left or the right. Blood flow through the kidneys is about 25 percent of cardiac output. Although the flow pattern of any particular volume element of blood cannot be predicted, on average about 1.5 liters of blood flow into and out of the kidneys every minute, assuming a total blood volume of 6 liters. On average, it takes four complete circulations of the entire blood volume, or about four minutes, for all the blood to be filtered through the kidneys.

Stochastic behavior in biological systems can be understood by partitioning the system into biologically meaningful compartments where rates of compartment input and output are determined experimentally. Input and output rates are the probabilities associated with the stochastic process. The gastrointestinal tract, blood plasma, kidneys, and liver are key compartments controlling the behavior of food substances ingested by mouth. The intestines absorb the substance with a characteristic absorption rate into the blood. The blood transports the substance throughout the body. The kidneys remove the substance with a characteristic removal rate. Knowledge of kinetic behavior permits calculation of excretion rates for a particular substance in the body. The reverse calculations are particularly useful when it is desirable to know how much substance was absorbed by measuring the urine concentration (a measure of excretion) at a known time after ingestion, injection, or inhalation.[20]

An important everyday application of stochastic behavior is dose scheduling for medical prescriptions. Instructions to patients about when and how much medication should be taken are based on pharmacokinetic data for the drug. The key is maintaining an appropriate blood plasma level of the drug as required for therapeutic benefit. When a drug is ingested, inhaled, or injected, levels build up in the blood plasma but are cleared constantly, usually by the liver or kidneys. The plasma half-life of most drugs is usually measured in hours and is drug specific. Half-life is proportional to the probability of plasma clearance (Table 5.3).

Table 5.3 **Plasma Half-Lives of Some Common Prescription Drugs**

Generic Name	Trade Name	Class	Plasma Half-Life*
Ibuprofen	Advil, Motrin, and other names	analgesic	2 hours
Amoxicillin	Amoxil	antibiotic	1 hour
Vincristine	Oncovin	cancer drug	80 hours
Atenolol	Tenormin	antihypertensive	6 hours
Atorvastatin	Lipitor	cholesterol/blood lipid control	14 hours
Amphetamine	Adderall	attention deficit hyperactivity disorder	10 hours

*Approximate plasma half-life. Impaired kidney or liver function may increase half-life.

The shorter the half-life, the higher the rate of drug clearance per unit time. If 8 mg of a drug are in the plasma at some time and the plasma half-life is one hour, then 4 mg will be in the blood after one hour, 2 mg in the blood after the second hour, and so on. The absolute amount of drug cleared is proportional to the amount of drug currently present. In theory, the drug is never completely cleared because a constant fraction is being removed in any defined time interval. In reality, however, the drug may be considered cleared after ten half-lives (twenty hours for ibuprofen) since only 1/1000 of the original dose is still present after that time.[21]

Therapeutic benefit is dictated by the dose and frequency of drug administration. Two competing processes determine how much and how frequently a drug is administered to sustain desirable blood plasma levels. Blood plasma uptake is a linear function of the amount of drug ingested or injected. Doubling the amount of drug ingested or injected doubles the amount of drug entering the blood. Clearance is more complex and is represented by a negative exponential function, the clearance rate being proportional to plasma half-life (Figure 5.4, upper left). The exponential clearance can be understood more easily by a logarithmic transformation of the blood plasma concentration (Figure 5.4, lower left). Half-life can be determined directly from the left upper or lower curves.

The right upper and lower curves of Figure 5.4 illustrate blood plasma levels after multiple drug administrations. When the drug is administered once every drug half-life, wide swings in plasma levels around the therapeutic dose range (shaded area) occur (Figure 5.4, upper right).

If the drug is administered multiple times during a drug half-life interval (Figure 5.4, lower right), variations in blood plasma levels are reduced, and better control of the blood levels of drug can be achieved. Many drug prescriptions are now available as slow-release formulations, reducing the need for multiple administrations.

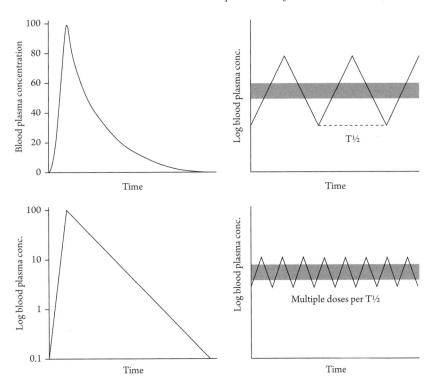

Figure 5.4 Plasma half-life dictates frequency of dose administration. More frequent administration or continuous administration gives better control of drug concentration in the blood. The shaded areas in the right upper and lower graphs represent the desired therapeutic dose range.

The Wisdom of Nature

Life is contingent on adaptation to an ever-changing environment through processes involving feedback loops, oscillations, robustness, and reserve capacity. Homeostasis as conceived by Bernard and refined by Cannon and others thus seems too narrow a term to account fully for adaptive behavior. A broader view suggests that homeostasis is the capacity of the body to maintain a highly organized internal environment fluctuating within acceptable limits. Thus, adaptability requires the organism to be open thermodynamically and to exchange matter and energy with the environment. The internal environment is not static but represents a spectrum of states reflecting continuous external environmental change.

Disease may be viewed as a spectrum of physiologic states that represents deviations from homeostasis. As aberrations in normal structure and function, diseases are themselves complex. Signs and symptoms of disease reflect the body's efforts to maintain homeostasis. Stabilizing the internal environment is constrained by known macroscopic laws of physics. A key homeostatic parameter is organ blood perfusion. When blood flow to tissues is reduced, the body responds by raising blood pressure to maintain blood flow. Hypertension is, thus, an adaptive systemic change. But biological complexity leads to potential problems. Unmanaged hypertension can lead to chronic injury to fragile blood vessels and to permanent damage to the kidneys, heart, and brain.

Pathology derives from biological complexity. Complex systems are highly integrated such that diseases in one system have impacts and lead to failure in other systems. Homeostasis is a systemic phenomenon that involves the interplay of multiple feedback loops. Altering one loop may impact, in a negative or positive fashion, one or more other loops. The interconnectivity of feedback loops, degenerate biological processes, and other homeostatic controls complicates disease management and identification of causes of disease. Manipulating complex systems without fully understanding the system that is manipulated often leads to unintended consequences. Effects of medical interventions, including errors by doctors, account for about 225,000 deaths annually in the United States—but roughly half of these deaths occur as a result of untoward effects of properly prescribed medicines. The leading causes of adverse drug reactions are antibiotics (17 percent), cardiovascular drugs (17 percent), cancer drugs (15 percent), and analgesics and anti-inflammatory agents (15 percent).[22]

Administration of drugs leads to perturbations in homeostasis. Without knowing specific perturbation pathways, it is difficult to predict what the countervailing risks might be. Statin drugs are powerful medications to control blood cholesterol but, in some patients, may lead to severe liver damage and muscle weakness. Certain pain medications raise blood pressure. Complications often occur in systems seemingly unrelated to the disease being treated. Drug complications and drug-drug interactions pose serious practical problems in medicine. Of course, there is little argument that many medications are effective in reducing pain and discomfort and manage many diseases successfully. Millions of lives have been saved by antibiotics alone. But cancer and other life-threatening diseases require toxic treatments, and in some cases the treatment is worse than the disease. Sometimes medical intervention is tinkering with the wisdom of nature. We ignore or override nature at our peril.

Homeostasis is a concept used in medicine and physiology to refer to equilibrium or balance among various elements of the organism. The idea of balance is not new and can be traced back to the ancient Greeks who thought that a person's health, mood, and character were determined by four humors circulating through the body—blood, phlegm, black bile, and yellow bile. Illness was thought to be a consequence of an imbalance of the four humors. Cancer, for example, occurred because of an excess of black bile in spite of the fact that black bile was never observed or adequately described by the ancients. The theory of humors was a powerful yet inexact tool in early medicine for centuries.[23]

Claude Bernard's constancy hypothesis and the introduction of the principle of homeostasis by Cannon ushered in the era of quantitative medicine in the twentieth century. Development of reliable clinical laboratory methods facilitated quantitative characterization of the *milieu interieur*. Diseases could be described in terms of measurable physiological parameters such as blood counts and serum electrolyte concentrations. The progress during a course of therapy could be easily tracked by serial laboratory tests.

The Western medicine model characterizes disease as a deviation from homeostasis, and the goal of disease treatment is to recover physiologic stability by returning to homeostasis. There is now considerable interest in viewing human disease as aberrations in complex dynamic processes. A dynamical perspective focuses on the nonlinear behavior of physiological systems. Changes in oscillatory behavior may be important signs of disease. Cheyne-Stokes respiration is an abnormal pattern of breathing characterized by alternating periods of the absence of breathing and rapid breathing. The abnormal oscillatory behavior is seen in patients with heart failure, strokes, and brain tumors. Clarifying the underlying nonlinear dynamics in abnormal oscillatory processes may help further our understanding of disease pathogenesis and develop more effective treatments.[24]

Historically, disease refers to a bodily structure or function that is not normal. But what is normal, and who decides? Can normal simply be defined in the context of homeostasis, or is it more complex than that? As discussed in the next chapter, disease is more difficult to define than one might think. Diseases have cultural, national, and social dimensions. A disease in one setting may not be considered as such in another. Disease manifestations can be highly variable; depending on the disease, patient response to treatment is unpredictable. Variability and unpredictability are hallmark features of complex systems.

6

Altered States

John Gonzalez, a fourteen-year-old middle-school student in Phoenix, Arizona, recently moved with his family from New York. His teacher estimated his cognitive abilities to be within the average range, though his performance on tasks was inconsistent. Sometimes, John completed assignments, and sometimes he did not because his focus appeared to be elsewhere. His teacher also noticed he tended to daydream. At a parent-teacher conference, the teacher suggested that the school psychologist evaluate John. Based on behavior scales and other tests, the results suggested an attention deficit disorder. John's parents were concerned with these findings and arranged an evaluation by a pediatrician, who reviewed the data provided by the school and visited with the teenager. The pediatrician concluded that John does not have an attention deficit disorder but was having problems adjusting to his move from New York, which had exacerbated his propensity for daydreaming. The pediatrician found no reason for medical intervention and instead advised brief counseling to assist the young man with his recent transition; the doctor also suggested that psychologists at his new school use redirection and structure to address John's daydreaming in class, as well as finding ways to help him integrate socially. The parents were comfortable with this approach and, as it turned out, the pediatrician's suggestions proved an effective remedy for John's difficulties.

The case raises two difficult issues. First, diagnosis and treatment of behavioral disorders are difficult and challenging. The brain is a complex system, and behavioral disorders derive from neural complexity. Complexity means that neural networks are highly interdependent and that system behavior cannot be predicted. Second, complexity blurs the line between what we mean by "normal" and what we mean by "disease." Complex system functions cannot be easily quantified, making distinctions between extremes of normal and disease states difficult to make. In effect, behaviors characterized by extreme shyness may be difficult to distinguish from some sociopathic disorders.

This chapter examines chronic, degenerative human diseases in the context of system complexity. The manifestation of disease and the effectiveness of therapy depend on the nature and extent of the physical abnormality and perceptions of the disease by the patient and others. How the patient perceives disease and responds to it is influenced by cultural and social factors that cannot be easily separated from the physical characteristics of the disorder itself.

In a complexity context, disease creates chaos. Small changes in a localized area of the body lead to system-wide effects. Type 1 diabetes, for example, is a disease characterized by the inability of beta cells in the pancreas to produce the hormone insulin necessary to regulate blood glucose. If blood sugar remains at chronically high levels, blood vessel damage can occur that subsequently compromises normal functioning of the eye, the kidney, and other tissues and organs.

We will also look at the blurry line that separates disease from normalcy. In traditional medicine, disease is usually distinguished from normal by comparing individual test results with a range of values obtained in a population of normal subjects. This "normal" range reflects homeostasis, a property of complex systems reflecting stability by maintaining a constant internal environment. Contemporary medical practice defines disease in a mechanistic way as a deviation from homeostasis. But who declares what is normal? Ultimately, what we decide is normal is a question that goes beyond the boundaries of science.[1] Science alone cannot provide the answers, because disease has social and cultural dimensions in addition to scientific ones.

Schrödinger's Cat

The human body occupies a wide spectrum of system states. The state of your body now as you read this paragraph will be different from the body state when you finish the chapter. Differences may be imperceptible, but, nonetheless, changes have occurred. For one thing, your heart rate may be quickened by reading this because the ideas excite you (I hope so!), or your heart rate may be slowed because you are bored and about to go to sleep (I hope not!). The idea of "states" was introduced in chapter 2 and refers to a physical description of the system. The state of the human body at a given time can be described by vital signs and other physiological parameters.[2] The state of the whole system is a nonlinear combination of all subsystem states. Descriptions of subsystem states and the state properties of the entire body cannot be known exactly because of uncertainties inherent in complexity.

In a quantum theory context, the body occupies several possible states simultaneously, and the state of the system is known only at the time we observe it. Possible states have probabilities that are determined by the conditions of the system at the time of observation. Erwin Schrödinger, the Nobel Prize–winning physicist, created an interesting thought experiment to illustrate the idea of multiple states. The Schrödinger's cat paradox imagines a cat housed in an airtight enclosure. Also in the enclosed space is a device consisting of a tiny amount of a radioactive substance, a Geiger radiation detector with an electronic circuit attached to a mechanical motor that operates a small hammer, and a small ampoule of hydrogen cyanide gas next to the hammer. The cat cannot interact with the device. The cat dies if the gas is released. The hammer will break the gas vial if an atom in the radioactive sample decays and emits radiation that causes the Geiger tube to discharge. The discharge establishes an electric current that causes the hammer to break the vial.

Death of the cat is determined solely by the probability that an atom decays during the time interval of the experiment. Since radioactive decay is a stochastic process—that is, it involves chance—one cannot know ahead of time what the fate of the cat is. Quantum theorists talk about superposition, the idea that matter can occupy multiple states simultaneously. Until the observer opens the container and looks inside, the cat is both dead and alive. The process of observation, opening the box and looking inside, uncouples the superposition and fixes the observed state.

Superposition is an interesting problem in quantum theory and the behavior of matter at the subatomic level, but there are important analogies in the real world of biology and medicine. State probabilities are determined by biochemical and physiological processes. Embryonic stem cells occupy many states simultaneously. They have the capacity to become any cell type in the body. The probability of occupying any particular state is determined by the local chemical and physical environment. Adult stem cells in the bone marrow have the capacity to become red blood cells, white blood cells, or platelets. In an anemic individual, erythropoietin forces the choice of state by committing the stem cell to become red blood cells. Very small lesions called ductal carcinoma in situ or DCIS in the female breast occupy multiple states simultaneously. We do not know whether these lesions will grow to cause a cancer requiring treatment or remain stagnant as pseudodisease and not cause any clinical problems. One of the significant challenges in cancer screening is uncoupling these states so the disease trajectory can be predicted. Knowing a lesion is not destined to grow means that no treatment is necessary. However, knowledge that disease is likely means early treatment will probably be successful.

Life is a progressive state of nature. The human body is a complex system subject to an arrow of time. Growth and maturation occur in only one direction from birth to adulthood. Biological complexity moves forward in time. Although Jaques's monologue "All the world's a stage" in Shakespeare's *As You Like It* would have us believe that later life is a reversion to early childhood, in fact, old age is a degenerative process reflecting failure of components in complex systems. Death is an irreversible state. People who report death-like experiences were never dead to begin with. The near-death state may reflect certain characteristics of death, but timely medical interventions preserve life.

In disease, the human body assumes numerous metastable states defined as transient perturbations from the normal. Everyone experiences some minor ailments during life. These may include bacterial or viral infections or perhaps a broken bone. Others have the misfortune of experiencing more serious problems like diabetes or cancer. Each of these conditions represents an array of metastable states. As the disease progresses, the body moves through states that are removed further from normal. The clinical horizon can be quite far off. Chronic diseases like cancer and heart disease often take decades to develop into clinically recognizable states. They involve a series of metastable states extending over years or decades. Microbial infections are often short-term perturbations lasting a few days or weeks. The primary goal of medical intervention is the reversion of metastable states to the normal state.

The relationships among key system states and medical interventions to detect and modify states are presented schematically in Figure 6.1. The transition from

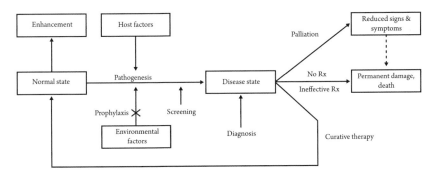

Figure 6.1 Medicine and health. The relationship between health and disease is complex. Medical interventions such as screening, diagnosis, curative therapy, palliative therapy, and prophylaxis are defined by the presence or absence of disease.

normal to disease is complex, and, for many diseases, the process is poorly understood. For illustrative purposes, the figure depicts the shift from normal to disease as a transition from one distinct state to another, with a bright line separating the two. In fact, no bright line exists. The clinical manifestation of disease is a result of gradual changes in normal structure and function. Although signs and symptoms might appear abruptly, the process of getting there may have been going on for days, weeks, or years. Symptoms of a cold or the flu may appear suddenly, but exposure to the offending virus occurred days before. Lung cancer in a smoker does not occur immediately but requires years or decades to develop into a clinically recognizable pathology.

Disease is a consequence of a combination of intrinsic system characteristics (host factors) and environmental factors. "Host factor" is a catch-all term for genetic, endocrine, immune, and metabolic determinants of disease. It also includes spontaneous failures of components in complex systems that occur for no reason at all. The shift from the normal to the disease state is system specific. The term "system specific" means that individuals respond differently. Why is it that some heavy smokers get lung cancer but others do not? In general, the transition to a pathological state involves some combination of host and environmental factors.

Too Many Things Can Go Wrong

The upside of biological complexity is that the human body can respond to a wide variety of environmental challenges while maintaining optimal functionality. The downside is that complexity means there are more opportunities for things to go wrong. Every component, every interconnection in the body is subject to malfunction or failure. This includes spontaneous failures where no causes can be identified. The body has the capacity for repair or replacement of some damaged parts, but this capacity is limited by the extent of damage. During human development, order and complexity are built from a single cell to a fully formed body containing more than one trillion cells in about thirty-eight weeks. During this time of very active cell proliferation and differentiation, all sorts of developmental processes can go awry, leading to developmental anomalies and death. Prenatal development presents the highest risk to life.[3]

Disease may be defined as a collection of signs and symptoms that reflect a physical or mental state judged to be abnormal. The key word is "judged." Many women live with DCIS that goes undetected in the breast during life because it causes no symptoms. In these women, DCIS is discovered following death due to unrelated causes. If there were no signs or symptoms of cancer, did these women have disease? The cancer-cell population never grew to a point where signs or symptoms became evident, thus requiring medical intervention, and the women lived long enough to die of something else. Indeed, a substantial reservoir of DCIS is undetected during life. How hard doctors look for the disease is an important factor in determining how many cases of DCIS are diagnosed. This has important implications for what it means to have the disease.[4]

The number of human diseases is not known but is probably ten thousand or more. There are at least two thousand categories of diseases based on classifications of disease in the International Classification of Diseases (ICD) manual.[5] Most diseases can be grouped into one of four main classes: (1) Pathogenic diseases like the common cold and whooping cough are caused by bacteria, viruses, and other microbial agents. Disease prevention and management involve either avoiding or neutralizing exposure or eliminating the offending microbe via therapy. (2) Deficiency diseases result from the absence or reduced levels of a biologically important molecule because of dietary deficiencies or metabolic abnormality. Type 1 diabetes is a consequence of little or no insulin production by the pancreas. Scurvy results from a deficiency of vitamin C in the diet. Replacement therapy or dietary modification can ameliorate or correct the problem. (3) Genetic diseases involve one or more genetic mutations that occur in body (somatic) cells or in germ cells. Cancer is a collection of more than one hundred distinct diseases characterized by genetic damage to body cells. If the genetic damage is in the germ cells, the damage can be passed on to future generations. For some inherited diseases like Tay-Sachs or cystic fibrosis, there are genetic tests available to determine the likelihood a couple will have a child with the disease. Finally, (4) physiological diseases, such as heart or kidney disease, are characterized by functional abnormalities in specific tissues and organs. They usually have multiple causes and frequently affect multiple organ systems. Reduced blood flow to the kidney because of a lesion in the renal artery can raise blood pressure, leading to a stroke. Syphilis is one example of many diseases that fit in more than one category. Syphilis has a microbial cause or etiology but also has a physiologic component in its late stages when brain function is compromised.

The complex nature of biological systems makes diagnosis and treatment of many chronic diseases exceedingly difficult. Complexity means that system behavior is irregular and that changes in one tissue or organ can have unpredictable consequences for other tissues and organs. We cannot predict exactly how the human body responds to a particular disease state or treatment. Even when the diagnosis is the same, no two patients will present symptoms or respond to treatment identically. The macroscopic laws of physics can be used to make general predictions of response, but exact predictions in individual cases will remain elusive because of the nature of complexity. Hypertension or high blood pressure is a good example. Vasoconstriction or narrowing of blood vessels increases blood pressure. The causal relationship between vessel lumen diameter and blood pressure is well known and can be described by classical equations in fluid dynamics. These equations predict how much of an increase in blood pressure should occur for a given level of vasoconstriction, but provide no additional information to predict accurately blood pressure readings in individual patients. The equations apply to an isolated blood vessel and ignore other physiological factors that modify response. In spite of the availability of numerous drugs to treat high blood pressure, many diagnosed patients have inadequate responses to therapy.

System complexity also means that diseases can involve multiple tissues and multiple causes. Although most diseases emerge in a single or small cluster of tissues, the presentation of the disease in terms of signs and systems reflects the whole body. Multiple factors that perturb different physiological systems in the body can lead to complex disorders like hypertension. Psychological stress can cause vasoconstrictions, leading to high blood pressure. So can physical obstructions within blood vessels. If they show up together, these unrelated causes may interact nonlinearly to increase the probability and severity of disease. Understanding disease causality and the complex interactions occurring among causal agents is important in disease prevention.[6]

The historical fight against human disease has been marked by the pursuit of two distinct medical problems. The identification, treatment, and control of microbial diseases are examples of simple medical problems characterized by a direct linkage between readily identifiable causal factors and specific signs and symptoms of infection. For example, the Spanish flu pandemic of 1918 killed tens of millions of people; signs and symptoms were generally uniform in infected individuals, and the course of the disease was predictable.[7] Approaches to controlling infectious diseases that once ravaged humanity for centuries are straightforward because of the linear, uncomplicated relationship between pathogen (the specific cause) and disease. If the "bug" caused the disease, then getting rid of the bug was the key to a cure. The solution to simple medical problems is obvious once the pathogen is known and pathways of infection are identified. However, although the way forward may be clear, finding an effective solution may be difficult. Controlling pathogen spread and pathogen inactivation after infection continue to be scientific and medical challenges.

The remarkable success of medicine and public health in controlling contagious diseases began in the nineteenth century. Social progress and prosperity drove the rates of infections down. As Western societies became richer, the conditions that allowed for infectious diseases like tuberculosis started to wane. Concurrently, nutrition, sanitation, and housing improved. Also key advances in science and medicine were made, particularly the introduction of rigorous scientific methods to isolate and characterize pathogenic bacteria and associate them with specific signs and symptoms of disease. Based primarily on the work of Robert Koch, the study of infectious disease was placed on a secure scientific foundation, which ultimately made possible rational treatment and control. Koch formulated a set of criteria that could be used as a framework to identify the pathogen responsible for a specific disease.

Koch's postulates consisted of four criteria: (1) The organism must be regularly associated with the disease and its characteristic lesions. (2) The organism must be isolated from the diseased host and grown in culture. (3) The disease must be reproduced when a pure culture of the organism is introduced into a healthy, susceptible host. (4) The same organism must be reisolated from the experimentally infected host. Koch applied his criteria to demonstrate that anthrax, a common disease in cattle, is caused by the bacterium *Bacillus anthracis*.[8]

The successful control of infectious diseases in the nineteenth and early twentieth centuries is arguably the crowning achievement of Western medicine and public health. Millions of lives have been saved by the introduction of antibiotics, clean water, and other public health practices. The average life span of Americans at the turn of the twentieth century was only about forty-five years, and most people alive then had their lives cut short by preventable infectious diseases like cholera, tuberculosis (consumption), and typhoid fever. Today, the average American life span is seventy-five to eighty years. Although microbial diseases still take the lives of millions, particularly in poor and underdeveloped countries, they are no longer at the top of the list of health concerns in Western countries.

A new set of challenges has emerged with the control of contagious diseases and extension of the human life span in Western countries. Late twentieth-century and early twenty-first-century medicine is now focused on chronic diseases like cancer, heart disease, type 2 diabetes, and Alzheimer's disease. These diseases were known prior to the twentieth century but occurred infrequently and did not rise to the level of concern for tuberculosis and other communicable diseases. The cost of our success in battling infectious diseases has been the emergence of chronic, complex diseases that have offered and continue to offer serious challenges to modern medicine and public health. Heart disease and cancer are the two leading causes of death in the United States. Treating and controlling complex diseases represent the second type of medical problem. These challenging medical problems involve complex systems that exhibit unpredictability because of the nonlinear dynamics of biological and pathological processes.

What makes diseases like cancer, Alzheimer's disease, and heart disease complex? First, complex diseases are evident at every scale of organization. In cancer, the disease is initiated at the subcellular level with the activation of cancer genes. As the disease progresses, tissues and organs become involved and, eventually, the entire body. The disease even impacts the patient's family and extended social networks. Second, complexity means there is a multiplicity of pathogenic mechanisms. Hypertension can result from aberrations in different blood pressure regulatory pathways, including stress, water retention, and vasoconstriction. Third, a disease may occur spontaneously (i.e., there is no identifiable cause) or can be caused by a multiplicity of factors. Causal factors rarely act independently. The resulting nonlinear interactions mean that the combined effect of all of the causal factors is more (or less) than a simple summation of effects attributed to each agent alone. Fourth, complexity means that disease progression is unpredictable and that the disease is highly individualized. Even the smallest error in describing initial conditions in a patient leads to unpredictable disease behavior. It is not possible to predict disease trajectories in the individual patient any more than is it possible to predict the future value of a stock in the market. Two patients with the same diagnosis will have unique clinical presentations and different clinical courses. Fifth, complexity means that there are multitudes of ways to attack the disease. Attacking different disease vulnerabilities increases the probability of successful disease management, but it is always preferable to get to the disease as early as possible. In cancer therapy one drug might be used to kill cancer cells outright while a second drug might starve the tumor by cutting off its blood supply. Sixth, patients respond to treatment differently. Complexity means that patient responses to identical treatments are different and cannot be predicted. Management of hypertension is, to some extent, a guessing game involving trial and error with different classes of antihypertensive therapies. One patient responds to a diuretic, while another does not.

Since 1950, Western medicine has had remarkable success in treating complex diseases such as cancer, cardiovascular disease, and diabetes; but there is still a long way to go to solve all the disease-management problems. Unfortunately, we know relatively little about neurodegenerative diseases, including Alzheimer's disease. Currently, these disorders are very difficult to manage and are essentially incurable.

Search and Destroy

Preventing disease is always preferable to treating disease. But diseases cannot always be prevented, and early diagnosis and therapy are essential for successful medical management.

Cancer offers one of the clearest examples of benefits of early detection and therapy (Table 6.1). In general, advanced disease is difficult to treat and results in poor outcomes. Cancer becomes increasingly complex as the disease progresses. The disease starts as a collection of a few abnormal cells and grows into a tumor with billions of cells and the capacity to metastasize to distant sites. Selected cancers are listed in Table 6.1 and include four of most common types—breast, colorectal, lung, and

Table 6.1 **Percentage of Five-Year Cancer Survival Depends on Early Diagnosis**

Cancer	All Stages	Localized	Regional Spread	Distant Spread
Breast	83.2	96.1	74.9	19.8
Colorectal	61	91	62.8	6.9
Lung	13.4	47.4	17.2	1.7
Melanoma	86.6	93.8	59.8	15.9
Ovary	44.1	90.9	49.5	23.3
Pancreas	3.6	12	4.8	1.6
Prostate	85.8	98.6	92.1	29.8
Uterine cervix	68.3	90.9	49.9	8.6

Source: Scientific American editors. Twelve major cancers. *Scientific American* 1996;275(3):126–132.

prostate. Survival statistics depend strongly on cancer type. But regardless of cancer type, early diagnosis offers the highest probability of survival. Lung cancer and pancreatic cancer are particularly difficult diseases because even early detection offers meager chances of survival. Sophisticated technologies including medical imaging (CT and MRI), advanced surgical techniques, and new powerful drugs introduced in the latter half of the twentieth century have been critical to early detection and treatment.

Two general approaches are used to search for and detect disease. Diagnostic tests, such as medical imaging and blood tests, are performed when there is preliminary evidence of disease-like symptoms reported by the patient or clinical information obtained on a physical examination. The purpose of diagnostic tests is to confirm disease, while disease screening is conducted in populations of asymptomatic individuals. The goal of screening is to find disease in people who have no indication of disease. The idea is that, if the disease is caught early, the probability of treatment success will be high, and disease mortality rates should decrease. A positive screening test then triggers diagnostic tests to confirm disease. Screening tests identify individuals who might have disease; diagnostic tests rule out or confirm presence of disease. Often the same test is used for screening and diagnosis. Mammography and the prostate specific antigen (PSA) test are used to screen for or diagnose breast cancer and prostate cancer, respectively.

The clinical value of diagnostic and screening tests is based on rates of decision errors. The false-positive rate is the percentage of tests that are positive in individuals without disease. The false-negative rate is the percentage of tests that are negative in individuals with disease. Common cancer tests and their false-positive rates are shown in Table 6.2.

Ideally, the false-positive and false-negative rates should be as close to zero as possible. However, this is unrealistic because reducing one rate causes an increase in the other rate. If every mammographic lesion were called a cancer, that would mean the false-negative rate would be zero because there would be no negative tests. The consequences are that the false-positive rate would be increased because a test positive for cancer would be found in individuals without disease. The predictive value of the test (how good the test is at identifying disease in persons with disease) increases as the false-positive rate decreases. Reducing false negatives increases confidence that a negative test really means no disease. The predictive value of mammography is

Table 6.2 **False-Positive Rates in Common Cancer Tests**

Test	Target Cancer	False-Positive Rate (%)
Fecal occult blood	Colon	8–16
Mammography	Breast	~ 5
Pap smear	Uterine cervix	15 (adolescents); 5 (> 60 years)
Prostate specific antigen (PSA)	Prostate	11–17

Source: Welch HG. *Should I Be Tested for Cancer?* Berkeley: University of California Press; 2004:39–41.

quite high since the false-positive rate is about 5 percent. Mammography can detect about 90 percent of breast cancer in women with disease.[9] PSA and other screening tests are less effective at finding disease when it is present.

Usually the false-positive rate is given more weight than the false-negative rate in determining clinical utility of a screening and diagnostic test. The false-positive rate is typically set below 10 percent to minimize the probability that disease is detected when, in fact, there is no disease. The weighting toward the false-positive rate derives from the idea that one can prove or confirm the presence of disease but cannot confirm or prove its absence. Absence of evidence is not evidence of absence.

Interfering factors are a significant contributor to decision errors in screening and diagnostic tests and are particularly important in determining the false-positive rate of the test. The PSA test simply reveals how much of the prostate antigen a man has in his blood. Infections, over-the-counter drugs like ibuprofen, and benign swelling of the prostate can all elevate PSA levels, but none of these interfering factors signals cancer. Men with low PSA levels might still harbor potentially dangerous cancers, while those with high readings might be completely healthy.

Interpreting screening results is also complicated by disease complexity. In mammography, detection of early stage lesions like DCIS does not necessarily mean the patient will go on to have a disease that requires treatment. The behavior of early lesions is unpredictable. In many instances, the lesions remain static, cause no symptoms, and require no treatment. Recent analyses of breast-cancer screening protocols in the United States illustrate how screening tests can lead to overdiagnosis and unnecessary treatment and other costs. The value of mammography as a cancer screen has been questioned in women younger than fifty years because screening costs (including pain, discomfort, and unnecessary additional diagnostic testing and treatments) greatly exceed the probability of early breast-cancer detection.[10]

PSA testing also reflects a complexity process. The clinically important evidence in PSA testing is the trends over time in PSA blood levels, rather than a single measurement. Increasing levels of PSA, along with a positive physical rectal exam, are a strong justification for prostate biopsy to confirm cancer. PSA levels in the blood at any particular time, however, reflect only the instantaneous production rate and removal rate of PSA. If the two rates are constant, then blood PSA levels are stable over time. But that is not the picture seen in the clinic. Even in disease-free individuals, PSA levels fluctuate in an unpredictable way because the rates of PSA production and removal are not constant. If the production rate and removal rate depend on the prior value of the protein in the blood, then blood levels will assume an oscillatory pattern. Careful analysis of temporal trends in PSA levels is necessary to distinguish real increases in PSA levels against normal fluctuations.

Although a negative cancer screening or diagnostic test does not mean that cancer is not present, a positive screening test confirms the presence of cancer. The key is what counts for a positive test. The false-positive rate has a significant impact on cancer screening tests. When disease rates in a population are fairly low (as is the case for most cancers), the number of false positives given by a screening test can easily exceed the number of true positives, thus limiting the value of the test. If the number of true positives and false positives is the same in a screened population, an individual's positive result has little meaning. It is a toss-up whether cancer is

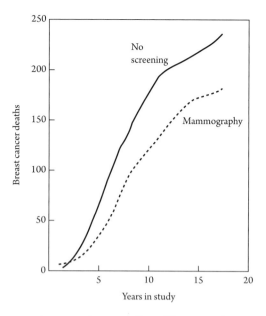

Figure 6.2 Mammography screening saves lives. Women undergoing screening mammography have 25–30 percent lower mortality rates. Increased survival in the screening population is attributable to earlier detection of disease. *Source:* Figure is modified from Figure 4 in Shapiro S. The status of breast cancer screening: a quarter of a century of research. *World Journal of Surgery* 1989;13:9–18. Figure reprinted with kind permission of Springer Science and Business Media.

present or not. Nevertheless, appropriate deployment of screening tests by identifying at-risk populations likely to benefit from screening can have significant public health benefits (Figure 6.2).

Studies conducted since the 1980s show that breast cancer death rates are reduced by 25–30 percent as a result of screening with mammography and physical examination. Given the high frequency of breast cancer, a 25-percent reduction in mortality corresponds to saving the lives of over ten thousand American women each year. The real benefit of mammography, however, is difficult to ascertain in these studies because a portion of the mortality reduction is due to better cancer treatment, not mammography. When treatment benefits are accounted for, about 15 percent of women whose cancer was detected by mammography actually benefited from the test.[11] Whatever the mortality benefit, women screened on a regular basis have lower mortality than women not screened, as shown in Figure 6.2.

Chronic degenerative disease management is medically complex. Diseases are unstable states that tend to progress unless medical interventions are introduced. In some instances (for example, certain neurological diseases or cancers), the diseases can reach a static stage and remain dormant or unchanged for unpredictable periods. Although many of these diseases can be treated effectively without knowing fully the causal factors, treatment is not always straightforward, and treatment outcomes and disease progression are not predictable. In about 90 percent of patients with hypertension, for example, the causal factors are not understood fully. Disease treatment amounts to a trial-and-error approach involving a series of classes of drugs that reduce blood pressure by various mechanisms, including vasodilation and reduction in blood volume. Usually a drug from one class is tried. If that does not work, either the dose is increased or a drug from another class is tried. The trial and error continues, often combining different classes of drugs until an effective therapeutic regimen is identified. Unpredictability means that what works in one patient is not guaranteed to work in another. Managing complex diseases is challenging, but the very nature of complexity offers multiple strategies to treat disease.

Mortality from heart disease has been reduced significantly since 1950 with the introduction of medications to control blood pressure and blood lipid levels, non-surgical interventional procedures to open clogged blood vessels, and surgical techniques to repair or bypass damaged blood vessels. The oncology community has seen similar successes. We can now successfully treat most cancers such that the five-year survival rates exceed 90 percent if the disease is diagnosed early enough. But all is not rosy, and significant clinical challenges remain. Lung cancer and cancer of the pancreas have proven to be exceedingly difficult to manage. These diseases, even when diagnosed early, have a relatively poor prognosis (Table 6.1). Alzheimer's disease has emerged as a very serious concern and is destined to become a worsening public health problem as the American population ages. This ravaging disease has no clearly definable cause and no effective therapies. In fact, the definitive diagnosis of Alzheimer's disease can only be made at autopsy.

Twentieth-century medicine has been marked by the emergence of medical specialties and the focus on an organ systems approach to treat disease. This local systems approach is now giving way to an integrative methodology to medical management. A sick patient does not represent a biochemistry problem or an anatomy problem or a genetics problem or an immunology problem. Instead, each person is the product of multiple molecular, cellular, genetic, environmental, and social influences that interact in complex ways to determine health and disease. The human body is a highly integrated set of subsystems. Changes in one tissue or organ can lead to physiological effects in other subsystems. Integration also means therapy can have broad-ranging effects. Treatment of disease in one tissue may have complicating effects in another tissue.

Therapy can be curative or palliative depending on the condition of the patient and goals of the intervention (Figure 6.1). Therapy for cure is intended to return the patient to normal by eliminating the pathogen (the causal agent), removing diseased tissues, or otherwise correcting the pathophysiologic abnormality. Successful curative therapy is associated with eliminating signs and symptoms. Palliative or supportive therapy ameliorates signs and symptoms without correcting or improving the underlying condition. Palliation improves quality of life and is used in cases of advanced or incurable disease or in patients who cannot tolerate curative treatment because of age or intervening disease. Prophylaxis is distinguishable from curative and palliative therapy by the absence of disease (Figure 6.1). Whereas prophylaxis is an intervention to prevent disease from occurring, curative and palliative therapies are interventions introduced after disease diagnosis to manage disease. Prophylaxis is always preferable to therapy and cure. We are all better off not having disease than having disease and then treating it.

Patients respond differently to therapy. A population of individuals given the same dose of aspirin will experience different levels of pain relief. Diversity of responses is not due entirely to genetics. When genetic factors are controlled for by using genetically identical experimental animals, the heterogeneity of responses persists. Biological complexity and the unpredictability of nonlinear systems to therapy play an important role in system response.

The sigmoid curves in Figure 6.3 illustrate the relation between drug dose and response. The left curve refers to beneficial effects of the drug, the right curve to side effects or complications of the drug. The steepness of the curves reflects the degree of homogeneity of the population. The flatter the dose-response, the more heterogeneous is the population. Some individuals respond to a low dose of the drug, while others respond only to higher doses. A dose-response reflecting a homogeneous population would be square-shaped and would mean that everyone experiences the full effect at the threshold dose and that no one experiences an effect at a dose lower than that.

Medical therapy has two goals that are often at cross-purposes. First, the physician strives to rid the patient of her disease or alternatively to reduce signs and symptoms of disease. Second, the physician strives to avoid harming the patient. In treating difficult diseases like cancer, patients often experience significant side effects in the effort to treat disease successfully. The principles of medical therapy are reflected in the relative positions of the two sigmoid-shaped curves in Figure 6.3. The idea is to separate the cure and complication curves in order to widen the range of doses for effective therapy. The goal of medicine is to optimize the ratio of benefits (cure) to costs (complications).

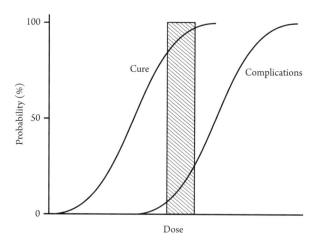

Figure 6.3 Dose-response for cure and complications. Therapeutic efficacy as measured by the ratio of benefits (cure) to costs (complications) improves as these curves are separated along the dose axis. The shaded area identifies the therapeutic or optimal dose range. Doses in this range provide for an acceptable level of cure and an acceptable level of complications.

The relative position and steepness of the cure and complications curves dictate the dose range for acceptable therapy. In the optimal therapy range, an acceptable level of cure is balanced by an acceptable level of complications. If the drug dose is too high, cure may be achieved with 100 percent probability but at the price of unacceptable complications. If the dose is too low, complications may be avoided at the price of uncontrolled disease. In medicine, there is no free lunch. Every treatment and every diagnostic test carries some risk. The balance of risk and benefit is a clinical and patient judgment and is disease dependent. Life-threatening diseases like cancer require very aggressive therapies often accompanied by terrible side effects. The amount of risk a patient is willing to accept is dictated by the real and perceived benefits of the intervention. Cancer patients usually are willing to accept a higher probability of serious complications associated with life-saving therapies.

Therapeutic medicine is guided by the principle of normal-tissue tolerance. Patient safety is the primary goal in medicine. In the United States, new drugs go through several phases of clinical testing before government approval. Phase 1 is a toxicology evaluation that establishes the maximum tolerated doses and dose schedule used in all subsequent phases of evaluation. If drug efficacy can only be achieved at doses exceeding tolerance, then the drug is removed from further evaluation.[12] Pharmaceutical companies emphasize risks in marketing products in print and broadcast media. If the patient experiences side effects, she is advised to stop taking the drug and talk to her doctor.

Complications from medical therapy arise for two principal reasons. First, drugs may act in a nonspecific way. The drug may control or eradicate the disease, but it may also damage healthy tissues. This is a very common problem in cancer medicine. Classic cancer drugs like the antimetabolites 5-fluorouracil and methotrexate are effective against specific cancers but produce serious side effects, particularly in rapidly dividing tissues like the bone marrow and gastrointestinal mucosa.[13] These cancer chemotherapeutics cannot distinguish cancer cells from normal cells: they kill both normal cells and cancer cells with about the same efficiency. As a consequence, normal-tissue injury occurs, the severity of which impacts therapy. Second, treating disease in one part of the body may have adverse effects on tissue function in another part. As a complex system, the human body adapts to therapy-induced changes. Vioxx is a good example of how treatment for one condition leads to untoward effects in an unrelated subsystem of the body. Vioxx is a nonsteroidal anti-inflammatory drug that is effective in the treatment of arthritis and related inflammatory conditions. However, high doses of this drug increase the risk of cardiovascular disease in some patients through mechanisms involving high blood pressure and tissue swelling.[14]

An important goal of research and development in diagnostic and therapeutic medicine is separation of the complication and cure curves, as seen in Figure 6.3. Moving the cure curve leftward increases the response to therapy. Improving drug potency means that the drug is effective at lower doses. Shifting the complication curve to the right protects normal tissues. But if the diseased tissue is protected to the same degree, no therapeutic advantage is realized because the cure and complication curves have not been uncoupled. Separation of the cure and complications curve means that the dose range for therapeutic effectiveness is widened. At the high end of the therapeutic range, high disease response is achievable without unacceptable normal-tissue injury.

Targeted therapy can avoid serious complications. Most chemotherapeutic drugs are administered by mouth or through the veins. Sensitive normal tissues are exposed because drug uptake results in whole-body exposure. In recent years, some drugs have been packaged to facilitate delivery directly to the disease site. Monoclonal antibody systems have been developed that bring the drug directly to the tumor because of the specificity of the monoclonal antibody for the tumor. In radiation, therapy advances in medical physics have led to methods of delivering high-energy radiation directly to tumors, thus substantially sparing normal tissue, which gets much smaller doses.

The mapping of the human genome in the year 2003 promised new opportunities to diagnose and treat disease based on genetics. Detailed knowledge of the 23,000 genes and the three billion base-pairs in the human genome was expected to lead to the development of a cornucopia of new drugs and an era of personalized medicine in which treatments would be tailored to an individual's genetic makeup. Drugs would be developed that specifically target the disease's molecular defect, thus sparing any damage to healthy cells and tissues. Personalized medicine would identify which patients would benefit or be harmed by a particular therapy based on genetic makeup.

Unfortunately, in the decade since the sequencing of the human genome, these expectations have yet to be reached, and the actual results have been disappointing. In retrospect, the problem of biological complexity had not been fully appreciated. The development of better diagnostics and therapies lies in understanding the complexities of how phenotype emerges from genotype. Many diseases are caused by or are a consequence of the proteins made by genes, not the genes themselves. The processes by which the genome regulates itself either by genes telling other genes what to do or by manipulating key molecular targets in the cell are vastly more complicated than anyone expected. The way genes are switched on and off via epigenetic processes are at least as important as the composition of the genes and their gene products. The keys to success are the connections between genetic information and how that information is ultimately expressed.

One potentially exciting application of genomics is the identification of genetic variations that might put an individual at higher risk for a degenerative disease like cancer or Alzheimer's disease. Knowing the genetic component of disease risk can lead to identifying at-risk individuals and implementing environmental risk-reduction strategies, because, while the genetic component of the risk is irreducible, the environmental risks can be altered. But predictive medicine is controversial, and genomic information must be interpreted cautiously. A positive genetic test does not necessarily mean the individual will get a certain disease, just as a negative genetic test does not eliminate the possibility of that disease. Because our understanding of the link between genomic information and disease expression is limited, disease risk estimation is highly uncertain.

However, genetic biomarkers do have the potential of identifying disease in its earliest stages. Therapeutic intervention before symptoms appear increases the chances of successful disease management. There is considerable effort underway to develop biomarkers of Alzheimer's disease so that early treatment can delay the onset of symptoms or reduce signs and symptoms, giving patients more years of quality of life. Currently, treatment begins late in the disease process when little can be done to delay disease progression or ameliorate signs and symptoms.

Identifying effective therapies in a personalized medicine context also requires understanding of genes and their RNA and protein products in health and disease and the link between genetic variation and disease. Managing complex diseases like diabetes and cancer also requires an understanding of systems biology beyond the complexities of molecular medicine. Although the molecular defect in type 1 diabetes is well known (lack of insulin production by the pancreas), the consequential loss of regulatory control of blood glucose has profound effects on system-wide physiology.

Our current understanding of the genotype-phenotype dynamic is limited because of poorly understood complexities at the molecular and systems level. The information contained in DNA is encoded in the linear arrangement of DNA bases. But in the cell, DNA is folded three-dimensionally such that genes located a distance apart linearly are really adjacent to each other in the folded configuration. These genes can cooperate with each other. Human disease may be a reflection of the altered cooperativity of these distant genes. Simple linear analyses of the genome may miss the importance of the separated genes. An unknown but large number of genes code for RNA as a final product, rather than for DNA. These RNA products play a regulatory role by controlling the function of other genes. RNA genes are observed in a number of cancers and may have clinical significance in developing therapies. How the environment influences disease incidence and progression is poorly understood, but the process involves complex networks and controls all the way down to the molecular level. Epigenetic processes (discussed in chapter 7) regulate gene expression by turning genes on or off in response to environmental cues.

In the Eye of the Beholder

Disease is more than just numbers and objective measurements. There are also social and cultural dimensions that are important in defining disease. How we distinguish the normal state from the disease state is primarily a cultural and social problem. What counts for disease depends on what counts for normal. As we saw in the case study at the beginning of the chapter, normal and disease conditions are not always separable. Our visceral sense of what is normal depends on what we experience and what we become used to. Poor dental hygiene is the statistical norm in the United Kingdom, but it is an still an abnormal physical condition.[15] Our concept of what is normal changes as technology evolves because technology impacts our experiences and our expectations. Eyeglasses have been around for centuries; so many people now wear eyeglasses that it is no longer considered unnatural. In fact, for some celebrities like Elton John, eyeglasses are part of their personal identity. Disease has social and cultural dimensions beyond the mechanistic perspective of traditional medicine.

Ideally, what is normal should rely on quantitative, objective assessments. Even so, many biological traits vary with age and gender, so different normative standards may apply. Normal testosterone levels refer to what is normal for men in their twenties. But even among younger men, testosterone levels can vary markedly over the course of a day. Many men in their sixties have testosterone levels below presumed normal levels but do not experience signs or symptoms that would justify hormone replacement therapy.[16] A statistical approach to normality avoids subjective assessments of normality but cannot distinguish between what is truly abnormal from what is merely unusual or rare. Athletic talents good enough for a professional career are unusual but not abnormal. Subjective assessment of normality is problematic because standards are sensitive to cultural and social influences.

Normative standards are established through assessing objective and subjective biometric criteria in a well-defined sample population that is assumed to be representative of the whole population. Intrinsic physical and behavioral traits (for example, blood pressure, height, IQ) are normally distributed such that most people are clustered around the mean value and relatively few people are at the ends with values that are either significantly higher or lower than the mean. Standards are often expressed as a range of values inclusive of the population average. The range of normal values reflects the natural variations of the trait in the population. The wider the range, the greater is the natural variation of the trait. But should the population average always function as a norm? Normative standards are based on a statistical analysis of the bell-shaped distribution or by comparing measurements in individuals with and without disease. Mental retardation is an example of a human disease that is defined by the statistical distribution of a biological characteristic. IQ is an intelligence metric that is normally distributed in the population with a mean value of 100. Individuals with measured IQs one or more standard deviations below the mean (below 85 IQ points) are considered to have below-average intelligence. Blood pressure is another example; it is also normally distributed, but the range of normal is bounded by values associated with blood pressure-related diseases such as coronary artery disease or stroke (Figure 6.4).

Distinguishing physiological states occurring as a result of natural variations from those due to pathology can be difficult. When biological traits are continuously variable (like blood pressure and height), the presence of disease may not depend solely on abnormal parametric values but on contributions of predisposing (genetic) factors and environmental risk factors. In such cases, setting standards of normality is difficult because standards are subject to environmental or social circumstances. Normal function is also linked to the individual and her circumstances. Individuals near the lower end of the normal distribution may be considered disadvantaged for that trait and, therefore, unhealthy compared to others. But people who fit into the average range may equally regard themselves as disadvantaged with regard to those who are above average or at the upper end of the distribution. In which cases of traits distributed "normally" should the average also function as a norm, or is the norm itself appropriately subject to alteration?

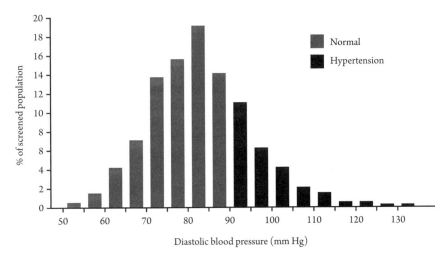

Figure 6.4 Distribution of blood pressure in a screening population of 159,000 persons ages 30–69 years. Hypertension is somewhat arbitrarily defined as diastolic pressure greater than 90 mm Hg. At this pressure and higher, cardiovascular disease risks may be elevated. *Source:* The data are from the US National Institutes of Health, Department of Health, Education and Welfare. The figure is modified from Hypertension Detection and Follow-up Program Cooperative Group. Hypertension Detection and Follow-up Program: a progress report. *Circulation Research* 1977;40(Suppl. 1):I-106–I-109.

Medicine Without Borders

The notion that medicine is international and knows no borders has become almost commonplace. Throughout the world, the medical profession has roughly the same principles and speaks to some extent the same clinical and scientific lingua franca. Because of this, the diagnosis and treatment of most diseases, including appendicitis, pneumonia, and rheumatism, are similar in different countries, and therapeutic success depends on the skill of the healthcare provider and the cooperation of the patient. Nevertheless, it is a gross oversimplification to assume that the practice of medicine is at all homogeneous in the Western world. Even within the United States, the use of diagnostic tests, especially imaging studies, varies considerably from one region of the country to another, with higher costs but no better patient outcomes associated with the highest-use regions.[17]

Disease and what we consider to be normal are culturally and socially constructed but are also deeply rooted in a mechanistic and systems perspective of human function. The biomedical model of medicine and disease emphasizes disease as physical or mental states that are quantifiable and objective deviations from homeostasis. Since the body is treated as a collection of parts, diagnoses and treatments are focused on specific tissues, organs, and organ systems. The goal of therapy is to return homeostatic parameters (like red blood cell count, blood pressure, blood glucose levels) to values within the normal range. In medicine, as it has been practiced, support by the patient's family is recognized as important to the overall success of therapy but is not considered central to diagnosis and management strategies. The cultural model of medicine and disease, on the other hand, argues that disease and its diagnosis and treatment represent more than alterations in specific body tissues and systems. Instead, medicine is a holistic art and science that involves the whole person both spiritually and physically. In this model, the disease boundary extends well beyond the patient to include the immediate family and extended social networks. The cultural model considers the broader socioenvironmental contexts in which health, disease, health-related behavior, and normal development are embedded.[18]

Patients with the same disease are likely to be treated in much the same way under an evidence-based biomedical model but may be treated and managed quite differently under the cultural model. Consequently, a disease in one culturally and socially defined community may be viewed differently than in another community with different social and cultural perspectives. Although medicine as practiced in the United States is still based primarily on the biomedical model, the importance of cultural and social dimensions of health and disease is increasingly recognized.

Medicine is shaped by its specific cultural or national setting. Cultural influences are pervasive and involve every aspect of healthcare, including public health and prevention, disease diagnosis, and disease management. The behaviors of patients and healthcare providers are influenced in particular by local organizations such as hospitals and clinics, malpractice lawyers, and imaging centers. These are, in turn, influenced by institutions in the larger society, including the media, healthcare plans, and the government. National cultures are keys to understanding normality and disease and explain why a condition in one country is a disease requiring treatment but in another is a variation of normal. The same disease in France, Germany, Great Britain, and the United States may be managed in entirely different ways because of different cultural norms.[19] Mental health is particularly sensitive to cultural and social perceptions. That the mind lives in the brain, the brain lives in the body, and the body lives in the community are keys to understanding mental health in all cultural and social contexts.

The line separating health and disease can be easily blurred. Among the Navajo, for whom the prevalence of congenital hip disease is relatively high, treatment is not seen as necessary, even when the disorder may eventually become painful. Resulting limps carry no stigma for the Navajo, but they do for American society in general. Ideas about the visible signs of health also differ. In the United States women strive for thinness, while in Jamaica a plump body is much more appealing.[20]

Medical management of blood pressure is an example of how "normal" is interpreted in different countries. Hypotension (low blood pressure) is a German disease. It is not considered a disease in the United States, however, and is viewed by some American healthcare professionals as advantageous for long life. American physicians would treat low blood pressure only if it resulted in serious signs and symptoms (for example, a vital sign in a medical emergency, fainting because of orthostatic hypotension), but Germans treat hypotension in even asymptomatic patients. Hypertension or high blood pressure, on the other hand, is aggressively treated in the United States. Americans with a diastolic blood pressure greater than 90 mm Hg are likely to be treated, but diastolic pressure would probably need to exceed 100 mm Hg to warrant treatment in the United Kingdom.[21]

In addition, whether an individual is considered to have a disease depends on the normative standards established in the community. A member of the deaf community is considered normal and part of the deaf community. The same person is viewed as sensory deficient in the hearing world. For some in the deaf community, the cochlear implant to improve hearing is an affront to their culture. As they view it, the hearing majority is a threat to the deaf minority. The deaf community feels that its way of life is fully functional and that using American Sign Language instead of oral English puts them at no disadvantage in society. On the other hand, the hearing community considers deafness a social disadvantage and a quality-of-life issue: this sensory deprivation needs to be corrected in order to be fully functional in society.

Beyond Therapy

Complex systems are flexibly adaptive. Physiological systems respond to a wide variety of environmental conditions by either increasing or decreasing function. Under normal circumstances, the body operates at the edge of chaos such that external factors trigger an adaptive response, but, in time, the system returns to a stable state. In disease states, adaptive responses do not result in a return to stability; rather, medications and other medical interventions are forcing agents that return the body to the stable state. Often medications (for example, insulin) must be taken for long periods to sustain stability.

Some diseases are characterized by a lack of a constituent substance that is responsible for the disease state; for example, type 1 diabetics produce too little or no insulin. Certain drugs work by increasing the deficient substance. But what happens if a "normal" person takes the drug, that is, a person who does not lack the necessary substance? In this case, the drug can cause an enhancement of functioning such that the individual performs tasks at levels beyond normal. Neuroenhancement and blood doping are common examples in American society. Drugs like Adderall and Ritalin are frequently used by students to enhance cognitive functioning. These prescription drugs treat attention deficit and other behavioral disorders but, in individuals who do not have these conditions, can enhance time-on-task and attention span to improve cognitive functioning. Neuroenhancement drugs work by altering brain levels of neurotransmitters like dopamine and serotonin. When serotonin levels are low, problems with depression and attention arise. Adderall increases levels of serotonin so that, in the normal individual, raising serotonin levels can enhance cognitive functioning.

Blood doping has been used by competitive athletes to improve physical performance. Increasing the number of circulating red blood cells delivers more oxygen to metabolically active tissues, such as skeletal muscle. Erythropoietin is a hormone produced by the kidneys to stimulate the bone marrow to make more red blood cells. Erythropoietin, produced by recombinant DNA technology, is an approved drug for the treatment of anemia from kidney failure and bone marrow toxicity from cancer chemotherapy. In normal individuals, however, erythropoietin increases red blood cells levels beyond normal levels.[22]

Enhancement is defined as the alteration of characteristics, traits, and abilities beyond what is considered to be normal. The distinctions between therapy and enhancement rely on notions of disease, normalcy, nature, and naturalness. There is no bright line that separates therapy from enhancement. Not surprisingly, enhancement technologies have emerged as a natural outgrowth of medical advances for the diagnosis and treatment of established diseases, such as bone marrow failure and kidney disease. Because concepts of therapy and enhancement are difficult to separate, the justification and acceptability of enhancement cannot be easily uncoupled from concepts of health and therapy and, therefore, cannot be adequately clarified. However, it can be said that enhancement and treatment are at opposite poles of the medical intervention spectrum.

The therapy-enhancement dynamic shifts according to culturally determined norms. Aggressive therapy as practiced in the United States leads to the availability of medical interventions for enhancement purposes. The diagnosis of attention deficit hyperactivity disorder (ADHD) is higher in the United States than in other countries. In fact, there is widespread concern that ADHD is seriously overdiagnosed; children who may not need them are prescribed stimulants. American consumption of psychotropic drugs for treating ADHD (and other mental disorders) and for enhancement of cognitive function far exceeds use in other countries.[23]

Nothing Is Simple

Complexity is a central feature of human biology and disease. The human body consists of a large number of interconnecting systems. Normal physiology is contingent on integrating specialized systems and coordinating specific functions. Flexible adaptation means that small changes occurring in one system lead to a cascade of responses in other systems. When an insect bites or stings and deposits a small quantity of venom, the nervous system, endocrine system, circulatory system, and local tissues respond to neutralize the venom, prevent its spread, and begin repair of the local injury. When the body detects a survival threat, the flight-or-fight response is elicited to reduce or eliminate the threat. Sensory inputs trigger the nervous system and endocrine systems to initiate a cascade of cardiovascular, immune, digestive, and musculoskeletal system responses. Changes in these systems are transient; once the threat has dissipated, the body quickly returns to a stable state.

Diseases result when systems fail to maintain stability or are unable to respond appropriately to environmental stresses. In this context, the study of diseases has been critical to understanding normal function. Historically, physiology developed and matured as a medical discipline based on the concept that we learn about what is normal by studying what is abnormal. The understanding of the normal function of the endocrine pancreas and the role of insulin in regulating blood glucose derived from studies of type 1 diabetes. These patients cannot produce insulin and have unregulated blood glucose levels. Disease and what we call "normal" mutually inform. We define disease in terms of what is considered normal (including all the cultural and social dimensions that apply to the perception of normalcy), but understanding disease also defines normalcy.

Most diseases represent a complex web of conditions that are connected via underlying biological mechanisms and processes that emerge over a lifetime. Chronic diseases pose some of the most challenging public health problems because the relationships among the environment, epigenetics, genetics, and other host factors are poorly understood. Many important illnesses like cancer and cardiovascular diseases are characterized by a chronicity that makes it nearly impossible to comprehend fully the relationship between disease-causing agents early in life with the clinical appearance of the disease in mid- to late adulthood. Early-life exposure to environmental risk factors and immune-inflammatory insult or dysfunction play key roles in many chronic diseases, but the details of the pathogenesis process are not fully understood.

The importance of unraveling the complex web of interactions among epigenetic, genetic, other host and environmental factors and cultural and social dimensions of disease cannot be overstated. The problem is extraordinarily challenging and will require a complex biology approach that takes into consideration how diverse physiological systems coordinate to deal with insults that occur throughout a lifetime, from the moment of conception onward. If we are to solve the heart disease problem, we need a better understanding of how adolescent dietary and social behaviors increases arterial disease risk and heart disease. Evidence of atherosclerosis is observable in young people.[24] Although the biochemistry and pathophysiology of atherosclerosis is now well understood, a more complete understanding of cardiovascular disease will require a complex systems perspective. Risk management depends not only on resolving host and environmental factors but also on understanding how these factors are influenced by cultural and social factors. Nonlinear interactions among disease factors are an inherent feature of biological complexity.

In the next three chapters, we explore biological complexity in the context of specific chronic degenerative diseases. Cancer cannot be explained simply as an aberration of normal cells gone wild. Alzheimer's disease cannot be explained simply as an aberration or dysfunction of nerve cells or their connections. These diseases are manifestations of a higher level of complexity. In the next chapter, we explore etiology in three closely linked diseases—heart disease, diabetes type 2, and obesity. This trinity shares a multiplex causality that is not well understood. Isolating single causal factors in complex systems is difficult because of the complex nature of the diseases and the fact that etiologic agents interact nonlinearly and cannot be easily separated. The resulting impact on disease prevention and public health strategies is considerable.

The Trinity

Bill Miller is a physically active fifty-eight-year-old Caucasian male who complained of chest pain while exercising. On occasion, the chest discomfort was so severe it forced Bill to stop his workout. Bill described the chest pain as diffuse and radiating down both arms. Chest discomfort disappeared a few minutes after he rested. In September 2006, soon after he first noticed the symptoms, Bill visited his family doctor to determine the cause of his discomfort. Bill's physical examination and clinical tests suggested significant heart disease risk factors, including high levels of low-density lipoprotein cholesterol (LDL cholesterol), low levels of high-density lipoprotein cholesterol (HDL cholesterol), high levels of triglycerides, and high blood pressure. Bill is 5'6" and overweight (210 pounds), but he does not smoke or drink alcohol excessively. Bill admits to significant job stress that he does not seem to be handling well. He also has a significant family history of coronary artery disease. His father had a coronary event when he was sixty years old, and his mother also had coronary artery disease and was treated for coronary artery blockage at age seventy. Bill's mother also had a history of high blood cholesterol levels that could not be managed by diet (statin drugs and other medications available today to manage high cholesterol were not available then). Based on the physical examination and medical history, Bill's physician arranged for a cardiology consult for additional tests. The cardiologist did a complete evaluation of the cardiovascular system including a stress echocardiogram to rule out coronary artery disease.[1] In spite of Bill's risk profile, the stress echocardiogram and heart workup revealed no unusual findings. The cardiologist prescribed medications to control blood pressure and blood lipids. Bill was advised to see a behavioral specialist about his job stress and to schedule a follow-up appointment in three months or sooner should symptoms get more severe.

During the next two months, the chest pains did get worse. A stress echo study was repeated in December 2006, and this time significant abnormalities in heart motion were observed consistent with poor blood flow to the heart (coronary artery disease). In late December, Bill had a left heart catheterization to evaluate blood flow to the heart. Findings were remarkable with significant triple vessel disease: The left anterior descending coronary artery was 90 percent occluded, the circumflex artery was 80 percent occluded, and the marginal artery was 75 percent occluded. Bill did not know it, but he was a walking time bomb and could have a serious heart attack at any time.

One day after the coronary angiogram, a triple coronary artery bypass graft was performed. The surgery involved grafting two segments of the internal mammary artery and one saphenous vein graft to bypass the occlusions in the diseased arteries. Bill tolerated the procedure well and was discharged five days after surgery. A stress echocardiogram six weeks after surgery was negative, indicating successful reestablishment of blood flow to the heart muscle. Bill experienced no chest pain during the test. He has returned to work and began a moderate exercise schedule. He manages his heart disease risk factors by taking medications to control blood pressure and blood lipids. He also watches his diet and is working to reduce job stress.

Heart disease remains the number one killer in the United States, claiming 800,000 lives annually (one in three deaths from all causes). Since 1950, remarkable progress has been made to reduce morbidity and mortality. In the 1950s and 1960s, doctors could do little more than wait until heart attack and stroke victims were rushed to the hospital and then try to keep them alive. As knowledge deepened of important causal factors, including smoking, blood pressure, and diet, the emphasis has shifted from treatment to prevention through risk management.[2]

Bill Miller exhibited several cardiac risk factors, including being overweight, elevated LDL cholesterol, low levels of HDL cholesterol, high blood pressure, and stress. Which of these factors was the primary cause of Bill's disease cannot be determined. In another person with the same diagnosis, a different set of etiologic agents might be involved. When multiple causal factors are at play, their relative importance cannot be determined in the individual but can be in well-designed epidemiological studies involving large populations where control groups and exposed groups are well characterized.

In this chapter, etiology or cause is discussed as an important dimension of disease complexity. The complex nature of biological systems means diseases are a consequence of seemingly unrelated causal factors acting in concert. It is difficult to isolate or change a single variable in the system without affecting other system parameters in unanticipated ways. This is particularly true for chronic, degenerative diseases where complexity predicts that disease-causing factors act in spatially and temporally distinct ways. Heart disease is primarily seen in middle age or later, but the initial stages of pathogenesis begin in the early twenties or perhaps in the teen years. The disease process takes years or decades and involves causal factors acting at various points along the way. The vascular lesions established early in life are exacerbated later in life by the long-term effects of smoking, diabetes, and high blood pressure.

Three Diseases

The focus in this chapter is the disease trinity linked to the metabolic syndrome—heart disease, type 2 diabetes, and obesity (Figure 7.1). The metabolic syndrome (also called Syndrome X and Insulin Resistance Syndrome) is a multiplex causal factor. In recent decades, metabolic syndrome and the associated disease trinity have emerged as significant public health problems.

Type 2 diabetes is associated with insulin resistance, central obesity, hypertension, and dyslipidemia, as shown in the figure above. Although these linkages are

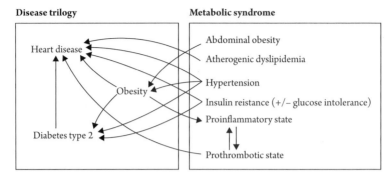

Figure 7.1 Metabolic syndrome is a name for a group of causal factors and risk factors that occur together and increase the risk for heart disease, type 2 diabetes, and obesity. Abdominal (central) obesity is both a key element of the metabolic syndrome and a disease linked to metabolic syndrome. *Source:* Figure based on Grundy SM, et al. Definition of metabolic syndrome: report of the National Heart, Lung, and Blood Institute/American Heart Association conference on scientific issues related to definition. *Circulation* 2004;109:433–438.[3]

well established, their pathophysiological basis remains unclear, and no unifying feature of the metabolic syndrome has emerged. Metabolic syndrome was first described in type 2 diabetic patients, and the broader concept of a metabolic syndrome was introduced by Gerald M. Reaven in 1988, who suggested the common factor was insulin resistance and not diabetes. More recently, central obesity (as measured by waist circumference) has been proposed as the central feature of the metabolic syndrome. The lack of a clear unifying feature has hampered defining the metabolic syndrome as a clinical entity. Nevertheless, the metabolic syndrome has clinical utility. The clinical construct has brought a heightened appreciation of risks of heart disease in type 2 diabetes. A broader risk perspective results in better disease management of people with type 2 diabetes, given that 75 percent of them will die of cardiovascular disease.[3]

The two most important factors in the metabolic syndrome are excessive weight around the abdomen (central obesity), making the body look apple-shaped, and insulin resistance in which the body cannot use insulin effectively to help control the amount of sugar in the body. In insulin resistance, the body does not respond to insulin, and blood glucose cannot enter cells. As a consequence, the body produces more insulin, and blood sugar and insulin levels rise. Chronic high levels of blood sugar damage blood vessels, affect kidney function, and raise levels of blood lipids, including triglycerides. Lack of exercise, aging, and genetic factors predispose the individual to metabolic syndrome.[4]

Heart disease, type 2 diabetes, and obesity are closely linked degenerative diseases. Glucose imbalance and related metabolic perturbations, along with diet and generalized inflammatory responses, bridge these diseases. Obesity is a comorbid condition for heart disease and type 2 diabetes. Heart disease is often a comorbid condition in diabetes, and type 2 diabetes is often a comorbid condition in heart disease. Thus, the presence of one disease increases the risk of the other two.

Human degenerative diseases are divided into four major pathologies. (1) Cardiovascular diseases involve damage to the heart and blood vessels and include hypertension, heart disease (primarily coronary artery disease), and strokes. (2) Neoplasias are tumors characterized by uncontrolled proliferation of abnormal cells and include benign growths and malignant tumors. (3) Neurodegenerative diseases involve the central nervous system and include Alzheimer's disease and Parkinson's disease. Finally, (4) metabolic pathologies are diseases related to abnormal metabolism and physiology and include diabetes and obesity. This chapter focuses on obesity, heart disease, and type 2 diabetes. To a lesser extent, cancer causation is also discussed; however, chapter 8 is devoted entirely to the cancer problem because it is one of the most thoroughly studied chronic degenerative diseases. Alzheimer's disease as an example of neurodegenerative disease has a unique complexity involving the most complex organ in the body—the brain—and is discussed in chapter 9.

All degenerative diseases are characterized by long clinical horizons. The clinical manifestations surface at the end of a long pathogenesis process that often begins decades earlier with subtle, imperceptible changes in a cluster of target cells. The degenerative process means age is an important risk factor. Go to any medical clinic treating degenerative diseases (like a cancer clinic); the waiting rooms are typically populated by seniors. These diseases are usually not observed in younger populations, but after about age fifty, disease risk increases significantly with age.[5] The chronic nature of degenerative diseases means that causal factors are difficult to identify because initiating events cannot be easily linked to the clinical appearance of disease. Nor can degenerative diseases be distinguished by the agents that cause them: heart disease is clinically similar in smokers and nonsmokers.

Evidence of obesity, type 2 diabetes, and heart disease is observable at every scale of biology—from individual cells to the whole organism to social communities. Changes seen at one level of biology are a consequence of the complexity at lower levels of organization. Emergent phenomena at the organ or organismal level cannot be predicted by analyzing changes at the subcellular or cellular level. In heart disease, the atherosclerotic plaque begins as a small lesion in the vascular wall. Over time, inflammatory processes and cellular proliferation lead to a hardened mass that protrudes into the blood vessel lumen. The growth and behavioral trajectory of the lesion cannot be easily predicted. The lesion may remain stable or mature into a complicated mass with a high probability of rupture and thrombus formation. Physiological consequences and clinical outcomes range from minor to life threatening.

Obesity

An individual is considered obese if the body mass index (BMI) exceeds 30 kg/m^2.[6] This is a somewhat arbitrary definition but is linked to BMI values associated with increased risk of disease. Obesity has become a serious public health problem in the United States after several decades of skyrocketing growth. Obesity was relatively stable in the United States between 1960 and 1980, when about 15 percent of people fell into the category, and then it increased dramatically in the 1980s and 1990s. The estimated prevalence of overweight and obese individuals in the United States in

2008 was 149 million. About one-third of American adults are obese. Approximately 17 percent (or 12.5 million) of children and adolescents aged two to nineteen years are excessively overweight. High rates of childhood obesity are likely to translate into higher rates of extreme obesity when those children reach adulthood. But obesity is primarily an adult disease. Very few children are born obese. Although there are developmental risk factors for later obesity, infant risks do not explain most adult obesity, and obesity in early childhood usually disappears.[7]

The alarming rise in obesity in the United States is a result of the confluence of forces that have led to an enormous increase in available calories. Many environmental factors from economic interests of the food and beverage industry to the ways urban communities are planned and built contribute to unhealthy nutritional behaviors. Vending machines, fast food restaurants, and processed foods laden with calories from fats and sugars conspire to make it easier for people to consume huge numbers of calories. Key determinants of body weight gain are high absolute metabolic rate, low rate of fat oxidation, and socioeconomic factors. If trends continue, 75 percent of Americans will be overweight or obese by 2020. The health consequences would be staggering—eight million more cases of diabetes, seven million more cases of coronary artery disease, and about 500,000 new cases of cancer.[8]

Obesity is an independent risk factor for hypertension, high levels of blood cholesterol, type 2 diabetes, heart disease, and certain cancers. The location of excess body fat is an important risk determinant. Central obesity is associated with higher risks as opposed to peripheral excess body fat (particularly in the buttocks). The reasons for this remain unclear.

Obesity is a multifactorial disorder. No single cause explains all cases. The primary problem is an imbalance in energy intake and expenditure. Body weight increases if caloric intake exceeds caloric expenditure. Genetic factors, abnormal glucose metabolism, and the in utero environment that predisposes the individual to excessive weight gain in childhood also contribute.

Weight loss has long been considered an eating behavior problem, but there is now compelling evidence that obesity is a genetic and biological disease. The genetic factors predisposing to obesity are poorly understood. A genome-wide search for type 2 diabetes-susceptibility genes identified a common variant in the *FTO* (fat mass and obesity-associated) gene that predisposes a person to diabetes through an effect on BMI. Obesity risk is about 30 percent higher in individuals carrying one copy of the *FTO* variant and 60 percent higher risk if two copies are present. *FTO* is among the strongest known genetic factors for obesity. The gene product is part of a family of enzymes important in DNA repair and fatty acid metabolism. *FTO* appears to influence obesity risk by increasing energy input.[9]

The body's response to changes in caloric intake and expenditure is a dynamic process. Weight loss will occur if energy expenditures exceed energy intake, but the general rule of thumb that burning 3,500 kilocalories results in the loss of one pound of body fat seriously overestimates actual weight loss. Some people can lose weight faster than others even when eating the same foods and doing the same exercises. Body weight can slowly rise even when eating and exercise habits have not changed. The static weight-loss rule does not account for dynamic physiological adaptations that occur with decreased body weight.[10]

For decades, the guiding principle of weight loss has been anchored in the idea that a calorie is a calorie. It did not matter what kinds of food you ate as long as you burned more calories than you took in. Obesity has always been thought of as an imbalance of calories-in versus calories-out. But this view has recently been challenged.[11] How much we eat is important, but, in terms of weight loss, a calorie of protein might not generate the same amount of energy as a calorie of carbohydrate. If obesity is an energy-storage defect, the trigger for weight gain might not be the quantity of food but the types of food ingested. But where calories come from as a strategy for weight management may be an illusion. A calorie is a calorie, and, based on the laws of thermodynamics, the number of calories taken in must exactly equal the number of calories leaving the system when fat storage is unchanged. This assumes all calories, regardless of source, are completely burned.

Control of body weight by some combination of diet, exercise, and behavioral modifications is an effective strategy to reduce BMI in most people. In extreme cases, surgical removal of excess fat may be indicated. But keeping weight off is a challenge for almost everyone who wants to control his or her weight. Physiological changes occur during weight loss that make it difficult to keep the weight off permanently. Compounding biological inertia are constant exposures to appetite stimuli. We are constantly surrounded by food messages and opportunities to eat.

Diabetes

Type 2 diabetes is a metabolic disorder characterized by insulin resistance and the inability to metabolize glucose properly.[12] About eighteen million people have been diagnosed with diabetes, and an estimated seven million people have undiagnosed diabetes.[13] Vascular damage involving the vascular endothelium is the primary and most common complication associated with diabetes and is a cause of inflammation and prothrombotic conditions leading to atherosclerosis. Diabetes is linked to high rates of premature death from infectious diseases and cancer and other chronic degenerative disorders.[14] The progression of the disease is determined primarily by how well blood glucose levels are controlled, but the clinical course in the individual patient cannot be predicted. A fifty-year-old with type 2 diabetes will lose an average of six years of life as a result of the disease. By comparison, a smoker of the same age would be expected to lose seven years of life. A type 2 diabetic is twice as likely to die of cardiovascular disease as someone without diabetes and 25 percent more likely to die of cancer. Type 2 diabetics are also more likely to die of kidney disease, liver disease, pneumonia, and other infectious diseases. These data are alarming because of the rapid increase in type 2 diabetes among Americans. About twenty-five million Americans have diabetes (8 percent of the US population), ten million more than two decades ago.[15]

The mechanisms of heart failure in type 2 diabetics are not fully understood, but perturbations in metabolic pathways appear to be important. In a healthy individual, the heart muscle cell metabolizes many substances to generate energy, including free fatty acids (FFAs) and glucose. The heart muscle cell (cardiomyocyte) has limited flexibility to switch from FFAs to glucose as a carbon energy source, resulting in increased free fatty acid exposure and accumulation. When the heart is in a resting state, metabolism of FFAs is preferred because the energy yield is higher. However, during stressed conditions (for example, ischemia, cardiac hypertrophy, or exercise), the heart switches to metabolize glucose as an energy source due to the metabolic efficiency. Type 2 diabetes is distinguished by the increased amount of FFA uptake and oxidation by the cardiac muscle cells, as well as insulin resistance. In a type 2 diabetic, there is an increased amount of FFA uptake and oxidation because of the high supply of FFAs that are circulating in the blood due to the insensitivity of insulin. Although there is excess glucose circulating, the cells are not able to use it as an energy source. The inability of these cells to switch over to glucose metabolism from FFA metabolism is primarily due to insulin resistance. Since there is a reciprocal effect on FFA and glucose metabolism, when the FFA metabolism increases, glucose metabolism is inhibited. The extended exposure to excess FFAs eventually leads to an increase in the formation of fat (lipogenesis) within cells. This contributes to excess fat deposits and FFA accumulation. While FFAs are inhibiting the uptake of glucose, they are also promoting the development of lipids in the blood (dyslipidemia).[16]

Type 2 diabetes should be considered a cardiovascular disease equivalent. For the growing population of type 2 diabetics, cardiovascular disease remains the number-one cause of morbidity and mortality. Not only are diabetics more likely to experience a cardiovascular event, but they are also at higher risk of a fatal outcome. About three-fourths of all type 2 diabetic mortality is due to cardiovascular disease.[17]

Heart Disease

Cardiovascular disease is the leading cause of death in the United States. Coronary artery disease (CAD) accounts for roughly half of deaths (or 400,000) annually from cardiovascular disease. CAD involves the buildup of atherosclerotic (fatty) plaques in blood vessel walls that have sustained unrepaired chronic injury to endothelial cells that line the interior walls of blood vessels. When these fatty plaques get large enough, they impede or completely block blood flow. In complicated plaques, portions break off, causing blockages downstream. Heart myocytes, or muscle cells, require a constant supply of blood because they are metabolically active and have a high rate of oxygen consumption. If blood flow is cut off, myocytes die quickly. Depending on the number, size, and location of atherosclerotic plaques, severe heart damage or death occurs unless blood flow can be restored quickly.[18]

Death rates from cardiovascular disease have declined, yet the disease burden remains high because control of traditional causal factors remains an issue. About seventy-five million adults (about one-third of United States adult population) have hypertension. Smoking remains a serious public health problem in spite of extensive efforts since the 1960s to reduce cigarette consumption. About 20 percent of the US population continues to smoke. An estimated thirty-three million US adults have high blood cholesterol levels.

Causes and Risks

Disease probability is determined by risk factors and causal factors. A risk factor is an agent or condition associated with an altered probability of disease occurrence. The key word is "associated." Risk factors are useful as biomarkers of disease that can be used to identify at-risk populations. An individual with one or more risk factors for a particular disease has an increased probability of having that disease now or sometime in the future. In theory, knowledge of risk factors should lead to behavioral modifications and heightened medical surveillance (including screening tests) to reduce disease risk or to detect disease in early stages. In reality, however, many individuals fail to take appropriate actions to manage their risk. The second factor, causal, is mechanistically linked to disease, that is, through a direct line of agency. If an agent is causal, then reducing exposure through avoidance behaviors changes disease incidence. Causal factors and risk factors impact public health and disease prevention in different ways. Causal factors are the keys to prevention and public health strategies; risk factors are keys to identifying at-risk populations and to detect disease in its early stages.[19]

Causal factors include environmental agents that can be manipulated to modify disease incidence. Preventing disease by reducing exposure to biological, chemical, and physical disease-causing agents is a key objective in public health. Evidence for causality derives from large-scale epidemiologic studies comparing exposure profiles in individuals with disease and without disease. These case-control studies establish correlations between agent exposure and disease. But evidence of correlation by itself is insufficient to establish causality. The possibility that an association may be causal can be strengthened by evidence of consistent findings across studies, a dose-response relationship showing that disease risk increases with increasing dose of the agent, and evidence of biological plausibility. Meaningful dose-response information is usually difficult to obtain because of the requirement for large study populations exposed to large gradations of agent doses. Only experimentation designed to establish a functional relationship between disease incidence and agent dose and mechanisms of action can provide definitive proof of causality. Animal studies are conducted in lieu of human experiments because of obvious ethical and practical limitations. Animal studies can provide definitive causal evidence if the animal model chosen is representative of the human response. An inappropriate experimental animal system can lead to false conclusions about disease risks in humans.[20]

Age and gender are risk factors, not causal factors, for disease. The association between age and most degenerative diseases, including cancer and heart disease, is striking. These diseases occur infrequently in young individuals, but the incidence increases markedly after age fifty. Risk factors are disease markers in that they reflect some characteristic of the disease but cannot be manipulated to modify disease risk.

Heart disease and other complex disorders result from nonlinear interactions involving multiple agents. Complexity is such that contributions to disease from specific etiologic (causal) agents cannot be determined in individual cases. In heart disease, some factors such as high levels of LDL cholesterol have a defined role in pathogenesis and are strongly linked to disease incidence and mortality; other factors such as high levels of C-reactive protein in the blood, a marker for inflammation, show evidence of correlation, but causality has been difficult to establish. It is unclear what role C-reactive protein itself plays in atherosclerosis, but the inflammatory process is a key contributor. Individuals with human immunodeficiency virus (HIV) infection have higher rates of cardiovascular disease than do uninfected subjects. People with HIV have more than four times the risk of sudden heart attack than their uninfected peers. The most likely explanation is that both the virus and the drugs to treat HIV infection cause chronic inflammation.[21]

Currently, scientists believe that disease results from some combination of genetic mutations and environmental factors (see Figure 6.1). It has been assumed genes and the environment interact in a linear fashion because genes and environmental agents do not share disease mechanisms. The ability of the environment to influence or promote disease does not generally involve DNA mutations because the DNA is chemically stable and resistant to most environmental stressors. If the DNA were not stable in the face of common environmental stressors, life would have quickly died out.[22]

Mutations are permanent changes in the information content of the DNA and increase or decrease disease susceptibility. For most diseases, the link between genotypes and phenotype is unclear. How do alterations in the DNA sequence lead to a specific pathologic phenotype? Manipulating genetic factors affects susceptibility to diseases, but, in the absence of agents that actually cause disease, genetic factors are not likely to influence disease incidence.[23] Nevertheless, genetic information serves a useful public health strategy. The genetic signature of a disease can be used to develop screening tests to identify at-risk populations. Several cancer tests to detect specific cancer genes are already available and in widespread use. About 10 percent of women with breast cancer are positive for the cancer genes BrCa1 and BrCa2. Since these genes increase susceptibility to disease, women who test positive can reduce their chances of disease by making lifestyle choices that reduce environmental risks, including managing their diet and not smoking.

Environmental factors increase the probability of disease occurrence. Exposure to environmental factors does not mean that disease will always occur but that the probability is assumed to increase monotonically with increasing dose of the agent. Public health strategies to reduce incidence of disease focus on environmental factors because exposure can be controlled by the community or by the individual. Genetic factors load the gun; lifestyle (environmental factors) pulls the trigger.

Unfortunately, the gun metaphor is too simplistic. The genotype-phenotype relationship and interactions between environmental influences and genetic information have turned out to be very complex. The successful mapping of the human genome in 2003 was supposed to usher in an era of personalized medicine whereby disease treatment could be tailored to the individual patient based on personal genetic information. That promise has yet to be realized in part because of our limited understanding of the relationship between genotype and phenotype and the role of complex molecular processes, including regulating gene expression. Knowledge about personal genetic information alone is simply not enough to predict disease susceptibility, outcomes, or therapeutic effectiveness.

A new paradigm has emerged recognizing a more complex and diversified role for the environment in chronic disease pathogenesis. The environment affects disease in essentially two ways. First, environment may be a proximal cause of disease; examples include cigarette smoking and alcohol consumption. Some environmental factors, such as cigarette smoke, cause more than one disease, but the combination and interactions of genetic and environmental factors are likely to be unique for each disease. It is well established that the environment can act independently of genetic influences and affect normal physiological processes. Hypertension can be triggered by emotional stress and can be controlled in part by removing the source of stress.[24] Second, the environment can impact pathogenesis by modifying biological processes that increase susceptibility to disease. Epigenetics is a common pathway for this. The environment influences gene regulation and determines which genes are turned on or turned off without changing the information content of the DNA, but how genetic factors cooperate and interact with environmental factors to cause disease is not fully understood.

The role of the environment in disease etiology is facilitated by the capacity of cells to regulate gene expression by switching genes on or off through epigenetic mechanisms (Figure 7.2). Whether a gene is switched on or off depends on an array of physical factors. In the living cell, DNA is tightly packaged and spooled by specialized proteins called chromatin and histones. This "epigenome" controls the differential expression of genes in specific cells by gating the access of the transcription machinery to transcriptional regulatory regions. Gene transcription occurs when the local DNA is unpacked, exposing transcription sites. Incomplete chromatin remodeling or methylation along strategic points in the DNA prevents transcription, resulting in gene silencing. Epigenomic regulation is influenced by local environmental factors and controls genomic activity without affecting genetic information.[25]

Environmentally controlled epigenetics starts during fetal life and is important in establishing susceptibility to disease later in life. The environmental factors operate as nutritional cues. The embryo and fetus are susceptible to these cues from conception to the immediate postnatal period. Developmental plasticity is affected in part by epigenetic processes and enables the developing organism to respond to environmental cues and adjust its phenotype to match its environment. Epigenetic processes alter genome activity associated with the differentiation programming of cells or organ systems. Altered program and gene expression profiles can promote an abnormal physiology and disease at the later adult stage of development. Mismatch in the form of disruption of the balance of epigenetic networks to turn genes on

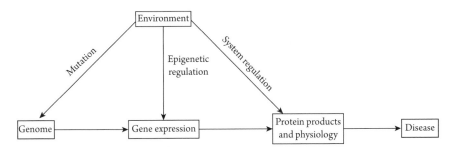

Figure 7.2 Disease results from perturbations in the genotype-phenotype dynamic. The genotype-phenotype dynamic is complex and involves modification of genotype by environmental factors that turn genes on or off. Epigenetics is a multifaceted control system. Environmental factors can also bypass genetic mechanisms and influence physiology and human disease processes directly.

or off between the early and mature environments may result in inappropriate patterns of epigenetic changes and gene expression. These patterns of expression increase subsequent susceptibility to disease, including cardiovascular disorders and diabetes, later in life.[26]

A large number of epidemiology studies support the belief that the environment is a major factor in disease etiology. Geographic regions around the world generally have distinct disease profiles and frequencies. North America has high rates of prostate disease and low rates of stomach disease, whereas eastern Asia has low rates of prostate disease and high rates of stomach disease. Migration from one region of the world to another often results in the adoption of the new region's disease profile. When identical twins grow up in different geographic regions, they also have different disease frequencies, suggesting environmental influences independent of genetic factors.[27]

Early evidence that the fetal environment influences subsequent susceptibility to chronic disorders came from experimental studies and epidemiological research that showed increased rates of cardiovascular disease in groups with high rates of infant mortality. Other studies showed an inverse relationship between birth weight and susceptibility to chronic diseases. Intrauterine growth retardation has been correlated with elevated rates of hypertension, cardiovascular disease, type 2 diabetes, and obesity. Collectively, these observations generated the idea that fetal metabolic adjustments in nutritionally adverse circumstances that serve to restrict growth and thus safeguard brain development may result in an increased risk of chronic diseases later in life. But increased risk of chronic disease has also been observed in situations when the fetus has been exposed to high nutritional environments. Apparently, the influence of environment on the phenotypic expression is quite complex, and the relationship among genetics, development, and environment is poorly understood. Untangling the genetics from the environmentally determined developmental processes is not straightforward.[28]

The ability to switch certain genes on or off in response to environmental cues is a key process in normal human development. Epigenetics is involved in many normal cellular processes and plays a key role in differentiating cells into various distinct cell types, such as neurons, liver cells, pancreatic cells, muscle cells, and inflammatory cells. All human body cells contain the same DNA but are structurally and functionally different because certain genes are turned on or turned off. Epigenetic changes determine which proteins are made. The combination of expressed and inhibited genes leads to a suite of cell proteins characteristic of specific cell types. Epigenetic mechanisms enable the developing organism to produce different yet stable phenotypes mapped from the same genotype. This helps explain how identical twins with the same genotype can behave differently when exposed to different environments because of altered phenotypic expressions.

Epigenetic traits are stable phenotypes resulting from changes in a chromosome without alterations to the DNA sequence. Epigenetic processes do not result in gene mutations. An epigenetic phenotype is initiated by an environmental signal that triggers an epigenetic pathway. The environmental signal activates DNA-binding factors or noncoding RNA that define the specific area on the chromosome where the epigenetic chromatin state is to be established. The epigenetic state can be "fixed" by remodeling the chromosome through histone protein modifiers. Epigenetic traits are primarily the result of turning off genes. Gene silencing occurs through the processes of chemical alteration of DNA, involving the addition of a methyl group to cytosine bases, called methylation, preventing transcription of the genetic code close to the chemical alteration; chemical modifications of histone proteins, the proteins that package DNA into chromatin; and the gene-regulating and chromatin-organizing activities of noncoding RNA.[29]

Epigenetics plays an important role in the development of disease, its pathogenesis. The pathogenesis of cardiovascular disease and diabetes type 2 begins before birth in the uterine environment. During the very early phases of human development, the genome is wiped clean of most epigenetic changes in DNA. Epigenetic modifications are progressively reestablished during the process of development. For example, development evolves to match the uterine environment. Mismatches between the current environment and the phenotypic outcome of developmental plasticity leads to cardiovascular disease, type 2 diabetes, and other chronic diseases that become clinically evident decades after birth.[30]

The pathogenesis of type 2 diabetes is an example of how epigenetic activity during in utero development can influence disease risk later in life. The timing of a critical period during in utero development determines the capacity for transfer of phenotypic information between generations. The maternal phenotype embodies a record of the mother's cumulative environmental experiences, and this information is transferred via nutrients, hormones, and other signals.

Type 2 diabetes is a disorder of complex genetics influenced by interactions between susceptible genes and the environment. Intrauterine growth restriction (the developing baby weighs less than 90 percent of other babies at the same gestational age) is linked to the development of the disease in adulthood. An abnormal metabolic milieu within the uterus affects fetal development by permanently modifying the activity of key genes regulating pancreatic beta cell development and glucose transport in muscle. Pancreatic beta cells produce insulin that regulates uptake of glucose by muscle and other tissues. Epigenetic regulation of gene expression is one mechanism by which genetic susceptibility and environmental insults can lead to type 2 diabetes.[31]

It is well known that the maternal environment can have a permanent effect on the physiology of offspring. Children of Dutch women who were pregnant during the "Hunger Winter" of 1944 suffered much higher rates of obesity, diabetes, and cardiovascular disease than those born a year or two earlier. Although disease causality is multiplex, one possible contributing factor is the fetal response to maternal nutrition. Epigenetic adjustments (through cytosine methylation, as discussed above) lead to changes in gene regulation (switching genes on and off) in the developing embryo/fetus. Offspring of starving mothers adjust their metabolism to hoard calories. If hard times go away, a result is a tendency to put on weight. The tendency to become overweight or obese increases the risk of heart disease and other chronic degenerative diseases.[32]

A role for epigenetics in cancer has been established where cancer cells have the capacity to turn selected genes on or off depending on the stage of disease development and local tissue microenvironments. Tumor cells with metastatic potential have the capacity to turn off genes that control cellular adhesion properties. When these genes are turned off, cancer cells can easily move from one part of the body to another and cross blood vessel walls to seed secondary growth sites.

Cancer cells can modulate their gene expression as disease progression and local tissue environments dictate. Colon cancer was the first human disease to be linked to epigenetics. Diseased tissue from patients with colorectal cancer has less chemical modification of the DNA than normal tissue from the same patients. Genes that are chemically modified by methylation are typically turned off, and this loss of DNA methylation can cause abnormally high gene activation by altering the arrangement of chromatin. Disruption of the ordered pattern of DNA methylation is a hallmark of the cancer phenotype. Thus, turning genes on or off alters the phenotypic profile that can lead to disease. Colorectal cancer arises as a consequence of the accumulation of genetic alterations (for example, gene mutations, gene amplification, and so forth) and epigenetic alterations (for example, aberrant DNA methylation, chromatin modifications, and such) that transform colonic epithelial cells into colon adenocarcinoma cells. The loss of genomic and epigenomic stability and the resulting gene alterations appear to be key molecular and pathogenic steps that occur early in tumor growth and permits the acquisition of a sufficient number of alterations in tumor suppressor genes and oncogenes in a clone of cells to result in their ultimate transformation into cancer. Epigenetic alterations are common in many cancers and affect the formation and behavior of the tumors.[33]

Large individual variations in probability and severity would be expected in an epigenetic model of disease. At any time, individuals have unique epigenetic profiles (that is, different system states). Epigenetic differences are linked to gender, lifestyle, and past and current environments. An array of clinical outcomes is expected when exposed to disease-causing agents, depending on the nature of the exposure and the interplay of factors such as cell communication, microenvironment, tissue infrastructure, and a whole host of systemic variables.

Where's Waldo?

All human diseases are caused by some combination of genetic and environmental factors. This includes microbial diseases for which almost all the risk can be assigned to the infectious agent. Although everyone diagnosed with cholera has been infected with *Vibrio cholerae*, not everyone infected gets the disease, in part because of host conditions that confer resistance. The relative contribution of genetic and environmental factors for some important chronic diseases is shown in Table 7.1. The contribution of genetic factors and the environment is highly variable and disease specific.[34]

Genetic contribution refers to inherited risks; these risks do not necessarily mean that the genetic marker is a cause of a disease. Environmental factors include a broad array of controllable agents ranging from diet and exercise to exposure to

Table 7.1 **Nature and Nurture**

Disease	Genetic Contribution to Risk (%)	Environmental Contribution to Risk (%)
Alzheimer's disease	62	38
Breast cancer	73	27
Colon cancer	35	65
Heart attack (female)	62	38
Heart attack (male)	57	43
Lung cancer	14	86
Melanoma	21	79
Multiple sclerosis	48	52
Obesity	67	33
Prostate cancer	42	58
Rheumatoid arthritis	53	47
Stomach cancer	21	79
Type 2 diabetes	64	36

Source: Agus DB. *The End of Illness.* New York: Free Press; 2011:79–80.

toxic agents such as cigarette smoke. The percentages shown in the table above are expressed as point estimates that suggest a level of certainty not borne out by our current understanding of the highly variable genetic and environmental components of risk. In reality, the relative contributions of genetic and environmental factors are not well known for most chronic diseases.

Genetic and environmental components of risk for each disease add up to 100 percent, but this should not be interpreted to mean risks are simply additive. Epigenetic phenomena strongly suggest that genetics and the environment interact in complex ways. Part of the total disease risk is due to genetic and environmental factors acting in concert. Environmental factors can influence gene expression, but the removal of environmental risk factors, including changes in personal behaviors that contribute to risk, does not necessarily eliminate the disease because of the complex interplay between genetics and biochemical and physiologic factors (called host factors) that influence disease development. Lung cancer can occur in someone who has never smoked because of the individual's set of host factors that increase disease risk.[35]

Disease complexity makes it difficult to identify causal factors, and there are several reasons for this. First, cases may arise simply because of spontaneous failure or perturbations in a metabolic pathway—a consequence of complexity. Some cancers, like prostate cancer or brain cancer, have no identifiable causes and seem to occur for no reason at all.[36]

Second, nonlinear interactions complicate teasing out the contributions of individual agents, particularly when one of the agents has predominance. Smoking is the overwhelming cause of lung cancer in the United States, accounting for about 90 percent of the disease burden. But other agents, including naturally occurring radon gas, a ubiquitous, naturally occurring radioactive substance produced by the radioactive decay of uranium in the Earth's crust, also cause the disease. In studies of lung cancer in uranium miners who smoke, the contribution of radon gas exposure in the mines has been difficult to assess because smoking and radiation interact in a nonlinear fashion. When both agents are present, the smoking effect easily masks the much smaller contribution of radon.[37]

Heart disease pathogenesis involves nonlinear interactions of several causal factors. How agents interact is part of the inherent complexity of the disease. Complexity is evident when manipulating one causal factor leads to unrelated changes in the body. Use of statin drugs to control blood lipids reduces heart disease risk but may increase risk of liver disease. Nonlinearity occurs when agents have overlapping mechanisms of action. Removing one factor (for example, cigarette smoking) reduces disease incidence, but we can't predict by how much because other sufficient causal agents are still in play. If two agents combine in a linear fashion, on the other hand, removal of one agent leads to a predictable reduction in disease that is attributable to the effects of the remaining agent.

Hypertension and hyperglycemia (high blood sugar) are mutually reinforcing. Hypertension is especially common among type 2 diabetics. Over 70 percent of type 2 diabetics are affected by hypertension, which increases the risk for cardiovascular disease. The insulin resistance characteristic of the diabetic state (hyperglycemia) leads to vascular changes that promote hypertension. Uncontrolled high blood pressure causes vascular injury and promotes atherosclerotic plaque formation. As abnormal glucose levels progressively increase, so does cardiovascular mortality. Poor glycemic control is a very strong predictor of future cardiovascular disease. It is a significant problem because diabetics are already at elevated risk for cardiovascular disease.[38]

Third, causal factors for complex diseases are neither necessary nor sufficient. There are some twenty factors associated with heart disease, including hypertension, cigarette smoking, total blood cholesterol, low levels of high-density lipoprotein cholesterol, high levels of low-density lipoprotein cholesterol, diet, homocysteine and C-reactive protein levels in the blood, personality type, physical inactivity, obesity, diabetes, and stress.[39] Cigarette smoking is clearly a causal factor because there is ample evidence that decreasing cigarette consumption reduced incidence of disease.[40] However, which other of these factors are really important as public health controls and how factors interact are poorly understood. Some factors, such C-reactive protein, may not be causal at all but may serve as a biomarker for an inflammatory state that contributes to disease. Complexity of disease means that some factors might look causal but, in fact, are not because they are not proximally or directly involved in the pathogenic process. If factor A causes disease B and factor C is correlated with factor A, then it is a spurious conclusion to claim that factor C causes the disease B.

Fourth, if an agent is causal, then reducing or removing it should be ameliorative. But that is not always the case in complex systems. Robustness in complex biological systems raises important questions about redundancy and degeneracy that can make identification and manipulation of causal factors difficult. Can the behavior of the system with multiple components organized in a robust network be reduced to a sequence of simple causes each separately contributing to the overall complex effect? It is not always easy or possible to isolate linear causal pathways. The traditional approach of deconstructing complex systems into simple modular component causes and then analytically reassembling them does not work in a straightforward way in complex systems. If changes in one factor induce corresponding changes in another, the first factor is the candidate for being the cause of the second. The requirement for causes to be explanatory in the cause-effect relationship never varies; it is stable.[41]

Although insulin signaling is the fundamental defect in diabetes, the complexity of the disease cannot be fully understood by manipulating the defective process. Insulin replacement and weight management are effective stop-gap measures but do not address the ultimate cause of the disease. Teasing out the precise contribution of individual causal factors is not just difficult: It may be impossible. The endlessly ramifying network interconnections characteristic of the complex disease process are too complex to yield readily to empirical, mathematics-based analysis.

Fifth, evidence for causality is often inconsistent because diseases are multifactorial and causal factors act together. As noted above, not all smokers get lung cancer or heart disease. Individuals with lung cancer or heart disease may be never smokers. Diet and nutrition have been implicated in many diseases, but their role in pathogenesis is far from clear. The Japanese eat very little fat and suffer fewer heart attacks than the British or Americans. On the other hand, the French eat a lot of fat and also suffer fewer heart attacks than the British or Americans. The Japanese drink very little red wine and suffer fewer heart attacks than the British or the Americans. The Italians drink large amounts of red wine and also suffer fewer heart attacks than the British or the Americans. There is more to disease than diet and nutrition.

Many patients at risk for heart disease present with a diverse risk profile including dyslipidemia (abnormal levels of plasma cholesterol), high blood pressure, and insulin resistance. These three factors act in concert to increase the probability of heart disease by contributing to the formation of atherosclerotic plaques. LDL cholesterol is a key component of vascular plaques. Hypertension exacerbates vascular wall injury, and high blood sugar due to insulin dysregulation compromises the integrity of the vascular wall. Which of these factors is the primary proximal cause in the individual cannot be determined, because causal factors are interdependent. A complexity model predicts that reducing two or more disease-causing factors should have a significantly greater impact than reducing one factor. Heart disease risk-management strategies frequently involve drug combinations to control blood cholesterol and reduce high blood pressure. At-risk individuals are also encouraged to control weight as a way to prevent or manage type 2 diabetes.

Sixth, because of biological complexity, there is an inherent uncertainty in determining what causes a disease in a particular case. For many diseases causation is nonspecific, because diseases themselves are complex with multiple pathogenesis pathways. Causes can be identified in well-designed, large-scale epidemiologic studies, but identification of cause in the individual is not possible.

It is no longer sufficient to focus on agent effects on single tissues or organs. Causal agents can have multiple effects on the body, and complex systems biology requires a multiscale approach to understanding disease causality. X-rays at sufficiently high dose affect every level of biological organization, from whole-body effects down to damage to the DNA. Long-term exposure to disease-causing agents increases the probability for interaction with other disease-causing agents. Many causal agents exert their effects by similar mechanisms (for example, DNA damage). This means that nonlinear interactions are likely and that individual health outcomes are not predictable.

Seventh, causation in chronic disease is problematic because agent exposure precedes clinical appearance of the disease by years or decades. Clinical effects are separable from exposure to causal factors in space and time. Nonspecificity and long latency means that causation cannot be easily assigned in the individual case.

One of the main risk factors for cardiovascular disease in type 2 diabetic patients is diabetic dyslipidemia. Dyslipidemia is distinguished by hypertriglyceridemia, high levels of LDL cholesterol, and low HDL-cholesterol levels. Dyslipidemia can occur before diabetes is even diagnosed, and up to 50 percent of patients have complications by the time of their actual diagnosis. This means atherosclerotic disease is already developing years before diagnosis. Even in the absence of a significant risk of diabetes, coronary atherosclerosis begins at a young age. About one in six teenagers already have atherosclerotic plaques in their coronary arteries based on detection of vascular lesions using intravascular ultrasound imaging.[42]

Identification of causes is particularly problematic for cancer, Alzheimer's disease, and other complex diseases where pathogenesis is not fully understood and many candidate causal factors have been identified through statistical association. Effective public health programs require detailed understanding of disease causality. Tobacco control is an effective public health measure because cigarettes are an overwhelming cause of heart disease and cancer. There is considerable and compelling epidemiologic evidence, and mechanisms by which cigarette smoke damages the body are known, although not fully understood. The cause-effect problem becomes significant and difficult to resolve when agent exposures are small, the spontaneous incidence of the disease greatly overwhelms the disease incidence due to agent exposure, and understanding of disease mechanisms is incomplete. In 2011, the World Health Organization's International Agency for Research on Cancer (IARC), after review of the published epidemiological literature, added radiofrequency electromagnetic radiation (a form of nonionizing radiation) from mobile phones to its list of possible causes of human cancer. The decision is controversial because of limited epidemiological evidence in support of causality and the lack of a mechanism that explains the link. But, of course, complex diseases like cancer do not have simple explanatory causes. Mobile phones have been linked to two rare brain cancers—gliomas and acoustic neuromas. Little is known about how these tumors develop or what might cause them.[43]

Western medicine has generally failed to identify causes of chronic degenerative diseases that can be used to establish effective public health programs to reduce disease prevalence. Unlike microbial diseases where the link between an identifiable causal agent and a disease is clear, the problem is more difficult for complex diseases. The clinical horizon for chronic, degenerative diseases is very long, extending to years or decades. The pathogenesis of complex diseases involves a temporal uncoupling of agent exposure and clinical presentation. Cigarette smoking is a known cause of heart disease, but smokers do not get the disease immediately after their first cigarettes. Further, not all heart disease patients are smokers. Extensive epidemiological studies of smoking and heart disease indicate a delay of about twenty years. If a population begins smoking in 1960, the effects of smoking in terms of increased incidence of disease are not evident until about 1980. Temporal uncoupling of cause and effect complicates causal factor identification. For one thing, intercurrent disease or events can mask influences of candidate causal agents. A smoker may die in a car accident before lung cancer becomes clinically evident, thus masking the effect of smoking. This is rarely a problem with microbial diseases (HIV exposure and AIDS are well-known exceptions) or disorders resulting from physical trauma where the proximal cause of the disease is readily identifiable because the causal event and clinical outcome are tightly coupled in time.

Proximal causes of coronary heart disease, type 2 diabetes, and obesity include smoking, diet, and nutrition. The major elements of the metabolic syndrome—obesity, dyslipidemia, hypertension, and hyperglycemia—are driven by diet. Because of overlapping pathogenic pathways, targeting multiple risk factors simultaneously is an effective risk management strategy.[44]

Put the Gun Down

The primary goal of public health is to get people to avoid pulling the trigger and to prevent disease through preventive measures or prophylaxis. Prophylaxis prevents or retards pathogenesis by eliminating or reducing exposures to environmental agents or by interfering with the mechanisms whereby the environmental agent causes disease (Figure 6.1). Prophylaxis assumes many forms: vaccines that neutralize disease-causing viruses, oral hygiene for the prevention of tooth decay, public health measures to improve water and food safety, and physical barriers to reduce environmental exposure, such as sunscreens that block solar ultraviolet light exposure.

The fact that the cards have been already dealt before birth that affect health later in life has profound implications for disease risk management. An individual's likelihood of getting cancer, heart disease, or diabetes depends in part on the maternal environment during development. Knowledge of disease risks acquired early in life is critical to establishing personal behaviors that reduce risks. Successful risk management depends on how early an individual adopts protective behaviors. This is challenging because young adults tend to live in the now and are not concerned with behaviors that may have important health impacts later in life.[45]

Understanding causality is central to effective disease prevention and public health. But knowledge of causality is less important in the treatment of many diseases. Clearly, effective treatment of microbial diseases requires knowledge of the offending microbe, since therapy is microbe specific. But for chronic, degenerative diseases like heart disease, knowledge of causation is not critical to effective therapy. Coronary artery disease is treated essentially in the same way whether the patient is a smoker or nonsmoker. It is helpful to identify causal agents for long-term disease risk management, but the treatment of the disease per se often does not require such knowledge. A smoker successfully treated for heart disease would be wise to stop smoking to reduce the risk of recurrence in the future. Knowledge of mechanisms is important in establishing sound science-based public health policy, but the lack of full information should not retard development of policies for the protection of the public health. Utility is not necessarily linked to understanding. One does not need to know how a television or computer works in order to use it.

The key challenge for twenty-first-century medicine and public health is the prevention and control of chronic diseases, particularly neurodegenerative disease. To a large extent, we can successfully treat cancer and heart disease, but we do not have a good handle on disease prevention except for controlling smoking, reducing animal-fat content in the diet, and blocking exposure to certain disease-causing viruses. Disease prevention is always preferable to treatment and cure, and identifying and managing causal factors are keys to effective public health programs Treatments for heart disease, cancer, and other chronic, degenerative diseases are battles fought one patient at a time. The disease fight is frequently won without fully comprehending the disease itself or its causes. The costs and time and effort are staggering. In the United States, costs of cancer treatment and the socioeconomic impacts of cancer on the patient, her family, and the community exceeded $260 billion per year in 2010 American dollars. Disease prevention, on the other hand, is a population-based strategy that works efficiently at relatively little expense. Humankind has had remarkable success eradicating a number of communicable diseases, including polio and smallpox, but wiping out cancer and heart disease will not be achievable because of the intrinsic complexity of these diseases. However, understanding these diseases from the perspective of causality might lead to better ways to control disease prevalence. There is little question we have considerable understanding of the role of smoking and diet in disease causation but our knowledge of pathogenesis remains incomplete. Even if tobacco consumption were completely eliminated, a substantial reservoir of heart disease and cancer would remain.[46]

Complexity limits what is doable in public health. In theory, we can eliminate a substantial disease burden by eliminating cigarette smoking, modifying diet and nutrition, and reducing or eliminating exposure to disease-causing viruses. However, these diseases are likely never going to be eradicated, although they can be controlled if detected early enough. Some degenerative diseases, particularly cancer and neurodegenerative diseases, may occur for no reason at all. There is no identifiable cause, and no one or no thing is to blame. Early detection of complex degenerative diseases is the key to successful management. In the next chapter, we focus on arguably the most complex of all human diseases—cancer.

8

The Mother of All Diseases

Charles Vance is a sixty-year-old Caucasian male who works as an engineer for a software development company. He has been married for thirty-two years and has one daughter and three grandchildren. He does not smoke or drink alcohol (except for an occasional glass of wine with dinner), exercises regularly, and lives what most would call a healthy lifestyle. One day about three months ago, Charles began experiencing memory difficulties and had problems remembering the names of friends and common objects. Charles did not think much of this, attributing his cognitive problems to tiredness and job stress. But the problems continued to worsen. Finally, after a week of progressively declining cognitive function, Charles's wife urged him to see his doctor, who immediately arranged for a neurology consult. The neurologist ordered an MRI brain scan and blood tests to explore possible causes of his memory difficulties. The blood tests came back normal, but the brain scan revealed a large lesion in the left temporal lobe. Although the tumor had likely been growing for months, it did not create any clinically significant symptoms until it got quite large. When the tumor size reached a "clinical horizon," it was exerting enough pressure on healthy brain tissue to cause neurological effects. The neurosurgeon performed a subtotal resection and harvested enough tissue for a biopsy. The surgeon decided the tumor could not be completely removed because of its location in the brain: attempting total resection risked a high probability of permanent brain injury or death. A biopsy confirmed a diagnosis of a primary brain tumor (glioblastoma multiforme grade IV). The doctors told Charles and his wife that, while his disease is not curable, a combination of radiation therapy and chemotherapy might give him one to two years of life.[1] Without treatment, Charles was told, survival time for this disease is about three months.

The news was devastating to Charles's family, who could not understand how this happened. No lifestyle or other causal factors could be identified that might have increased Charles's cancer risk. He was healthy and active. Family members and friends felt hopeless because there was nothing they could do to improve his chances of survival. They supported Charles and each other in the best way possible.

Charles completed his cancer therapy but, after several months, gradually began to feel weaker and eventually was unable to care for himself. The tumor had partially responded to the therapy, but not all tumor cells were killed. Surviving tumor cells led to regrowth of the tumor, so that the tumor now was even more aggressive and resistant to therapy. Charles and his wife heard about experimental treatments but decided against further therapies when the doctor told them the available drugs were highly toxic and provided no guarantees for extended survival.

Charles's last two weeks of life were difficult to watch, yet he was in no pain or discomfort. He completely lost his appetite and refused all food. When he was healthy, Charles weighed about 170 pounds. At the time of his death, he weighed a mere 115 pounds because of loss of body fat stores and muscle mass. Charles died at home under hospice care about fourteen months after initial diagnosis.

Cancer is the mother of all diseases. It is arguably the most relentless and insidious enemy of human life. Cancers can grow quickly and end life within weeks or months of diagnosis. Or they can grow slowly and gradually erode quality of life. There is nothing like cancer to cause havoc within the patient's body and rippling effects throughout the patient's network of family, friends, and coworkers. A diagnosis of cancer is devastating to the patient and family. In some cases, as in Charles Vance's glioblastoma, the disease is particularly distressing because there are no known causes or cures. Often the patient and family feel helpless. Although cancer is primarily observed in older populations, it can strike at any age, often without warning. As the second leading cause of death in the United States, cancers start off as small innocuous and undetectable growths that, when left unchecked, grow and spread inexorably by consuming body energy stores and causing vital tissue dysfunction leading to death. Fear of cancer is unmatched by any other disease, including Alzheimer's disease and heart disease. Cancer and its treatments can result in pain and discomfort, and the progression of the disease to advanced stages can be slow and debilitating. But remarkable progress has been made, particularly since the 1960s, to prevent, diagnose, and treat many cancers. Indeed, about 65 percent of all cancers are now curable. Skin cancer, lung cancer, and cervical cancer are better controlled now by effective public health measures. Some cancers, including breast cancer and colon cancer, can be detected at an early stage resulting in high cure rates.

This chapter explores cancer as a disease of biological complexity. Typically, diseases are categorized on the basis of causality or pathogenesis or clinical signs and symptoms. Infectious diseases are categorized and described by the microbial agents that cause them. But for chronic degenerative diseases, pigeonholing based on whether the disease is infectious, causes inflammation, and so forth fails to capture underlying complexity phenomena. As we will see in this chapter, complex diseases present some of the most daunting challenges in contemporary medicine and public health.

A Brief Cancer Overview

Cancer is not a single disease. There are more than one hundred different types of cancer. It can occur in almost any tissue in the body, and disease incidence, mortality rates, pathogenesis, and treatments vary considerably across cancer sites. There are about 1.5 million new cases of cancer diagnosed annually in the United States (excluding nonmelanoma skin cancers); it is the leading cause of death in people under eighty-five years of age in the United States. The most common cancers are found in the lung, female breast, male prostate, and colon. About 500,000 individuals die of cancer each year, making it the second leading cause of death in the United States (cardiovascular disease is number one). Cancer is also a leading cause of death worldwide, accounting for about twelve million new cases diagnosed in 2012 and 7.6 million cancer deaths in 2012. Deaths from cancer worldwide are expected to continue to rise, reaching about twelve million deaths in 2030.[2]

Cancer remains one of America's biggest public health problems. Since the passage of the National Cancer Act in 1971, the United States has spent billions of dollars on the fight against this disease. Are we winning the war? The data in Figure 8.1 suggest we are not. Compared to 1950, cancer death rates have changed little; the cancer death rate in 1950 was 193 deaths per 100,000; in 2004, it was 186 deaths per 100,000. In the meantime, death rates from heart disease, cerebrovascular diseases, and pneumonia/influenza have fallen dramatically. But these statistics mask the remarkable advances made in understanding cancer, its treatment, and early diagnosis. Although significant challenges remain, the war on cancer is actually being won. Battles are ongoing against recalcitrant neoplastic diseases such as lung cancer, ovarian cancer, pancreatic cancer, and stomach cancer.

The dismal cancer statistics over the past sixty years primarily reflect the inability to control and manage lung cancer. Lung cancer mortality, particularly in males, rose precipitously from 1950 to 1990 (Figure 8.2). Cigarette smoking is the primary preventable cause of lung cancer and heart disease. Significant successes since 1950 in treating heart disease mean that people are living longer and are, consequently, at greater risk for lung and other tobacco-related cancers.

The fight against cancer looks more promising when the focus is the past twenty years. The year 1990 marked an important turning point in the war on cancer. Lung cancer mortality rates began to fall because of the delayed benefits of smoking-cessation

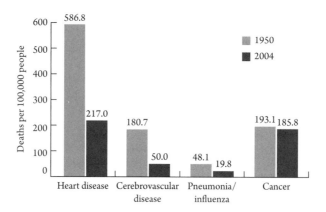

Figure 8.1 Successes and failures. The number of people dying from heart disease, cerebrovascular disease, and pneumonia or influenza fell sharply between 1950 and 2004. However, the death rate from cancer has remained largely unchanged over the same period. The data have been adjusted to reflect the US population in the year 2000. *Source:* National Center for Health Statistics (NCHS) and Centers for Disease Control and Prevention (CDC) (2004 data); CDC/NCHS National Vital Statistics System (1950 data).

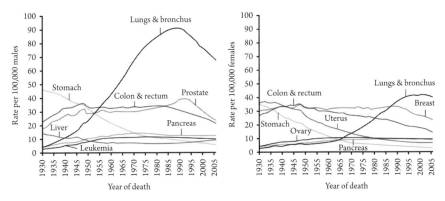

Figure 8.2 Annual age-adjusted cancer mortality rates for selected cancers in the United States, 1930 to 2006. Left panel, males; right panel, females. Rates are age adjusted to the 2000 US standard population. *Source:* American Cancer Society; and Jemal A, Siegal R, Xu J, Ward E. Cancer statistics—2010. CA: *Cancer Journal for Clinicians* 2010;60:277–300. The figure is reproduced with permission from John Wiley and Sons.

programs. Cancer death rates fell 21 percent among men and 12.3 percent among women from 1991 to 2006 (Figure 8.2). That translates to about 767,000 cancer deaths that have been avoided since the early 1990s. Among men, reductions in lung, prostate, and colorectal cancer rates account for nearly 80 percent of the total decrease. The decline in breast and colorectal cancer rates account for 60 percent of the total decrease in women. The number of new cancer cases is also waning—cancer incidence decreased 1.3 percent per year among men from 2000 to 2006 and 0.5 percent per year from 1998 to 2006 among women. The reduction in disease incidence is largely due to decreases in the three major cancer sites in men (lung, prostate, and colorectum) and the two major cancer sites in women (breast and colorectum). Yet winning the cancer war does not mean all the major battles are behind us. There is considerably more work that needs to be done. The single major contributor to cancer mortality—lung cancer—continues to defy effective management. We know how to prevent the disease but can't treat it very well. Cancer incidence rates (usually expressed as age-adjusted numbers of cancers per 100,000 population) are expected to rise as the baby boomer generation—those born after World War II between 1946 and 1964—move into their sixties and seventies. By 2020 baby boomers will constitute more than one-quarter of the US population and will likely account for one-third of all new cancer cases and more than one quarter of all deaths. The key to countering the growing numbers of cancers will be prevention and early detection.[3]

In the United States, improvements in early diagnosis and treatment have raised survival rates for all cancers combined from 50 percent in the mid-1970s to about 65 percent now. Lung, stomach, liver, colon, and breast cancer cause the most cancer deaths each year. Cancers of the lung and pancreas continue to be difficult to manage. These diseases are usually detected after they have spread, making localized treatments ineffective. Five-year survival across all stages is less than 15 percent for these cancers. However, there is remarkable success in treating early-stage breast cancer and prostate cancer; five-year survival rates are in excess of 90 percent if the disease is diagnosed early.

Because cancer is not a single disease, the war must be fought on numerous fronts. Cancers are highly heterogeneous. The disease behaves differently from one individual to the next; even within the same tumor, there are heterogeneous populations of cells. Cancers are also highly dynamic. The disease progresses from a benign to metastatic state, leading to spread of the cancer to new locations. As treatment progresses, cancers become more difficult to manage.

Although the causes of many cancers remain poorly defined, a number of cancer-causing agents have been identified, including tobacco, diet, solar ultraviolet (UV) radiation, and certain viruses. More than 30 percent of cancer deaths can be prevented by reducing or eliminating exposures to these agents. Tobacco, however, is the single most important causal factor for cancer.[4]

Cancer arises from genetic mutations in normal cells that become transformed and grow uncontrollably. Environmental factors can act on cancer cells to promote cancer growth. Cancers are clonal in origin and arise from a single cell. The mutation that initiates cancer may be spontaneous or may result from exposure to external agents.

Cancer cells differ from normal cells in several important ways and acquire certain capabilities characteristic of the neoplastic state. First, normal cell growth and proliferation are under tight regulatory control, but cancer cells do not respond to the normal growth-inhibitory signals that normal cells do. Second, cancer cells have their own growth stimulation signals necessary to sustain cell proliferation. Third, normal cells have a finite life span, but cancer cells are immortal with unlimited proliferative potential achieved by avoiding the process of programmed cell death (called apoptosis) carried out by normal cells. Fourth, unlike most normal cells, cancer cells are able to attract blood vessels to grow into the tumor mass. Pirating a blood supply by the process of angiogenesis is critical for the tumor to continue to grow. Fifth, most normal cells are fixed in place to carry out their functions, but tumor cells are not anchored to any particular tissue, allowing them to invade tissues and blood vessels or lymphatic channels, to spread to other areas of the body in a process called metastasis.[5]

Recent advances in cancer biology indicate that cancer is far more complex than previously imagined. The idea that this disease could ultimately be understood by mapping out the cancer cell's circuitry in much the same way as the behavior of a computer chip can be understood by mapping out the transistor circuits is too simplistic. Reducing the phenomenon of cancer to laws of physics and chemistry marginalizes the complexity of the disease and its dependence on the dynamics of tissue-environment interactions. Two new emerging areas of cancer biology reflect the complex nature of the disease. Cancer cells have the capacity to reprogram their metabolism to maintain their high rate of proliferation in the face of changing environmental and nutrient conditions. Tumors also have the capacity to evade the immune system.[6]

Much of what is known about cancer has largely been guided by a reductionist focus on cancer cells and the genes within them. An elementalist approach is limited by the complexity of cancer as a disease process. Tumors exhibit emergent properties that cannot be explained by focusing on cell and subcellular phenomena. Tumor growth trajectories cannot be predicted. Some tumors of the same cancer type will grow and metastasize to distant sites; others will grow to a certain size and, for no apparent reason, stop growing. Tumors establish a dynamic relationship with their hosts. In a process called tumor cachexia or wasting disease, tumors rob the host of vast amounts of energy to support their own growth. As a consequence, cachectic patients lose weight and muscle mass that cannot be explained by loss of appetite.

Cancer is more than a disease of cells. The view now is that tumors are more like tissues or organs than collections of aberrant cells. Remarkable progress has been made since the 1980s to understand the inner workings of the cancer cell, but key questions at higher levels of biological complexity remain unanswered. For example, the Epstein-Barr virus is a known human carcinogen, but why does it cause different cancers in different populations? Why are some tissues more susceptible to cancers than others? Why do patients with certain neurological diseases, including Alzheimer's disease and Parkinson's disease, have a lower cancer risk than the general population?

Cancers vary in shape and size. In the bone marrow and lymphatic systems, tumors are amorphous and do not have a well-defined structure. In other tissues, cancers form solid masses (Figure 8.3). These tumors may have well-defined margins that easily separate them from surrounding normal tissue or may be crab-like, infiltrating normal tissue in many directions (cancer gets its name from the Greek word for crab).

Cancer is defined as the abnormal growth and spread of abnormal cells. It is generally understood that cancers result from genetic mutations in healthy target cells. Genetic mutations in cancer are uniformly deleterious and generally perturb or inactivate important cellular control mechanisms. In a supportive tissue environment, mutated cells proliferate and acquire additional mutations that lead to a state of genomic instability. Eventually, some cancer cells acquire a metastatic phenotype that results in the spread of cancer cells to distant tissues (usually the lungs, bone,

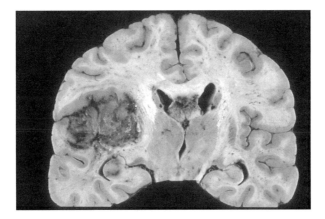

Figure 8.3 Glioblastoma is a rare and highly aggressive primary brain tumor that is usually fatal within one to two years of diagnosis.

liver, or brain). When treatment fails or the disease is diagnosed in late stages, death occurs as a result of physiologic failure of vital tissues or cancer cachexia.

For most cancers, proximal causes are poorly understood, in part because cancer is a chronic disease that requires years, if not decades, to become clinically evident. The molecular events associated with mutation induction occur as a result of normal metabolism (particularly free radical production associated with aerobic metabolism) and exposure to certain toxic agents in the environment. For certain common cancers, such as breast and prostate cancer, most patients have no readily identifiable environmental causal factors. For other common cancers, such as lung and colon cancer, environmental factors are well known and include smoking and dietary animal fat. As much as we would like to, we cannot turn the clock back to determine what caused a particular cancer. Complex systems, by virtue of their adaptive capacities, are endowed with an arrow of time—the future can be distinguished from the past. Dynamic memory erases itself as the tumor becomes increasingly complex.

Everyone has cancer, but relatively few people have the disease. During a lifetime, hundreds if not thousands of cancers cells are formed that could potentially lead to a tumor and metastasize. If the average number of such cells per individual is as small as one hundred, the probability that any individual will have no cancer cells in her lifetime is essentially zero (assuming a Poisson distribution of cancer cells among individuals). But the presence of cancerous cells does not mean a person will get the disease. Cancer cells are constantly being created through normal cell functions and exposure to certain toxic agents that cause genetic damage in cells. The prevalence of cancer in the United States is approximately twelve million. Assuming a population of 300 million, this means 3–4 percent of the population now has cancer—but 96–97 percent does not. If everyone in the US population has one or more cancer cells, this means that everyone has the potential to develop cancer but that only a small percentage actually will. Why is this? First, cancer cells must go through a bottleneck to become clinically observable tumors. Not all damaged cells can multiply; in fact, many of them die quickly. Those that have the potential to divide and form cancer are effectively destroyed by the various mechanisms available to the immune system. This process takes place continuously. Therefore, cancer develops if the immune system is not working properly or the number of cancer cells is too great for the immune system to eliminate. To maintain growth, cancers must establish and maintain a blood supply. This requires that the tumor recruit new blood vessels and establish connections to the individual's general circulation. Second, cancer cells must inhabit a tissue environment that promotes cell growth and division. If such an environment does not exist, tumors are unlikely to develop, even though damaged cells with cancer potential are present. When a cancer does appear, it is because a few cells have escaped death and can divide to form a tumor in a supportive tissue environment.[7]

Cancer is a modern disease with an ancient past. The early history of cancer is essentially unknown because cancers were uncommon and diseased tissues in ancient times could not be preserved as confirmatory evidence. However, since bone-related tumors may be preserved in the skeletal remains, one of the earliest confirmed cases of cancer is a lymphoma of the jawbone found in a skeleton dating to 4000 BCE. Another reason we have little information about cancer in ancient times may be that it is an age-related disease, and, in premodern times, people usually did not live long enough to express this disease.

So, we consider cancer a modern malady because it emerged as a serious public health problem only when infectious diseases were controlled and cigarette smoking became popular in the twentieth century. Did civilization awaken a sleeping giant? Civilization proved to be both a blessing and a curse: it unveiled cancer through technological advances that extended the human life span, but it also has had a hand in promoting cancer through cultural change, including tobacco smoking, alcohol consumption, and technological advances that introduced cancer-causing agents like asbestos and high-dose ionizing radiation.[6]

A Complexity Perspective

The human body is designed not to fail, but it is also not designed to go on forever. Cells die and are not replaced, and damage to tissues and organs is incompletely repaired as aging progresses. The features of complexity that make living systems efficient are the same features that produce complex disease. As we have seen, complex diseases arise when small errors or perturbations are not rectified and are allowed to accumulate. Because all tissues in the body are interconnected through a sophisticated distributive network of communication pathways, small changes in one tissue can have large effects in other tissues. These small perturbations can have disproportionate and unpredictable effects.

Cancer may be viewed as self-assembled systems embedded in the larger complex system of the whole body. Understanding tumor complexity is challenging because of the multiscale nature of the disease and the diversity of emergent properties that develop during disease progression. Reductionist approaches to the cancer problem have been fruitful but are necessarily limited because they cannot account for the multiscale spatial and temporal properties of the developing tumor.

Cancer is arguably the most complex disease in medicine. Advanced cancer defies prediction and is so variable from patient to patient that treatment outcomes are difficult to forecast even in patients with the same diagnosis. Uncertainty stems from the large number of parameters controlling the temporal and spatial behavior of tumors. Modeling tumor growth and disease progression is constrained by lack of knowledge of cancer's parameters and the physical rules that govern growth and spread of this disease.

Where does complexity come from? Based on the multistage model, tumors go through initiation, promotion, and progression to evolve from a single transformed cell to a full-blown tumor. These stages consist of a series of metastable states. At the cell and tissue level, metastable states describe cell interactions with the surrounding microenvironment. The local cell and tissue environment consists of various cell types, growth factors, and other chemical and physical cues to regulate cell and tissue function. The cell-environment dynamic is so complex that it is impossible to measure the properties of individual metastable states without disturbing the system. At the intracellular level, complexity arises from the heterogeneity of proteins, their spatial and temporal properties, and the multiplicity of regulatory networks, feedback control loops, and signaling pathways. Complex diseases like cancer exhibit several defining characteristics.

Disease Progression Is Unpredictable

In the case study at the beginning of the chapter, it was not possible to predict the course of Charles's disease. No one could have predicted how long he was going to live. Although the median survival time from diagnosis of glioblastoma multiforme grade IV is about fifteen months, two demographically similar individuals with the same cancer diagnosis and stage of disease will likely respond differently to treatment and have different disease trajectories. One patient might live three months after diagnosis; another might live two years. Differences in disease trajectories reflect the chaotic behavior and nonlinear dynamics of complex biological systems. The smallest difference in a biologic process (for example, a biochemical pathway) can lead to large differences in the growth and behavior of tumors. The progression of many infectious diseases, including the common cold, has much less uncertainty in their time course. Although individual variations occur, they are small, and the disease trajectory is predictable. On the other hand, the unpredictability of cancer means cancer statistics have limited utility and need to be interpreted cautiously. A median survival time of fifteen months tells you nothing about survival time of the individual patient and even less about his or her quality of life. Almost everyone would agree that survival well beyond the median survival time is not necessarily a good thing if the patient has little or no quality of life.[9]

Complexity Is Evident at Multiple Scales

Cancer is evident at every organizational level of human biology, from genetic changes in individual cells all the way up to impacts on families and communities. Effects observed at one scale are driven by changes in the scales below. The relationship among scales is not linear, however. Small changes at one level of organization can lead to dramatic, disproportionate changes at the next higher level. Complexity leads to emergent phenomena whereby effects at one scale cannot be predicted or understood by changes observed at lower scales. Thus, cancer cannot be entirely understood by applying a reductionist approach. Although studying cancer at the molecular and cellular level has provided valuable insights about the early events in carcinogenesis, this strategy leads to a limited understanding of cancer as a systems problem. The metastatic behavior of a particular tumor cannot be predicted by studying individual tumor cells. In addition, the response of the patient's family to cancer cannot be understood by limiting observations to the cancer patient.

Complex Systems Require Energy

The growth and spread of cancer occur if a substantial energy gradient exists. As a complex system, tumors may be considered dissipative structures operating in a far-from-equilibrium state. Growth and therapeutic responses of tumors are based on an understanding that tumors do not act independently of their hosts. Interactions between tumors (as a large population of interdependent cancer cells) and the host dictate tumor behavior. Tumors are complex systems that emerge from another complex system (the whole body).

Cancer cachexia is an important example illustrating how tumors interact with the host environment and behave as dissipative structures. Cachexia—the massive (up to 80 percent) loss of both fatty tissue and skeletal muscle mass—is a significant factor in the poor performance status and high mortality rate of cancer patients. Cachexia is a complex process leading to the depletion of the host's energy stores. Recently, major advances have been made in the identification of factors that act to break down host tissues, called catabolic factors, during the cachectic process. Although anorexia is frequently present, loss of appetite and decreased food intake alone are not responsible for the wasting of body tissues, as nutritional supplementation or pharmacological manipulation of appetite are unable to reverse the catabolic process, especially with respect to skeletal muscle.

Many tumor cells prefer to use glycolysis, a metabolic pathway that does not require oxygen, to breakdown glucose and use the metabolic products to support other tumor cell processes. In addition, some tumors have oxygen-deficient or hypoxic cell subpopulations because the tumor is located distant from blood vessels and rapidly growing tumors outgrow the available blood supply. When cells do not use or have access to oxygen or when other substrates necessary for cell metabolism are restricted, certain cell functions are modified and minimize entropy or disorder. The local environment changes the energy gradients, leading to energy reorganization of the tumor. Based on laws of thermodynamics, a system that is better organized (that is, it has less entropy while increasing the dissipation of matter and energy to the environment) is favored. Neoplasms are self-organizing dissipative structures in the multicellular organism formed out of the parts of the host. It is known that the environment has an active role in this process, since each self-organized system produces less entropy at the expense of increased entropy in the environment.

Cancers increase entropy through an inefficient anaerobic metabolism that leads to the incomplete breakdown of glucose and the generation of significant waste heat. In glycolysis, tumor cells partially metabolize glucose with lactic acid as the main metabolic product. The liver uses three times as much adenosine triphosphate (ATP), the molecule that stores energy, as the tumor makes in regenerating glucose from lactic acid in the lactic acid cycle. This imbalance of ATP production and its consumption leads to the wasting condition known as cachexia. The body is forced to use fat stores and proteins as a source of energy since carbohydrate stores are depleted by the tumor. The cachexia condition literally sucks energy from the host (the tumor's environment) for the tumor's benefit.[10]

The Root Causes of Disease Are Masked by Complexity

Even though the ultimate causes of cancer are not known with certainty, a large number of environmental and genetic factors have been linked to the disease.[11] How these factors actually cause cancer remains unclear. In the case of lung cancer, about

15 percent of the lung cancer burden in the United States is found in people who never smoked. What is cigarette smoke doing to elevate cancer risk in the remaining 85 percent?[12] We don't know because the processes that lead to cell transformation and the subsequent formation of tumors are not completely understood. A key obstacle to understanding the cancer process is the chronic, degenerative nature of the disease. Smokers do not get cancer immediately following first exposure to cigarette smoke; exposure to carcinogenic agents usually precedes clinical appearance of the disease by a decade or more, making a connection between exposures and disease difficult. Even in the case of potent cancer-causing agents like cigarette smoke, large epidemiological studies are needed to establish links between causal factors and the disease. In the case of acute diseases, such as blunt force trauma to the head, neurological signs and symptoms develop quickly and are easily coupled to the traumatic event. Fortunately, cancer treatments are not contingent on identification of causal factors.[13]

From a complexity perspective, ultimate causality is inherent in complexity itself. Cancer is an inevitable consequence of life and results when cells in complex tissue networks fail. Accumulated genetic damage, deleterious alterations in long-lived proteins, damage produced by reactive oxygen species, disruption and failure of cellular repair processes, diminished immune system function, and untoward changes in epigenetic expression are clearly important processes that make cells prone to failure, thus leading to disease. But cell failure can also occur for no apparent reason. Regardless of the failure mode, the creation of rogue cells leads to the creation of abnormal cells that divide and behave uncontrollably.

The increased cancer risk observed in a population as it ages is consistent with a complexity model of cancer. It is well known that cancer occurs primarily in older individuals.[14] Age is a significant risk factor for cancer. Age-dependency is consistent with the idea that cancer results from a failure of a key component in the complex biological system, leading to uncontrolled cell division and the development of a tumor. Components in this case are cells. But failure does not mean that cells wear out in the sense that mechanical devices like automobile parts break down. Either cells function normally or they do not. In cancer, transformed cells still function but lose the capacity to control proliferation and to respond to the body's regulatory controls.

Age-dependent mortality risks for several cancers, including breast and prostate, are well known because of the relatively high incidence of these diseases in the population. The cumulative distribution of risks over all ages is consistent with a Weibull distribution, a statistical distribution commonly used to estimate failure times of components in reliability engineering. The distribution model says nothing about the modes of failure or mechanisms of failure that lead to disease but can be used to estimate mortality probabilities at any given age.[15]

Cancer results when perturbations at the cellular level are unchecked, leading to tumor growth and distant spread. Identifying the failure mechanism is difficult because disease etiology is poorly understood for most cancers. When a threshold level of damage is reached that includes registration of DNA mutations, the normal cell is transformed and becomes a cancer cell. Cancer-causing agents like cigarette smoke and high-dose ionizing radiation increase the risk of cancer by exacerbating these naturally occurring processes. Isolating specific failure modes is difficult because biological processes have significant overlap.

A key failure mode involves the p53 tumor suppressor system. About 50 percent of all cancers are associated with this system that controls programmed cell death (apoptosis). When normal cells accumulate too much genetic damage, apoptosis is triggered, and the cell commits suicide. Cell death occurs all the time, and, in cell renewal systems, dead cells are replaced by new cells to sustain tissue function. In cancer cells, however, apoptosis programming is disabled, and the damaged cell continues to proliferate. Because these death-resistant cells contain genetic mutations, the process of cell division results in "daughter" cells having the same suite of mutations. Cancer cells continue to accumulate mutations as the tumor grows and metastatic potential develops.[16]

Complexity Offers Multiple Ways to Attack Disease

Disease complexity suggests multiple therapeutic approaches since there are many ways to attack the disease. Cancer treatments often involve a combination of strategies to control tumor growth and spread. Surgery physically removes all or part of a tumor; it is a local therapy and is of little value in the management of systemic disease. Radiotherapy is primarily used to treat local disease but may also be employed to manage regional spread. Chemotherapy is used primarily to treat spreading disease. Some drugs kill cancer cells outright. Other chemotherapeutic approaches limit or shut off blood flow, thus starving the tumor or stimulating the immune system to attack it. Still other cancer drugs target metabolic, protein synthesis, or signal pathways to limit tumor growth or interrupt cell-to-cell communications.

The clinical course in any patient is unpredictable, suggesting that advanced cancers are likely to be clinically unmanageable. Almost all cancers in advanced stages have poor prognoses. Cancer progression is not a simple, linear process. The nonlinear behavior of cancer looks disorderly and marked by irregularly timed events, characteristics frequently ascribed to chaotic systems. As such, disease progression is sensitive to small perturbations, and, consequently, disease trajectories can be neither predicted nor easily modeled. For example, as tumors grow there are periods of accelerated changes intermingled with states of inactivity; nothing can be predicted.

Even historical knowledge of the disease in a patient cannot be used to predict the future clinical course. As explained in chapter 1, the only way to predict the future—to have a straightforward, mechanistic disease—is to have a full and complete description of initial disease conditions, an impossible situation. The nonlinear dynamic behavior of tumors would also predict that combination therapies are not likely to interact in a simple linear fashion. Development of combination protocols cannot be easily modeled and requires a trial-and-error approach to identify effective combinations. A particular treatment protocol will not be equally effective for everyone. Doses may need to be tweaked, or different drugs might need to be used. A specific combination of drugs might work in one patient but have limited effectiveness in another patient with the identical diagnosis.

Other Perspectives

Complexity science and its applications in medicine are recent developments based on nonlinear dynamics analyses of physiological systems.[17] Other perspectives also provide important insights into the cancer problem and are based primarily on reductionist approaches. Cancer was first understood as an aberrant cell problem, and research naturally focused on understanding the inner workings of cells, especially the molecular genetics and molecular biology of transformed cells.

Cancer Development Is a Multistage Process

A multistage approach to understanding tumor growth and progression was first proposed in the 1950s.[18] Cancer is thought to occur as a consequence of two fundamental, independent events. First, normal cells at risk sustain genetic damage. Second, the mutated cells must exist in an environment that supports cell growth and proliferation. In the absence of an appropriate microenvironment, mutated cells will not grow, and tumors will not form.

In the tumor-initiation stage, cancer is thought to occur as a result of mutations in target cells that are unrepaired. One or two mutations are all that is needed to get carcinogenesis started. It is now known that two types of genes are involved in the initiation process—oncogenes and tumor-suppressor genes. Mutations of proto-oncogenes (normal constituents of the genome) into oncogenes lead to the accelerated growth of cells, often by amplification of protein products called kinases that catalyze the addition of phosphate groups to other molecules and are essential to signal transduction pathways. Mutations of tumor-suppressor genes lead to a loss of cell proliferation control by interfering with genome caretaker and gatekeeper functions. Accordingly, DNA repair and control of cell cycle progression are compromised.[19] As transformed cells acquire further mutations, they become progressively more aggressive and refractory to growth controls. This stage is called promotion and depends on a local tissue environment that promotes cell growth. As the tumor develops, further additional mutations are acquired that confer a metastatic potential characterized by the spread of disease. This last stage is referred to as metastasis. The "seed and soil" hypothesis suggests that cancer metastasis is analogous to colonization of a new habitat.[20]

The earliest demonstrations of multistage carcinogenesis are studies to investigate tumor initiation and promotion. Using a rat skin cancer model, R. K. Boutwell showed that both an initiator (an agent that causes mutations) and a promoter (an agent that promotes cell growth) are required for skin-tumor growth. If the skin is exposed only to the initiator (such as dimethylbenzanthracene, or DMBA), no tumors form; if the skin is exposed only to a promoter (such as croton oil), no skin cancers form. Only when the skin is first exposed to DMBA and subsequently exposed continuously to croton oil do tumors appear and grow.[21]

The multistage progression model has been useful in understanding the importance of various environmental risk factors in the carcinogenesis process.[22] This perspective has also facilitated development of important cancer preventive strategies. For example, there is now considerable evidence that reduction or cessation of cigarette smoking (understood to be primarily a promoting agent) leads to a reduction in lung cancer mortality. Among individuals who smoke fifteen or more cigarettes per day, smoking reduction by 50 percent significantly reduces the risk of lung cancer.[23] More recently, breast cancers have been observed to regress in a large population of postmenopausal women who stopped using hormone replacement therapy (HRT). Risk of breast cancer associated with the use of estrogen plus progestin declined markedly soon after discontinuation of HRT and was unrelated to changes in the frequency of mammography. The study suggests (it does not establish causality) that lack of exogenous estrogen (one of the components of HRT) removes the promotional stimulus necessary for tumor growth.[24]

The multistage carcinogenesis perspective has also been helpful in developing effective cancer therapies. For example, about 80 percent of breast cancers are estrogen sensitive. Estrogen, a naturally occurring hormone, promotes cell proliferation in the breast. In these women, use of tamoxifen, an estrogen antagonist, has proved to be an effective therapy. Tamoxifen binds the estrogen receptor in cells and prevents stimulation of cancer cell proliferation by estrogen.[25]

Cancer Is an Evolutionary and Ecological Process

Considerable interest has been generated in the evolutionary biology and ecology communities regarding cancer as a Darwinian process.[26] An evolutionary perspective was first proposed by P. C. Nowell.[27] Cancer can be viewed as a large genetically and epigenetically heterogeneous population of individual cells. Evolutionary processes are driven by two major factors—mutation of target cells and natural selection whereby the mutated cells gain a proliferative and survival advantage. Genetic drift, or random mutations that change allele frequencies over generations independent of environmental selection pressures, might also be important particularly in large tumors.[28] Mutational events contribute to the variation in heritable characteristics that populations of cells or organisms require in an evolutionary process. Natural selection is the competitive process whereby altered cells successfully compete for common environmental resources. The benefit or value of a particular mutation to a cell or organism is dictated by the environment in which the cell or organism functions.[29] Natural selection is believed to occur in cancers because mutations generate heritable variations, and some mutations confer a selective advantage to some cancer cells. Acquisition of the malignant phenotype is a process of natural selection by which mutant clones evolve to escape cell cycle checkpoints, cell death, and other host defenses.[30]

Cancers also exhibit fundamental ecological properties; here, "ecology" is the study of the dynamics of cellular or organismal communities and their interactions with each other and their environments. In the context of tumor biology, a mosaic of abnormal, mutated cells competes for space and common resources. The zero-sum game is played among different mutant tumor cell clones and with surrounding normal cells. Because resources are limited, a zero-sum game predicts that some players will be winners and the rest losers. Some tumors are able to grow and metastasize; other tumors show limited growth potential. When reciprocal signaling between cancer cells and their environment are disrupted, tumor reversion may be observed.[31] The importance of the environment as a support for cancer growth and spread has been observed clinically with lung cancer and breast cancer.

Evolutionary biology proponents argue that the tools of evolutionary biology and ecology are providing new insights into cancer progression and the clinical control of the disease. An evolutionary and ecological perspective suggests that interfering with clonal evolution and altering the fitness landscapes of cancer cells could provide the basis for novel treatment approaches. For example, evolutionary biology might provide important insights in overcoming the serious clinical problem of multidrug resistance. Chemotherapies that are toxic to cells select for cancer cells with resistance mutations. The result is that a course of chemotherapy with curative intent may leave a subpopulation of resistant cells that can cause regrowth of the tumor and patient relapse. Applying principles of evolution and ecology to tumor cell evolution and the problem of pharmacologic selection pressures may enhance our understanding of the multidrug resistance problem and its management in the clinic, including selecting for benign or chemosensitive cells, altering the carrying capacity of the neoplasm, and understanding the competitive effects of cancer and normal cells on each other.[32]

Methods in evolutionary biology can also provide useful directions in cancer research. For example, Richard Doll and Austin Bradford Hill demonstrated in epidemiological studies that cigarette smoking is a cause of lung cancer by using the idea of "tagging" developed by the geneticist Edmund Ford. Ford created a cohort of moths (by using visible tags or marks) to follow the population over time and document changes in wing shape, coat color, and other variables. These field experiments were some of the first to demonstrate Darwinian natural selection in real time. Hill and Doll used a cohort design to document the appearance of lung cancer in smokers versus nonsmokers.[33]

Cancer Is a Systems Biology Problem

A systems biology perspective involves understanding interactions among elements in a complex biological system. How do cells interact with each other and with their microenvironments? Cancer is viewed as complex interactive networks at the cell, tumor, and host level. Tumor behavior is also tissue specific. Cancer of the pancreas is an entirely different disease from primary brain cancer and, consequently, is managed clinically in different ways. But underlying all forms of cancer are common regulatory networks that are necessary for the normal control of cell proliferation and tissue function. Research has focused historically on individual genes and a small number of interactions between genes. But cancer can only be fully understood at the systems level, including elucidation of the regulatory networks involving key cancer genes.

The idea of a systems approach evolved from the growing understanding that cancer genes have important regulatory functions involving numerous gene regulatory networks. For example, the *MYC* proto-oncogene subnetwork is a central regulatory system in the cell (see Figure 4.7). This proto-oncogene is a transcription factor that regulates expression of 15 percent of all genes. When it is mutated, cancer results.[34] At the level of the cell, perturbations at one point in the gene regulatory network can have a rippling effect at other points in the network. Tumor cells also communicate with one another and elaborate various substances, including chemicals that stimulate the growth of new blood vessels for the benefit of the growing tumor.[35]

Epigenetics is an important process in gene regulation and plays a key role in many human diseases, including cancer.[36] Cancer has been viewed traditionally as a genetic disease, but it now appears that epigenetic factors are also important. Epigenetics involves extensive genomic reprogramming in cancer cells, including methylation of DNA, chemical modification of the histone proteins, and RNA-dependent regulation. Recognizing that carcinogenesis involves both genetic and epigenetic alterations has led to a better understanding of the molecular pathways that govern the development of cancer and to improving diagnosis and predicting treatment outcomes. Studies of the mechanism(s) of epigenetic regulation have resulted in the identification of novel targets that may be useful in developing new strategies for the prevention and treatment of cancer.[37]

A fascinating aspect of the epigenetic process is that it can be reversed. Epigenetic switching is like flipping the lights on or off in a room. When a cell adopts a new gene expression pattern as a result of an epigenetic change, the cell and its progeny retain the capability to revert back to a previous gene expression pattern. (Gene expression is a process whereby the genetic information in the gene is used to make a protein product.) Accordingly, cancer progression ought not to be considered a continual march toward an increasingly aggressive phenotype, but as a random process toward increasing aggressiveness in a two-steps-forward, one-step-back manner.[38]

A systems biology perspective of cancer may be helpful in solving some of the more difficult problems in cancer medicine. In cancer diagnosis, it is often difficult to identify which cancers require medical attention and which ones are pseudodisease and do not require medical intervention. This is a well-known problem in breast and prostate cancer screening. The detection of in situ lesions often leads to diagnosis of cancer, and the patient is treated even though these very small tumors were never destined to grow and require medical management.[39] Since it is not possible to identify which tumors represent pseudodisease and can be medically ignored, all detected tumors identified in the screening process are treated. This conservative approach leads to significant economic costs, but the real costs are the pain, discomfort, and patient anxiety resulting from additional tests and treatments.

Most tumors require years if not decades to develop, but the disease process does not appear to progress at a constant rate. Studies in colorectal cancer suggest that the early acquisition of cancer genes may take decades, but the subsequent mutations that lead to genomic instability and growth of the tumor may take only a few years.[40] Once the small population of cells has a sufficient and necessary complement of mutations, tumor growth and spread take off. Thus, aggressiveness and metastatic potential are likely to occur relatively late in the development of a tumor. Pseudodisease may represent those tumors that are not capable of "taking off." A systems biology approach to understanding the transition from tumor latency to aggressive tumor growth and spread might identify predictive factors to differentiate lesions that need attention from those that can be safely ignored.

A systems biology approach might also provide considerable insights into the drug-resistance problem. Many cancer chemotherapy patients develop resistance to cytotoxic drugs because cancer cells protect themselves constitutively by activating multiple drug resistance (MDR) transport proteins that reduce a cell membrane's ability to allow toxic drugs to pass through. As a consequence, a resistant subpopulation of cancer cells withstands chemotherapy treatments and survives to cause regrowth of the tumor and clinical relapse. The MDR transporter up-regulation is a regulatory network response to environmental stressors that is cancer (and normal) cell protective. If the stressor is removed, MDR transporters are not activated. One way to overcome the drug-resistance problem is to identify intervals of cell vulnerability when gene regulatory pathways are inactivated or down-regulated. One period of vulnerability may be the transition period when cancer cells enter the cell cycle.[41]

A Consolidated View

As a complex disease, cancer is best understood through multiple lenses. The four perspectives discussed above have overlapping features and are not mutually exclusive. Complexity provides the broadest perspective of the cancer problem, while the other views are more limited and can be considered subsets of complexity. A comparison of perspectives offers important insights into the major features of cancer.

Evolution reflects a reductionist view of cancer: cancer is viewed as a consequence of natural selection of cells that have acquired mutations, providing a proliferative advantage. Reductionism considers cancer as a collection of aberrant cells.[42] In cancer therapy based on this view, the cancer cell is the focal point since cell killing is the objective of therapy. On the other hand, systems biology and complexity models are holistic and consider cancer mutations as a part of the more general problem of cell and tissue dysregulation; these models view tumor and host tissues in a dynamic relationship. Complexity and systems biology approaches are more fruitful than an evolutionary model to understanding tumor growth and spread. It is the behavior of the tumor as a multicellular entity that dictates disease behavior.

The tumor cachexia problem is an example of how systems biology and complexity approaches differ from an evolutionary one. Darwinian evolution does not account for organismal complexity and cannot explain tumor behavior associated with cachexia. Complexity in living systems arises from a more fundamental process related to the capacity of systems to self-organize when operating far from equilibrium.[43] In cachexia, the host and growing tumor establish an energy gradient whereby the growing tumor sucks all the energy reserves from the host, leading to the wasting condition. The tumor and host compete for resources. When resources are limited, competition results in gains by one party (the tumor) and losses by the other (the host). Ironically, in the end, both the host and tumor lose because cachexia is incompatible with life.

Cancer as a complex dissipative structure predicts cancer reversion and cancer risk reduction by removal or reduction of environmental stimuli.[44] Environmental cues for cancer are important because they are linked to energy sources for the growth and maintenance of the dissipative structure. When the source of energy or the cues to process available energy are removed, the dissipative structure cannot be sustained. An obvious example is the dissipation of hurricane force winds when hurricanes pass over large land masses; thermal gradients that drive hurricane forces diminish, leaving the hurricane with no energy to feed on. The hurricane then simply disappears.

In general, it is unclear what the evolutionary perspective tells us about cancer that we already do not know. Cancer clinics do not employ Darwinian strategies in treating patients. For example, in multidrug resistance, the evolutionary perspective posits that the probability of treatment success is highest when disease is diagnosed at the earliest stages.[45] Tumor cell heterogeneity is minimal at early stages of tumor growth; accordingly, multidrug resistance is likely to be less of a problem. But for early-stage disease, drug therapy is usually not the treatment of choice, except for leukemia and other naturally disseminated cancers. Depending on the site of the disease, surgical excision and local radiotherapy are the preferred options. Traditionally, multiple drug regimens have been used to treat disseminated cancers when tumor heterogeneity is high. Combining two or more drugs is more effective than any single drug because tumor cell killing is enhanced by invoking multiple cytotoxic mechanisms and complication rates are decreased by using drugs with different normal-tissue toxicities. The idea is that a drug does not have to be entirely effective on its own but should have a unique mechanism of action that complements the effects offered by other drugs in the multidrug protocol. Multidrug therapies work well when spatial (normal-tissue toxicities) and temporal (time for repair and recovery) coordination is optimized. For cancer, there is no need for a single magic bullet. Cancer medicine has relied on knowledge of drug effects and toxicities, clinical experience, and trial and error in the design and fine-tuning of multidrug treatment protocols.

A Darwinian perspective paints an incomplete picture of cancer. First, the types of mutations that characterize cancer are unlike any mutations that contribute to evolution. Cancer mutations do not provide for an evolutionary advantage. Mutations of cancer genes result in a loss of cell regulatory control, and cells are able to divide uncontrollably. The loss of proliferative control is so powerful that cancer cells can grow just about anywhere.[46] In an evolutionary process, mutations occur that provide a proliferative and survival advantage under specific environmental conditions. The inherited mutation may be beneficial in one environment but detrimental in another. For example, sickle cell anemia is a genetic disease that provides survival advantages in a malarial environment but is of no real benefit and is often harmful in nonmalarial settings.

Second, evolution is a system that has order and patterns without agency. It is a natural process with no direction and no "arrow of time." It is unclear how evolution can account for increasing complexity, and that is precisely what is observed as tumors grow and disseminate. Cancers acquire more complex characteristics as they advance to later stages. As a consequence, late-stage disease is more difficult to manage clinically. As a complex disease, cancer can be viewed as a progressively degenerative process without order or predictable pattern. The cancer is the agency of degeneration. Complexity predicts an "arrow of time"—that is, a movement toward increasing entropy or disorder. Once disseminated, cancers do not revert to an earlier stage of tumor development.

Third, cancers develop as a consequence of self-organization and self-assembly of aberrant cells. Studies of social order and division of labor in insect societies such as bee colonies suggest that Darwinian selection may be a secondary phenomenon to self-organization and may serve as a fine-tuning mechanism to have the society best adapt to the environment. Perhaps it is self-organizing behavior rather than natural selection that is responsible for evolution.[47]

Fourth, neo-Darwinists claim that looking at cancer in an evolutionary context promises to lead to new insights about the disease and reveal strategies for disease management. For example, chemotherapy agents might be targeted toward preventing or delaying genomic instability in cancer cells or can be used to alter the competitive dynamics between normal and cancer cells. Alternatively, a nutrient or mitogen that selects for chemosensitive cancer cells can be administered, followed by agents that kill residual cells.[48] But it is unclear what the value of this approach might be. Genomic instability is a key process that occurs early in the clinical development of disease. Tumors are still small, and, if detected early, surgical excision or local radiotherapy are effective therapies in almost all cases. The key is early detection of cancer, not evolution.

In spite of these limitations, an evolutionary approach to cancer has important value. Neo-Darwinian principles may enhance our understanding of cancer incidence and patterns of disease. Most of the dynamics of evolution have not been measured in cancers, including mutation rates, fitness effects of mutations, generation times, and tumor-cell population structure. Analytical methods first developed to tackle problems in evolutionary biology may help us understand age of onset of cancer, genetic and environmental causes of disease, and the role of clonal cells and somatic mutations in tissue dynamics and tissue-specific carcinogenesis.[49]

Major questions remain about fundamental processes in cancer. Metastasis remains poorly understood. Are cancer cells endowed with metastatic potential, or is it a characteristic acquired by some cells as disease progresses? Why do lung and pancreatic cancers have such poor prognoses even when caught early? Are lifestyle changes the key to controlling cancer incidence? Genetic mutations and cancer genes are acquired over multiple generations, but individual risks are established within a lifetime.

Search and Destroy

Treatment aims to cure, prolong life, and improve the quality of life for patients. Some of the most common cancer types, including breast cancer, prostate cancer, and colorectal cancer, have high cure rates when detected early and treated according to best practices. The principal treatment methods are surgery, radiotherapy, and chemotherapy. Surgery and radiotherapy are the primary treatment modalities for localized disease. However, advanced cancers that have spread to distant sites have poor prognosis because surgery and radiotherapy cannot be used and available cancer drugs are generally ineffective.[50]

Combination therapies are frequently used to manage disease because single agents attack the disease in a limited way. Treatment strategy combines several drugs, each doing something different to the cell. Combination therapy overcomes the drug-resistance problem by attacking the cell from different directions. Combinations are also selected to manage local and clinically evident disseminated disease. Conservative cancer management frequently employs accompanying or auxiliary chemotherapy, called adjuvant therapy, to manage undetected micrometastases. Although the disease appears localized, there may be undetected spread. Disease complexity predicts that combination therapy produces a total effect greater than the sum of the effects of each agent alone. The *degree* of synergy is not predictable in the clinical setting. Accordingly, drug doses and timing are frequently adjusted during therapy to account for individual biological sensitivities.

The complexity model also makes certain predictions about the clinical behavior of cancer. Complexity evolves as the disease progresses. As the cancer grows, tumor cells acquire additional mutations because of genomic instability. These mutations may confer metastatic potential and other characteristics of aggressive growth that early tumors lack. Accumulation of mutations causes a breakdown of the cell's regulatory controls. Without these controls, the cells grow unchecked, and the cancer continues to develop unabated until it compromises vital physiological functions and kills the host. Thus, at very early stages of disease when tumors are genetically simple (that is, they contain relatively few mutations and are not very heterogeneous), there is a short time when minimally aggressive local therapies like surgery and radiation therapy can contain and destroy the tumor. The earlier the disease is diagnosed and treated, the higher the probability of cure.[51]

Understanding cancer pathophysiology from a complexity perspective and the nature of the interactions between cell-tissue systems provides new targets for combating disease. The novel seed-and-soil hypothesis suggests targeting the interaction between tumor cells and the local tissue microenvironment as a therapeutic strategy. Aiming at the microenvironment might be a more effective and important therapeutic strategy than targeting cancer cells themselves.

Tumors are moving targets; this fact poses significant challenges in cancer therapy. As the cancer progresses, the disease goes through a series of metastable states. Cancer cells acquire new mutations, local tumor environments change, and cancer cells spread to distant sites to establish new tumors. Changes in tumor cells and their local environments nullify the effects of treatment, and the tumor starts to grow again. Resistance to nonsurgical therapy is a monumental problem in cancer medicine. Even in successful targeted therapies acquired resistance is problematic. Gleevec is an effective treatment against chronic myelogenous leukemia (CML). The drug targets the protein made by the cancer gene characteristic of CML. But the gene can further mutate, thus rendering Gleevec therapy ineffective, and the cancer will continue to grow in the presence of the drug. Gleevec is one of the first successful targeted therapies. It is the product of a nontraditional approach to drug development—start with the disease and work toward an effective therapy. This approach works if sufficiently detailed knowledge of the disease is available.[52]

Development of targeted therapies represents a significant paradigm shift in therapeutic medicine. Molecular medicine focuses on understanding the disease, identifying "drugable" molecular defects or pathways, and matching appropriate therapies to it. Traditional approaches have been more of a fishing expedition— start with a drug candidate and identify diseases that might be treated by the drug. Such an exercise in random searching for matches between disease and treatment is highly uncertain because there is no theoretical foundation to guide identification of specific treatments with specific disease characteristics. However intratumor heterogeneity can lead to underestimation of the tumor genomics landscape as determined by single tumor-biopsy samples and may present major challenges to treatment biomarker development. In one study of four patients with disseminated renal cell cancer, the genetic makeup of cells from the primary tumor differed significantly from the genetic patterns in cancer cells taken from distant sites. All cells had descended from a common ancestor, but cells that had broken off from the main tumor mass and spread to distance sites had mutated in new directions presumably because of the influences of local tissue microenvironments. Cells at or near the primary tumor site shared about 30 percent of their genomes with tumor cells taken from metastatic sites. Cancer complexity as reflected in intratumor heterogeneity is associated with heterogeneous protein function, leading to tumor adaptation and therapeutic failure.[53]

Cancer can look similar under the microscope but have different genetic patterns and disease characteristics, thus requiring different treatment strategies. Relying solely on a tumor's genetic signature as a basis for developing personalized treatment strategies is limiting. The key to effective personalized medicine is the understanding of the relationship between genotype and phenotype. What is the nature of the cancer cells' aberrant proteins synthesized from cancer genes, and what are the roles of these proteins in the clinical behavior of the tumor? The success of Gleevec as a targeted therapy hinges on the fact that the BCR-ABL fusion oncogene is the single defining molecular defect of CML. Most cancers are more complex and cannot be defined by a single molecular lesion. Although personalized medicine approaches to disease diagnosis and treatment have in general had limited success, there appears to be promise in using genetic testing of familial cancers that can identify individuals in whom life-saving surveillance or treatment should be initiated.

Complexity and Public Health

A complexity perspective provides important insights into cancer control and prevention. Two public health principles are derivable from a complexity model. First, detection and treatment of disease in very early stages save lives, but not all early lesions are destined to cause disease requiring treatment because of unpredictability in disease trajectories. Second, if cancer is a result of the spontaneous failure of normal cells, then cancer will never be wiped out. But many cancers can be prevented by controlling known causal factors, including cancer-causing viruses, cigarette smoke, and solar ultraviolet light.

Public health measures such as population screening and control of environmental carcinogens are the best way to control the disease burden. Having the disease and then treating it amounts to an individual battle against cancer in a global war. Fighting the disease one person at a time is extraordinarily expensive because of the medical costs involved. Treating a cancer patient can easily cost upward of $100,000.[54] Preventing disease through public health measures is a far more efficient process because the battle is waged at the population level. Screening tests are easily administered to large populations, and costs are relatively inexpensive on a per capita basis. For example, a single mammogram to identify early-stage breast cancer costs about $300, whereas public health campaigns to warn the public about the dangers of smoking are relatively inexpensive and reach millions of consumers. The remainder of this chapter examines the importance of screening and prevention.

Screening

About one-third of the cancer burden could be wiped out if cases were detected and treated early. The aim is to detect the cancer when it is localized (before metastasis). Treatment of early-stage disease is associated with five-year survival of more than 90 percent for most cancers. Unfortunately, lung and pancreatic cancers are notable exceptions. For these cancers, early diagnosis provides little advantage because metastasis occurs early in the disease process. Diagnosis in the late stages of any cancer is linked with poor survival because of disseminated disease and the general ineffectiveness of drug therapies, as we have seen in chapter 6.[55]

The goal of screening is to detect disease in large asymptomatic populations using simple, inexpensive tests. Disease is not prevented but caught in an early enough stage that treatment is usually highly effective. Diagnosis and screening have different goals, although the same test may be used. In diagnosis, the appearance of symptoms drives the diagnosis of disease. The patient comes to the doctor because she does not feel well or is troubled by something. Screening, on the other hand, is used to detect early disease or precancerous conditions in asymptomatic and otherwise healthy individuals. A cytology screen (the "Pap smear") detects precancerous lesions in the uterine cervix; mammography, an X-ray imaging procedure, detects very small lesions in the breast.

Screening effectiveness as measured by the positive predictive value depends on the sensitivity and specificity of the test. Disease prevalence is also a key determinant of positive predictive value.[56] With increasing disease prevalence it becomes more likely that a person with a positive test result has the disease and the less likely that a positive result is a false positive (Figure 8.4).

The predictive value of a screening test is higher in at-risk populations compared to the general population because the false-positive rate is reduced—thus, it is more likely that a positive test really means the individual has the disease. A false-positive result can mean either there is no cancer or there is cancer but it is destined not to grow and cause disease that needs to be treated. Pseudodisease reflects the uncertainty in disease trajectory. A small cancerous lesion such as ductal carcinoma in situ (DCIS) of the breast may remain dormant or may grow and spread. In either case, conservative medicine dictates the patient receives additional tests and treatment to rule out cancer or remove questionable lesions.

The false-positive rate is at the heart of the ongoing mammography controversy. Breast cancer is the most common cancer in women in the United States, with more than 190,000 women receiving a diagnosis of invasive disease annually and more than 40,000 dying of breast cancer each year. Mammography detects early-stage disease, and early detection saves lives. The debate rests on whether women should have mammography screening beginning in their forties. Because the prevalence of

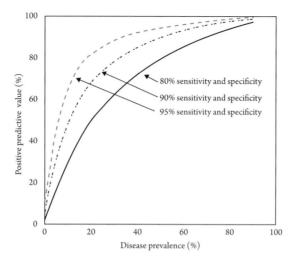

Figure 8.4 Screening effectiveness depends on disease prevalence. The positive predictive value (PPV) is the probability that a person with a positive test actually has the disease. PPV is contingent on disease prevalence. Screening tests are not very good for diseases that are rare in the population, even if the test's sensitivity and specificity are high.

breast cancer in women under age fifty is low, the benefits of screening do not clearly outweigh costs. The absolute benefit of mammographic screening in women in their forties is quite limited. More than 1,900 women must be screened for ten years to prevent one death from breast cancer, and there are approximately 60 percent more false-positive results and unnecessary biopsies than there would be if screening began at fifty years of age. False-positive results lead to anxiety, pain, discomfort, and higher economic costs associated with additional tests and treatments.[57]

Screening tests for ovarian cancer are also associated with a high false-positive rate that limits the utility of the test as a mass screening tool. An effective screening tool is particularly important for ovarian cancer because it is among the more rapidly fatal forms of cancer. By the time the disease is diagnosed, most patients are already in an advanced stage of the disease: the disease is fatal in about 70 percent of cases. Currently, there is no existing method of screening for ovarian cancer that is effective in reducing deaths. Screening consists of ultrasound examinations and detection of levels of the CA-125 protein that can be a sign of ovarian cancer. A high percentage of women who undergo ovarian-cancer screening experience false-positive test results that lead to unnecessary surgery and other painful and potentially harmful treatments. The high false-positive problem, common for most screening tests, derives from the nonspecificity of the test. Biological markers like the CA-125 protein can be elevated by noncancerous conditions. Imaging procedures like ultrasound cannot easily distinguish between cancer and benign conditions (like ovarian cysts). Biomarkers are important keys to early detection, but, as experience has shown, the clinical efficacy of biomarkers as screening tools rests on high cancer specificity. In 2012, an Expert Panel of the United States Preventative

Task Force recommended against screening in healthy women with an average risk for ovarian cancer. Screening remains advisable for women with suspicious symptoms or who are at high risk because they carry disease-related gene mutations or have a familial history of the disease. Screening women at high risk for ovarian cancer lowers the false-positive rate and increases the chances that a positive screen really means cancer is present because disease prevalence is higher in the at-risk subpopulation.[58]

Similar concerns have been raised regarding screening for prostate cancer in healthy males. Benefits of prostate specific antigen (PSA) screening have been called into question for years. Results from five well-controlled clinical trials suggest that PSA testing does not save lives and often leads to more tests and treatments that needlessly cause pain, impotence, and bladder incontinence in many patients. Prostate cancer is slow growing, and, for the forty-four million men age fifty years and older, it is probably better they never find out they have cancer. The anxiety of knowing they have cancer is far worse that living with a disease that is not likely to affect their lives. However, although questionable for the general population, males with a significant medical history should be screened and observed closely.[59]

Identifying at-risk individuals for screening is preferable to indiscriminate screening of the larger population. Populations at-risk have different risk profiles depending on cancer type. Age is a key risk factor for all cancers. The incidence of cancer rises dramatically with age because of a buildup of cellular damage. Damage accumulation is enhanced with the tendency for cellular repair mechanisms to be less effective as a person grows older. Some cancers, including breast cancer, have a genetic predisposition. Other cancers, including lung and colon cancer, are linked to tobacco use, alcohol consumption, diet (for example, high animal fat and low fruit and vegetable intake), or exposure to cancer-causing viruses. The challenge in cancer screening is defining the high-risk individual who can benefit from routine screening.

Use of screening panels ameliorates the false-positive problem. Although an individual test may have an unacceptably high false-positive rate, combined results from multiple tests based on different structural or functional disease parameters increases the collective positive predictive value. One of the earliest examples of this approach is the combined use of digital rectal examination (DRE) with PSA testing to screen for prostate cancer. Neither test alone is definitive, but, in combination, they provide important guidance on how to manage the patient. A patient's high PSA level might be explained by a benign enlargement of the prostate. Depending on the specifics of the clinical situation, simple monitoring of the patient may be all that is needed. If, however, the DRE suggests cancer (small nodules on the gland's surface are detected), an ultrasound examination of the prostate and tissue biopsy may be justified. The goal in cancer screening should be the development of a small number of clinical tests that provide useful information about tissue-specific disease. Each test should have demonstrated clinical utility and, in combination with other tests, provide powerful information to guide clinical decision-making.

Screening also presents significant public relations challenges. Recommendations to limit screening, although medically and scientifically sound, usually raise the ire of groups who have been diagnosed and treated successfully, who make the compelling argument that screening saves lives. But such arguments ignore the important distinction between personal and community health. Public health messages need to address conceptual differences between individual and collective probabilities. Cancer is not a lottery. A loser is not mandated. In a population of 1,000, statistics may say that one or two people are destined to have disease, but, in reality, it is possible that no one gets disease.

The difficulties with massive screening programs, particularly when false-positive rates are high, suggest that we should think about redefining "cancer." It is a catch-all term for a group of diseases that have high prognostic variability. The word "cancer" is synonymous with death in popular parlance, but not all cancers are death sentences. Early-stage breast cancer and prostate cancer are highly curable, but glioblastoma multiforme, a particularly aggressive type of brain cancer, is essentially untreatable. The idea that cancer is lethal goes back almost two hundred years to the work of Rudolf Virchow, a pathologist who described cells taken from tumors of patients who died of the disease.[60] Virchow studied several cancer types, including leukemia and various solid tumors, and noted the consistent aberrant cell structure. Because these cells came from patients who died from cancer, it was reasonable to conclude that the presence of cancer cells leads to death. Since Virchow's observations, the link between cancer and death has evolved into a powerful public message. It is arguable whether DCIS of the breast should be classified as cancer. Carcinomas are invasive lesions, but DCIS is not. Perhaps DCIS should be called something other than "cancer"; these lesions usually remain localized and do not grow or spread. Avoiding the term "cancer" as a catch-all term makes medical sense but, more importantly, will have a positive impact on the public psyche. Telling a patient she has a small dysplastic lesion in the breast that needs watching is preferable to a message of cancer and the fear of death.

Prevention

Cancer is a natural byproduct of life, a disease that occurs spontaneously. Human carcinogens—the biological, chemical, and physical agents that cause cancer—increase the cancer rate over and above the spontaneous rate in a dose-dependent fashion. An agent is causal in a public health context if reduction or elimination of agent exposure results in a diminution in disease incidence. Cancer causation is a stochastic process. No one is guaranteed of getting cancer or of not getting cancer. Carcinogens simply increase the chance. Some people who have never smoked get lung cancer, and some heavy smokers do not. But the chances of getting lung cancer increase as cigarette consumption does. Reduction in cigarette consumption reduces cancer incidence.[61] The fact that cancer cannot be totally eradicated should not deter public health efforts to control the disease.

Causal factors increase the probability of naturally occurring cellular failure or promote proliferation of transformed cells. Thus, in the absence of known causal factors, a complexity model predicts a residual cancer background. Eradicating smoking will not eliminate all lung cancer because it is a consequence of normal regulatory pathways in the cell going awry (so we see that about 15 percent of lung cancer is found in nonsmokers[62]). Normal cellular metabolism produces byproducts that are toxic and, if not neutralized, can cause genetic damage leading to cancer. Cells are transformed into rogue cells that divide uncontrollably. For many cancers, including most breast and prostate cancers (the leading cancers in females and males, respectively), there are no identifiable causes, and spontaneous transformation of healthy cells appears to be the key pathway to the cancerous state. The key to public health and cancer control is elimination or reduction of known causal agents and early detection. The idea that disease prevention is always preferable to treatment and cure is one of the few absolutes in contemporary medicine and public health.

A complexity model further suggests that disease causation can be multifactorial involving agent-specific effects. Genotoxic agents lead to mutations that perturb the regulatory control of cell division; many environmental agents serve to stimulate cell proliferation. Although causal factors are not known for many cancers, it is likely that most cancers result from nonlinear interactions among spontaneous cellular changes and genotoxic and environmental factors. When causal agents act interdependently, it is difficult to identify and isolate effects of individual causal factors. In the case study introducing the chapter, Charles Vance had no identifiable causal factors.

Knowledge about cancer causation and interventions in cancer control is extensive. Cancer can be reduced and controlled by implementing evidence-based strategies for cancer prevention. More than 30 percent of cancer could be prevented by modifying or avoiding key risk factors, such as tobacco use, alcohol use, sexually transmitted human papillomavirus infection, obesity, physical inactivity, and exposure to certain types of air pollution.

Richard Doll and Richard Peto, two well-respected British epidemiologists, analyzed the cancer epidemiology literature to determine the contributions of known risk factors to the US cancer burden (Table 8.1). The original study was published in 1981 before the HIV/AIDS pandemic. Although HIV infection contributes to the cancer burden, the relative ranking of the risk factors has not changed since 1981. Diet and cigarette smoking still account for about two-thirds of cancers. If infectious agents and sexual behaviors are included, about 85 percent of cancer *with known causal factors* is accounted for.[63]

The risk factors in Table 8.1 are listed in order of their contribution to the US cancer burden. The percent of cancer deaths attributable to each risk factor is a central estimate and does not reflect the large uncertainties in these estimates. For some estimates, the bounds of uncertainty may be an order of magnitude or more. Numerous epidemiological studies were evaluated to derive these estimates. It is not surprising that variability among studies is substantial. The annual number of cancer deaths shown in the last column assumes a total cancer mortality burden of 600,000 deaths annually. The number of deaths attributed to a particular risk factor is probably an overestimate because the total cancer burden includes deaths for which no known risk factors have been identified.

The Doll-Peto risk factor analysis does not fully explain the entire cancer burden. For example, prostate cancer has a very high incidence rate in the United States, striking about 180,000 males annually. But very little is known about what causes the disease. No specific causal factors have been identified. Some cancers, like female breast cancers, have a defined genetic component, but environmental factors are not fully understood. Ionizing radiation is a known risk factor but only

Table 8.1 **Ranking Cancer Risks**

Risk Factor	% of all Cancer Deaths	Annual Number of Deaths Attributable to Factor
Diet	35	210,000
Tobacco	30	180,000
Infections, reproductive and sexual behaviors	15	90,000
Occupational exposures (chemicals, radiation)	4	24,000
Alcohol	3	18,000
Geophysical factors (including natural background radiation)	3	18,000
Pollution	2	12,000

Source: Doll R, Peto R. The causes of cancer: quantitative estimates of avoidable risks of cancer in the United States today. *Journal of the National Cancer Institute* 1981;66:1191–1308; Mossman KL. *Radiation Risks in Perspective.* Boca Raton, FL: Taylor & Francis; 2007:110.

at high doses; doses typically encountered in mammography have not been associated with elevated cancer risk. It is generally believed that heritable factors account for about 10 percent of cancers in Western populations. This, however, does not mean that the remaining 90 percent of cancers are caused by environmental factors. The nongenetic component of cancers includes a wide spectrum of interacting elements that may be expected to vary over time with changing social and economic conditions. These include population structure and life style factors such as diet, reproductive behaviors, and certain types of infection (for example, the human papillomavirus).

Evidence for cancer causation comes from studies involving high doses of carcinogens. Populations of heavy smokers show a significant excess of lung cancer over nonsmokers. Japanese atomic bomb survivors exposed to high radiation doses have a significant excess of cancer compared to unexposed populations. At small doses of carcinogens, excess cancers are more difficult to observe because risks are proportionately lower. Individuals who smoke on average two packs per day have a significant increase in lung cancer rates, but, at two cigarettes per day, a twenty-fold reduction in smoking "dose," the evidence for lung cancer is not clearly evident. Ionizing radiation at high dose is carcinogenic, but smaller doses typically used in diagnostic medical imaging (like dental X-rays, chest X-ray, CT scans) have not been linked to increased radiogenic risks.[64] Although elevated cancer risks have not been consistently observed at low doses, it is assumed for the purposes of public health protection that cancer risk is a linear nonthreshold (LNT) function of a dose of a carcinogen. Under LNT, a risk is assigned to every nonzero dose, so doubling the dose doubles the risk.

The LNT assumption may not be valid in a complexity context, however. A dose of a carcinogenic agent may give rise to emergent phenomena by inducing small perturbations in many cells that result in big changes, such as cancer, in the tissue. If cancer is an emergent phenomenon of transformed cells, then the dose and dose rate would change the cancer risk in a nonlinear manner. Typical doses in environmental and occupational settings are much lower than those associated with direct observations of risks. Although risks cannot be measured directly, a risk is nevertheless assumed since the absence of evidence of risk is not evidence of absence of risk. The risk is theoretical and calculated using the conservative LNT assumption. Linking negative events—exposure to low doses of carcinogens with cancer—is nearly impossible. For complex diseases like cancer, cause and effect are not always clear. Probabilities of cancer induction from low-dose exposure to carcinogens are too small compared to spontaneous probabilities of disease to establish a clear relationship.

The problem in policymaking is that we can never know the actual risks. Risks are uncertain because of the inherent complexity of cancer. Complexity theory predicts a practical threshold at small doses of carcinogens. A practical threshold is not a threshold in the truest sense of the word. It does not mean cancer risk is zero at sub-threshold doses; it means that any real risk in the practical threshold-dose domain is too small to measure reliably. How well we control cancer in environmental and occupational settings is a guessing game because cancers associated with small doses are in the background noise and not easily partitioned from the spontaneous cancer rate. If cancer does occur, it is difficult to separate spontaneous causation from the carcinogen effect.

Public health policies to control exposures to synthetic chemicals in foods, personal care and cleaning products, toys, and household goods are questionable because there is no clear evidence of a linkage between chemical exposures and cancer. That has not stopped the European Union, however. Guided by the precautionary principle, the EU requires no proof to ban entire categories of chemicals from use in consumer goods.[65]

The problem is significant because there is little scientific or epidemiologic guidance to establish rules for allocating resources for cancer control when causality is uncertain. How much money should be spent to control a risk that cannot be measured reliably and is highly uncertain? Scientific challenges are considerable and focus on the complexity of identifying causal agents and the need to establish consistent standards for doing so. For some agents like cigarette smoking, the evidence is substantial, but, for others like nonionizing radiation from mobile phones, the link with cancer is questionable.[66]

There needs to be a stronger national emphasis on early detection and prevention of cancer. Society invests much more on research for treatments and cures for advanced cancers than on prevention and early detection because new cancer drugs are far more lucrative for industry than are new screening or diagnostic tests. Although treatment for advanced cancer can be enormously expensive, individual costs for treating advanced cancer have become acceptable. Development of new screening and early diagnostic tests will be challenging and expensive, but in the long term, a public health approach—detecting the disease in an early stage or preventing the disease from occurring in the first place—will have a larger payoff than developing treatments for advanced disease. There is no question that research on therapies for advanced disease must continue, but it is always preferable to prevent disease rather than to find and treat it. Cancer deaths can be reduced by more than 75 percent in the decades to come with improved efforts in early detection and prevention.[67]

The national goal in the fight against cancer should be to eliminate the need for chemotherapy drugs.[68] As we saw in Table 6.1, early diagnosis saves lives. When cancers are caught early, surgery and local radiotherapy are effective treatments. But reaching this goal will be challenging. We still have not tamed diseases like lung cancer and pancreatic cancer that have already spread even at an early stage. One of the central questions in cancer medicine is the problem of tissue-specific differences in cancer-growth characteristics: why are lung cancer and pancreatic cancer so lethal at early stages but breast and prostate cancers curable?

In the next chapter, we take a look at disease complexity centered in the most complex system in the Cosmos—the human brain. Unlike cancer, where rogue cells proliferate uncontrollably to form their own complex system, neurodegenerative diseases like Alzheimer's disease are consequences of perturbations in the complex neural networks themselves. Like cancer, neurodegenerative diseases are scalable, have unpredictable trajectories, and the characteristics of disease among individuals are highly variable.

9

Brain Drain

Charles Smith, a Caucasian male, had a remarkable medical history. He died in 1995 at age eighty due to complications from coronary artery disease and Alzheimer's disease (AD). Charles had smoked one to two packs per day for thirty-five years. He quit smoking in 1965, however, after his doctor told him about the hazards of smoking (the first surgeon's general report on smoking had just been released by the United States government). But it was too late. In 1970, Charles suffered a heart attack at fifty-five. The cardiac event did not stop him from working, but it had lasting psychological effects. He became a classic "cardiac cripple," eschewing his active, hard-working lifestyle for an increasingly sedentary one. Every day reminded him of his heart condition. He had difficulty climbing stairs and often had to pause for a minute or two because of angina. He was prescribed nitroglycerine to control chest pain but received no other medical treatment (coronary artery bypass grafting, angiography, and other high-tech heart procedures were unavailable in his community at the time). Worsening heart disease symptoms forced Charles to sell his business in 1982. In 1984, at age sixty-nine, Charles began losing cognitive function and exhibited early signs of AD. He became forgetful, would frequently misplace his house keys, and become disoriented in very familiar areas. These cardinal signs of dementia worsened to the point that he stopped attending weekly poker games with friends and became less communicative with his wife, children, and grandchildren. By 1989, Charles's heart condition had worsened to the point that he needed coronary artery bypass surgery to improve his heart function and reduce angina. The surgery was successful, but he remained in an anesthesia-induced coma for five days after surgery. When he regained consciousness and returned home, his cognitive decline accelerated noticeably. Within months, he completely stopped communicating with his wife and grown children and eventually was unable to recognize them. In the last two years of his life, Charles could not care for himself, requiring twenty-four-hour nursing care. During the last years of his life, Charles's wife had episodes of depression and anger because of frustrations with her husband's deteriorating condition. Counseling did not seem to help. The specter of watching her husband die and not being able to do anything about it was often too much to bear.

Much has yet to be learned about chronic degenerative diseases of the nervous system. Disease etiology remains poorly defined. Although Charles quit smoking about five years before his heart attack, it is likely the residual smoking risk contributed to his cardiac event, but the cause of his AD is unclear. It is possible that cardiac insufficiency and reduced blood perfusion of the brain contributed to his dementia. Years of poor circulation might have precipitated dementia. But no one knows. There are no clearly established environmental causal factors for AD.[1]

Charles Smith's case is tragic on several levels. Once the AD process has started, there is no effective way to stop it in its tracks. The best we can hope for now are treatments to slow the disease down and extend months or years of quality life by delaying progression. Diagnosis brings its own set of challenges because the disease cannot be easily diagnosed in its earliest stages when intervention is most effective. Moreover, the disease is not isolated to the patient. Family members and friends are negatively impacted because there is nothing they can do to retard the disease. Often, family members seek treatment to cope better with a difficult situation.

The graying of the US population will lead to increasing numbers of cases like Charles. People are living longer, but the big question is their quality of life in old age. The challenge for medicine and public health will be detecting these diseases early enough so permanent damage and loss of quality of life can be prevented or delayed. Chronic degenerative diseases will not be eradicated but, if detected early enough, can be manageable, so individuals can have quality years toward the end of their lives.

This chapter explores chronic neurodegenerative diseases from a complexity perspective, focusing on AD. The human brain has special complexity and exhibits unique emergent properties. Neurodegenerative diseases are perturbations of nervous system complexity that cannot be fully understood by reductionist explorations of brain structures or functions.

Complexity breeds complexity. Changes in complex systems are complex themselves. Management of neurodegenerative disease is one of the most difficult challenges in clinical medicine. Although disease mechanisms are becoming increasingly clear, causation remains unknown in the vast majority of cases. Diagnosis is often difficult to make because objective, quantitative measurements of signs of disease are lacking. There are no simple blood tests. In AD, confirmatory diagnosis can only be made after death. Disease progression is highly individualized. Hallmarks of neurodegenerative diseases have yet to be identified that mark a clear path of progression. The impact of clinical uncertainty is substantial for the patient, her family, and her social network.

Chronic neurodegenerative diseases reflect unique features of nervous system complexity. Clinical management of these diseases requires an understanding and appreciation for the uniqueness of the brain's complexity—analog and digital information processing, brain states and mind states, modularity and plasticity. Unpacking these features of complexity informs our understanding of disease processes and leads to development of markers for better diagnosis and treatment.

Unique Complexity

There is no tissue or organ in the human body as complex as the brain. How emergent behavior that characterizes higher cortical functions comes about is poorly understood, but it appears to be contingent on the number of component connections relative to the number of system components. The human brain has about 10^{14} synapses connecting 10^{11} neurons. Higher-order cortical functions are not simply a collection of brain cells that achieve a high level of cooperation. The brain's emergent properties are not demonstrated by individual cells or networks and cannot be predicted even with full understanding of the parts alone. Emergence is a type of gestaltism, the school of thought that the whole is greater than the sum of the parts. What we observe in the real world is the complex nature of life.[2]

The Brain as an Information Processor

The brain is a remarkable computation device. It can process about 10^{16} instructions per second because of its parallel, distributed computational structure.[3] The human brain's computational power far exceeds the capacity of today's most advanced computers. All brain activity boils down to the generation and transport of electrical impulses by neurons arranged in networks. Information processing has both analog and digital features.[4] Traditionally, neuronal operations in the cerebral cortex have been thought of as interactions of synaptic potentials in the dendrite and nerve-cell body followed by the initiation of an action potential. The firing of a neuron—the generation of the action potential—is an all-or-none phenomenon. The membrane voltage in the nerve-cell body must exceed a threshold value to produce the action potential. This would make neural functioning digital, because only discrete events are allowed. Digital processing in computers is based on this binary on-or-off phenomenon. However, brain function and the neural information processed are not based simply on the generation of action potentials. Neural information is coded in several ways. First, oscillating resting membrane potentials are overlaid by input voltages that determine whether an action potential is generated. Second, information is encoded in the variations in spatial and temporal frequencies of action potentials. Third, neural networks have plasticity. The number and sensitivity of synapses change as physiological requirements or external environmental conditions dictate. Fourth, synaptic membrane potentials are graded as a consequence of combinations of excitatory and inhibitory neurotransmitters.[5]

How the brain processes analog information in carrying out higher-order cortical functions remains one of the central questions in neuroscience. The laws of physics cannot explain consciousness.[6] We do know that the brain is more than a computer churning out thousands of trillions of operations per second. Emergent properties are somehow related to the very high degree of neural network connectedness and component interactions in multinetworks behaving in a highly nonlinear fashion.

The question whether the brain operates in an analog or digital mode has never been completely resolved. Part of the problem is the brain cannot be compared simply to a computer, where digital and analog operations are easily defined in terms of discrete or continuous signals. In fact, the brain has properties of each. The all-or-none action potential is digital in character, but information encoded in the temporal and spatial distribution of action potentials is analog.

Brain States and Mental States

Emergence is operationally linked to the coupling of brain states with mental states. A brain state may be defined as a measurable structural or physiological condition. Mental states refer to conditions of mind and feeling that are observable, such as fear, anxiety, and excitement.

Neuroscientists rely on two approaches to study the correlation between brain states and mental states. First, neuroimaging employs functional magnetic resonance imaging (fMRI) and positron emission tomography (PET) imaging to measure and quantify blood flow in specific brain areas (Figure 9.1). What blood flow changes signify is not entirely clear. Increased blood flow usually means there is an increase in local metabolic rate, but no one knows what blood flow changes mean for nerve-cell activity that ultimately influences mental states.

Second, behavioral disorders in which specific brain areas are diseased or injured can be correlated with observable behavioral changes. Disease states reveal a lot about what normal function is or ought to be. Understanding the relationship between mental states and the brain can be informed by study of subjects who, through disease or injury, lack or have significantly reduced specific mental capacities. Psychopaths or sociopaths have remarkable egocentricity coupled with a complete lack of concern for the suffering of others. Neuroimaging studies comparing psychopaths, nonpsychopathic criminals, and noncriminal controls reveal that psychopaths have significantly less brain activity in a region that controls emotion.[7]

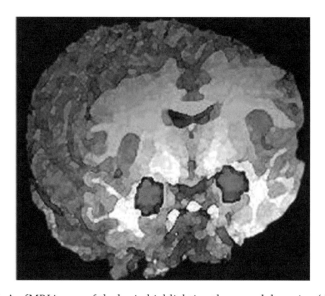

Figure 9.1 An fMRI image of the brain highlighting the amygdala region (the large paired regions outlined in bold). The amygdala is activated in a response to fear.
Source: National Institutes of Mental Health.

Modularity and Plasticity

Over the centuries, the brain has been compared to a hydraulic machine (eighteenth century), a mechanical calculator (nineteenth century), and an electronic computer (twentieth century). Many scientists now consider the brain to have modular features—specialized modules are believed to exist for vision, language, facial recognition, spirituality, and a host of other higher-order brain functions. But any modular construction oversimplifies the complex and intricate activities of the brain. Most regions of the brain serve multiple functions consistent with a distributive model. Brain plasticity, the capacity of healthy brain tissue to assume functions in damaged areas, depends on this multifunctional capability. When one sense is lost, the corresponding brain region can be recruited for other tasks. Brain-imaging studies reveal that blind subjects can locate sounds using both the auditory cortex and the visual processing center in the occipital lobe. A similar phenomenon has been observed in the deaf. When touch and vision responses are stimulated in deaf subjects, both senses were processed in the auditory cortex, suggesting that this part of the brain has been dedicated to other senses.[8]

The brain is not structured in a way that defined, isolated areas perform distinctive functions coordinated by a central control area. Certainly, there are areas of the brain with specialization (for example, the amygdala or the visual cortex), but these areas are not always dedicated to specific tasks. The complexities of the brain make interpretation of brain scans difficult. Correlations between image-identified brain states and mental states do not imply causality.[9]

Mind and Body

Is the mind separate from the body? French philosopher René Descartes in his *Discourse on Method* (1641) claimed that the physical attributes of the body could be explained by the laws of physics. Inspired by William Harvey's discovery of the circulation of the blood in 1628, Descartes reasoned that deterministic processes could explain muscle movement, sensory physiology, and other physical functions of the body. What could not be explained were the workings of the mind because the mind is a nonphysical substance. The mind is associated with self-awareness and consciousness, and the brain is the seat of intelligence. Descartes believed the rational soul, the basis for reasoning and speaking, cannot be explained as a physical entity. Intelligence is a distinctive feature of humans. Cartesian dualism is arguably the most significant formulation of the mind-body problem.

However, modern views of neurobiology and cognitive sciences call into question the separation of body and mind, suggesting that they cannot be easily uncoupled. The body, brain and mind, and environment interact in complex ways to shape our behavior, personality, and identity. The endocrine, peripheral nervous, and immune systems serve important coordinating functions that facilitate coupling the mind and body. It is well known that hormones like estrogen and oxytocin have behavioral influences, but how the brain and behavior are regulated remains a mystery.

Neurodegenerative diseases are a window on the mind-body problem. What the brain expects to happen in the near future affects its functional state. The placebo effect is an interesting case in point. The effect is the result of the patient's expectation that a treatment will help. But expectations can also be harmful: when a patient anticipates a pill's possible side effects, she can suffer them even if the pill is a fake. This nocebo effect has been largely overlooked by researchers, clinicians, and patients.[10] Understanding nocebo and placebo effects are important in designing and interpreting drug clinical trials that compare an experimental drug with a control substance. Our bodies begin to prepare for medicines when we expect to receive them. Patients with AD show diminished or extinguished placebo effects because they are unable to anticipate the future and, therefore, cannot prepare for it.[11]

Road to Oblivion

Age-associated neurodegenerative diseases are a major, heterogeneous group of diseases with mostly unpredictable and often overwhelming outcomes. A 2013 dementia study reports that nearly 15 percent of people in the United States ages seventy-one or older, or about 3.8 million people, have dementia. By 2040, that number will balloon to 9.1 million. The costs of managing dementia are also staggering. Direct healthcare expenses for dementia, including nursing home care, were $109 billion in 2010. In comparison, costs for heart disease totaled $102 billion and for cancer $77 billion. Alzheimer's is a form of dementia, a broad term for the loss of brain function that gradually worsens over time. Memory, speech, perception, judgment, personality, decision-making abilities, and cognitive skills are typically impaired. Actual AD prevalence is difficult to ascertain because of several important comorbidities. In the case study above, Charles Smith's AD was complicated by the presence of his cardiovascular disease. Although heart disease could not be clearly identified as causal in the case study, patients with a history of stroke are at increased risk for developing dementia or depression.[12]

A devastating neurodegenerative disease, AD affects older men and women, with the risk increasing dramatically with age. It is perhaps the classic illness of old age; it is the sixth leading cause of death in the United States, and about 5.3 million Americans now live with the disease. Although other major causes of death have been on the decline, deaths from AD have been rising dramatically. Between 2000 and 2008, heart disease deaths decreased by 13 percent, stroke deaths by 20 percent, and prostate cancer-related deaths by 8 percent, whereas deaths because of AD increased by 66 percent. As the population ages, the number of people suffering from the disease is expected to increase dramatically. By 2050, the incidence of AD is expected to approach nearly a million people per year, with an estimated prevalence of eleven to sixteen million people. And the costs are staggering. Total payments in 2011 for healthcare, long-term care, and hospice services for people aged sixty-five years and older with AD and other dementias are about $183 billion.[13]

Alzheimer's exhibits all the hallmarks of complexity. The disease is incurable, largely untreatable, and unpredictable in its behavior. Once a diagnosis has been made, disease progression is unknowable. Cognitive decline adheres to no particular arc since cognitive deterioration is highly individualized. The disease usually begins in a nonspecific way with memory loss, but this is a common occurrence as a person gets older. What distinguishes AD from natural aging or other forms of dementia is a combination of symptoms, including basic language problems, forgetting the names of everyday and familiar items, getting lost in familiar surroundings, becoming less sociable, changing personality, and difficulty in executing tasks that were previously easy. As AD worsens, these symptoms become more apparent and extreme in nature. Those with very advanced disease are unable to identify familiar people such as family and friends, comprehend their native language, or perform basic tasks such as eating. Usually, AD is defined by its more extreme symptoms to distinguish it from the dementia that comes with old age. Moreover, early symptoms of disease are not a harbinger of things to come. Whether a patient will exhibit a specific behavior (like violence) in advanced stages of disease cannot be predicted.

Clinical signs of the disease are not limited to cognitive dysfunction. The way people walk appears to be linked strongly to the way they think, so changes in a person's gait appear to be an early indicator of cognitive impairment. Studies suggest that thinking skills, including remembering, planning activities, or processing information, decline almost in parallel with the ability to walk fluidly. Evaluating a patient's gait may reveal early indications of cognitive impairment.[14]

A definitive diagnosis of AD can be made only at autopsy, when the brain can be examined directly. Currently, the disease cannot be characterized well enough to make the diagnosis while the patient is still alive. Nevertheless, careful charting of the patient's behavior and cognitive abilities and the use of brain-imaging techniques, including PET scans and MRIs to detect telltale pathologic changes such as the presence of amyloid plaques, can facilitate diagnosis. Brain-imaging studies need to be interpreted carefully, however. Imaging measures local blood flow and metabolism, but it is unclear how that is correlated with disease-directed neural changes. Uncertainties in disease diagnosis are reduced as the disease progresses since signs and symptoms become more severe.

Alzheimer's usually occurs late in life, but about 1–5 percent of victims get the disease at an early age. Early onset of the disease in an individual's early forties appears to have a strong heritable component. There is a large extended family in Colombia linked to an inherited form of the disease, presenting a useful model to study pathogenesis in the presymptomatic stages. If the disease can be identified at an early stage, it may be possible to introduce therapeutic measures to delay disease progression or reduce severity of the disease.[15]

Late-onset AD is characterized by the appearance of symptoms after the age of sixty-five. Of the more than five million persons in the United States with AD, about 4.8 million are diagnosed after that age. The average life span of someone diagnosed is typically twelve years after the symptoms begin. Like other diseases of complexity, the causes of this disease are not fully understood. The disease may occur spontaneously or could be associated with a combination of genetic and environmental factors.[16]

Age is clearly the most significant risk factor for AD. Whether the aging process itself is a key component of pathogenesis or is simply a correlational factor is unclear. Physical inactivity, smoking, depression, low level of education, hypertension, obesity, and diabetes have all been linked to AD. These factors might be linked to 50 percent of AD cases in the United States, and thirty-four million cases worldwide. However, a causal connection for any of these factors has not been established. A 2010 National Institutes of Health panel of experts concluded that there is no evidence of even moderate scientific quality to support the association of disease risk with modifying factors, including nutritional supplements, herbal preparations, dietary factors, prescription or nonprescription drugs, social or economic factors, medical conditions, toxins, or environmental exposures.[17]

Longitudinal studies of patients with cognitive impairment of variable severity (from none to moderate dementia) suggest the pathophysiology of AD starts at least ten years before the onset of the earliest clinical symptoms. This protracted clinical horizon is a hallmark of chronic degenerative disease. Early pathologic changes appear years or decades before signs and symptoms of heart disease and of most cancers. In the case of AD, signs and symptoms often consist of cognitive impairment that, in five to ten years, leads to disability and dementia and death within ten to fifteen years after that. By the time a patient has symptoms like mild cognitive impairment with memory decline, his loss of key neurons is profound.[18]

There is now considerable evidence that the underlying pathologic defect in AD is brain beta-amyloidosis, the precursor to extracellular plaques and intracellular neurofibrillary tangles that are the pathological hallmarks of AD. Plaques and tangles lead to neuronal cell death and neuronal injury (synaptic failure and neuronal degeneration). Mutations in the *APP* gene alter metabolism of the amyloid precursor protein. Individuals with this heritable mutation exhibit the same array of pathological characteristics as do people with the more common sporadic form, supporting the claim that amyloidosis is the primary molecular event in the disease.[19]

The occurrence of AD in Down syndrome patients provides additional support for the role of amyloid precursor protein in AD. Those with Down syndrome typically display characteristics similar to sporadic early onset Alzheimer's by the age of forty. The *APP* gene is found on chromosome 21, which is also the locus of the central genetic defect of Down syndrome, a disease characterized by three copies of chromosome 21, instead of the normal two copies (called trisomy 21). The link between Down syndrome and AD suggests that amplification of the *APP* gene product may be sufficient to produce the disease. Too much amyloid precursor protein may be just as detrimental as the more common *APP* mutation pathway.

While there may be many external causes of AD, the same pathological sequence of events is likely to occur in all cases (Figure 9.2). Mutations in the *APP* gene in combination with environmental factors lead to altered amyloid precursor protein metabolism.

The altered amyloid precursor protein leads to amyloid deposition. Plaques and neurofibrillary tangles subsequently formed are cytotoxic and lead to neuronal cell death. Once a threshold of neurodegeneration has been reached, signs and symptoms of dementia become apparent. The Alzheimer's schema in Figure 9.2 identifies key milestones in the development of the disease but fails to capture the complexity of the pathologic process. Amyloid deposition does not continually occur as the disease progresses. Plaque formation appears to level off as signs and symptoms progress.[20] This uncoupling suggests that the progression of signs and symptoms may be independent of the plaque burden or that plaques and neurofibrillary tangles develop independently or that plaques and neurofibrillary tangles are products rather than causes of neurodegeneration. Plaque-independent disease progression

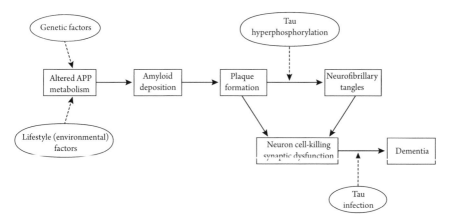

Figure 9.2 Pathway to dementia. Alzheimer's disease pathogenesis is complex and involves several sequential brain states (rectangles) and pathological processes (ovals). The entire process requires many years to play out. Current research focuses on modifying early stages of pathogenesis. Once plaque formation and neurofibrillary tangles are established, it is difficult to prevent or retard the progress of dementia. *Source:* The figure is based on the model proposed by Maccioni RB, et al. The revitalized tau hypothesis on Alzheimer's disease. *Archives of Medical Research* 2010;41:226–231.

might explain why drugs designed to control plaque formation have not been successful in treating AD. By the time patients get the drugs, sufficient and irreversible neurodegeneration has already occurred.

Intact amyloid precursor protein is located in the cell membrane of nerve cells and appears to have three major cell maintenance functions—protease inhibition, cell substrate adhesion, and regulation of cell growth. These functional properties are associated with different domains of the intact amyloid precursor protein molecule. Amyloid precursor protein itself is not the culprit in amyloid plaque formation. A subunit or fragment of amyloid precursor protein called the beta-amyloid protein is the putative agent. In AD, an alternative or abnormal pathway of amyloid precursor protein breakdown is hypothesized to liberate beta-amyloid, which is chemically "sticky" and tends to clump together to form plaques. How plaques interfere with normal nerve-cell functioning is not entirely clear, but small plaques may block cell-to-cell signaling at synapses. They may also activate immune system cells that trigger inflammation and devour disabled cells. Plaques also lead to the production of intracellular neurofibrillary tangles that have been identified in dying neurons, suggesting they play a role in cell killing. Local plaques create an environment promoting the production and spread of the tau protein.[21]

Neurofibrillary tangles derive from the intracellular tau protein in nerve cells. Tau proteins serve to stabilize structure within the nerve cell. But, in the presence of beta-amyloid protein and other damage signals, the tau protein is chemically altered by the addition of numerous phosphate groups to the molecule (a process called hyperphosphorylation). The hyperphosphorylated tau protein combines with other strands of tau to form neurofibrillary tangles. These tangles collect inside the nerve-cell body, which causes the cell skeleton to disintegrate. As the skeleton falls apart, the neuron's transport system collapses. When the neuron can no longer send and receive signals, it dies. Tau hyperphosphorylation is an important sequel to beta-amyloidosis and is the key final step in killing a nerve cell. Once neurons die, they release the tau protein. This process activates microglial cells that act as the immune defense for the central nervous system and remove the newly released tau protein. Activation of a local immune response also facilitates neural degeneration.[22]

There is a growing body of evidence suggesting that insulin deficiency and insulin resistance in the brain are important mediators of AD-type neurodegeneration. This suggests AD is a form of diabetes that selectively involves the brain and has molecular and biochemical features that overlap with types 1 and 2 diabetes. The brain produces its own insulin that is not affected by the level of glucose in the blood as in type 1 diabetes and type 2 diabetes. In brain diabetes lower-than-normal levels of brain insulin are produced. If the brain cells are deprived of insulin they eventually die, causing memory loss and other degenerative diseases. This new type of diabetes supports the belief that people with diabetes have an increased risk of AD by up to 65 percent. A link between insulin dysregulation and AD is intriguing because it suggests a connection between AD and other important chronic degenerative diseases— obesity, type 2 diabetes, and heart disease. However, any link between AD and brain insulin must be considered tentative until the role of insulin dysfunction in the development of molecular, biochemical, and histopathological lesions in AD is clarified.[23]

The pathology of AD starts out as a local disturbance. The entire brain is not affected at once. In time, however, the disease spreads to other areas of the brain. The question is how the disease is spread. Two hypotheses have emerged. First, AD seems to spread like an infection from brain cell to brain cell, but, instead of viruses or bacteria as vectors, hyperphosphorylated tau protein is the culprit. Second, the molecular defects are already in various regions of the brain, but these regions are somehow more resistant to tau invasion. Recent studies suggest that tau pathology spreads in the brain by a prion-like mechanism involving dysfunctional tau protein. Tau infection spreads from neuron to neuron via the synapses that connect neurons. The spread of the disease within the brain is not uniform and may reflect different responses of cells. The patterns of the spread of the disease may be explained by which cells take longer to succumb to the wave of infection.[24]

Numerous mutations in the *APP* gene have been identified, and some play a key role in the 1 to 5 percent of cases with the sporadic form of early-onset disease and the 1 percent of Alzheimer's cases that are inherited. Three mutations have received considerable attention and are being studied to elucidate disease mechanisms and characteristics of the disease in presymptomatic stages.

Some cases have no known cause, but most cases of early-onset Alzheimer's are inherited, a type known as familial AD. The familial form of the disease is caused by single-gene mutations on chromosomes 1, 14, and 21. Each of these mutations causes abnormal proteins to be synthesized. Mutations on chromosome 21 cause the formation of abnormal amyloid precursor protein. The exact role of the normal *APP* gene in the brain is not fully understood, but the mutated *APP* has long been suspected as the primary molecular defect in beta-amyloid deposition and subsequent plaque formation. A mutation on chromosome 14 causes abnormal presenilin 1 to be made, and a mutation on chromosome 1 leads to abnormal presenilin 2. *PSEN1* and *PSEN2* have been suggested to play a role in the fragmentation of amyloid precursor protein, which causes beta-amyloid to accumulate. Both forms of presenilin are also speculated to play a role in the control of tau phosphorylation. If presenilin mutations are present, the pathways that signal tau phosphorylation are disrupted. Mutations in the *PSEN1* gene may also lead to overproduction of amyloid plaques in brain cells.[25]

The mutations responsible for early-onset AD do not seem to be involved in late-onset Alzheimer's. In sporadic late-onset AD, the *ApOE* gene is thought to be a major contributor. Apolipoprotein E is a protein that binds to lipids and appears to regulate extracellular and intracellular clearance of beta-amyloid in the brain. There seems to be an inverse correlation—less apolipoprotein E means more beta-amyloid. Several mutations of the *ApOE* gene have been identified. *ApOE* ε4 is present in about 25 to 30 percent of the population and in about 40 percent of all people with late-onset Alzheimer's. People who develop Alzheimer's are more likely to have an *ApOE* ε4 polymorphism than people who do not develop the disease.[26]

As previously mentioned, a large Colombian family has been identified with the *PSEN1* mutation. Carriers of the *PSEN1* gene (identified through a blood test) are destined to get AD. These unfortunate subjects are a valuable resource in the fight against AD. Knowing the disease is inevitable, studying these individuals can clarify early disease progression before symptoms actually appear. Based on the mutation, scientists can predict accurately who will get AD and when disease onset will occur. Charting the course of plaque formation in presymptomatic patients will provide foundational data for how much the brain changes during early stages of disease. The hope is that studying disease carriers may result in the development of biomarkers of disease and drugs that can be used to treat individuals before they begin experiencing memory loss.[27]

Developing treatments to reduce or eliminate amyloid plaques presupposes amyloid protein is causal, but the causality question has not been completely resolved. As Alzheimer's is a disease of complexity, its causality rests on uncoupling plaque effects from confounding effects. Studies of individuals with gene mutations for AD provide important information in resolving the causality question.

Recent reports of a rare gene mutation in *APP* that protects people against AD provide the strongest evidence yet that excessive levels of beta-amyloid are a driving force in the disease. The protective mutation is highly uncommon, however; it is not the reason most people do not develop Alzheimer's. But understanding how the mutated gene product protects the brain would bolster efforts to develop drugs to treat or prevent the ravaging condition by blocking beta-amyloid plaque formation. The mutated genes that increase the risk of AD produce excessive amounts of beta-amyloid in the brain. The protective mutation, by contrast, slows beta-amyloid production, so people make much less of it and have lower disease risk. The protective mutation evidently decelerates the milder mental deterioration most elderly people experience. Carriers of the beneficial mutation are about 7.5 times more likely than noncarriers to reach the age of eighty-five without suffering any major cognitive decline, such as memory loss. They also perform better on cognitive tests. A drug that mimics the effects of the mutated gene product would be expected to slow cognitive decline and to prevent Alzheimer's. The beta-amyloid target is not the only way to fight the disease. As a disease of complexity, Alzheimer's has multiple vulnerabilities that can serve as therapeutic targets.[28]

Currently, the medical community can offer no effective treatment for AD. Once the disease has progressed to the symptomatic stage, there is little that can be done to slow or stop disease progression. Existing plaque-busting drugs have not proven effective at halting the progression of AD, presumably because the drugs have been administered too late (that is, the disease is advanced enough to cause symptoms). Any effort to develop effective drugs will be contingent on early disease diagnosis. This is a challenge because no reliable biomarkers for the disease exist. A biochemical marker would help identify those for whom early intervention would be advisable and help distinguish people with Alzheimer's from those with less aggressive forms of dementia usually associated with old age.

The cascade of events leading to AD (Figure 9.2) serves as a road map for development of biomarkers of the disease. There is considerable interest in developing biomarkers of brain beta-amyloidosis based on amyloid imaging using PET scanning. Recent tests have been developed using florbetapir (Amyvid), a tracer tagged with a radionuclide used in PET imaging, to measure the presence and density of beta-amyloid, and reports provide evidence that the imaging procedure can identify beta-amyloid pathology in the brains of individuals during life. Florbetapir binds beta-amyloid and allows imaging that highlights beta-amyloid deposition in the brain. Additional studies are needed to clarify appropriate uses of florbetapir-PET imaging in the clinical diagnosis of AD and for the prediction of progression to dementia. Results of biomarker tests like these must be interpreted carefully, however. The problem remains whether the plaques are a cause or a result of the disease. A negative test (no plaques) probably rules out Alzheimer's, but a positive test (presence of plaques) does not necessarily mean AD is present.[29] Other biomarkers measure functional states in the brain and rely on neuroimaging in specific regions of the brain as a way of detecting neuronal degeneration and synaptic dysfunction.[30]

Florbetapir-PET imaging is currently the most effective diagnostic tool for AD in living patients with signs and symptoms of dementia. Brain imaging can identify the telltale plaques that define the disease, but the ability to detect Alzheimer's has leapt far ahead of treatments. Given that there are no treatments that can stop or even significantly slow disease progression, is it wise to learn you have the disease and have no good options? Technology has its benefits, but there may also be significant drawbacks.

Drug development is proceeding on several fronts. Since the 1990s, the smart money has been on the theory that the disease is caused by brain beta-amyloidosis. But as more is learned about the disease, tau pathology and the spread of dysfunctional tau protein in the brain are also recognized as important disease processes. Regardless of the therapeutic approach, understanding how the disease gets started and spreads within the brain is key to developing effective treatment.

Most of the drug-development effort has been directed to synthesizing drugs that remove amyloid plaques. Drugs work by various mechanisms, including decreasing beta-amyloid production by changing the behavior of proteins that break amyloid precursor protein into beta-amyloid fragments. Another approach involves preventing beta-amyloid from forming plaques. An immunological strategy involves developing vaccines with antibodies to remove beta-amyloid from the brain altogether. Antibodies against beta-amyloid might stop Alzheimer's from getting started. Vaccines are also being developed to inactivate the tau protein and prevent its spread using blocking antibodies. Some of these approaches show promise, but so far researchers have not hit pay dirt. Another class of drugs focuses on modifying symptoms of the disease rather than correcting molecular defects. A palliative approach is not designed to cure or prevent the disease. Nootropic drugs mask cognitive and other deficiencies by enhancing other memory processes. Nootropics either interact with the informational process of storage and learning or enhance or mimic other important features of the brain that facilitate learning and memory, such as attention, sleep, and reward. A second type of nootropics includes caffeine, nicotine, amphetamines, glucose, and cocaine. Provigil (modafinil) and Ritalin (methylphenidate) are also nootropics. Palliation works best in the early phases of the disease when there is enough residual functioning to return the patient to or toward normal. As Alzheimer's advances, however, reduced drug efficacy is expected, since cognitive functioning becomes so severely compromised that enhancements are not likely to work very well.[31]

In theory, prevention should lead to eradication of a disease if all causal factors are identified and eliminated. Smallpox and polio have been eradicated because these diseases are known to be caused by single agents whose removal prevents the disease. Unfortunately, the likelihood of eradicating AD (and other chronic degenerative diseases) is slim to none because prevention requires an understanding of the relationship between underlying disease mechanisms and causal factors. Factors known to correlate with incidence of Alzheimer's are poorly understood. Causality is difficult to establish because of the complexity of the disease process and the presence of comorbid conditions, including heart disease and cancer.

Even if all external causal factors of Alzheimer's could be identified and eliminated, there is still a proportion of the disease burden that occurs spontaneously. The disease occurs for no apparent reason at all. Certain vulnerable biochemical pathways might be identifiable, and, if treatable with drugs, correcting defects might prevent the disease but at the cost of potentially serious complications. Tinkering with one biochemical network impacts the functioning of many others because of biochemical complexity tying the targeted pathway with many other unrelated biological processes.

In spite of these challenges, there is considerable interest in developing prevention strategies. Even if AD cannot be eliminated, any delay in disease progression and severity of signs and symptoms is worth the effort. Research on AD prevention is in its infancy; it has only been since the 1980s that dementia has not been considered a symptom of normal aging. Prevention studies can be complicated; controlled clinical trials are expensive and require long follow-up times. Resolving individual risk factors (for example, obesity and hypertension) can be challenging because mechanisms are often overlapping.

The best we can do now is to identify AD in its early stages and engage in personal behaviors that generally maintain good health. One of the anticipated payoffs of the Colombia family study is the identification of biomarkers that are predictive of disease. Delaying the onset of AD by even five years could have a profound impact. Perhaps half the people who would have suffered from its horrible symptoms might be spared.[32]

Solving AD hinges on clarifying the complex relationship between molecular manifestations (sticky plaques and neurofibrillary tangles) and the clinical presentations (dementia and other behavioral and physical characteristics). This is the problem of emergence. How do the loss of neurons and dysfunctional neural signaling translate into perturbations of higher cortical functioning? More generally, how is the mind-body dynamic altered in neurodegenerative diseases?

Successfully managing chronic neurodegenerative diseases is one of the biggest challenges facing medicine and public health in the coming decades. A key challenge in geriatric medicine is distinguishing between "normal" aging changes and changes brought about by disease. Distinctions particularly for behavioral diseases can be difficult because what is "normal" cannot always be made clear. Accurate assessment of AD before symptoms set in and at different stages of disease progression will become increasingly important with the growing elderly population.

Age-related memory loss appears to be distinguishable from AD. Recent studies using postmortem human brain cells and brain tissue from mice have found that deficiency in the RbAp48 protein in the hippocampus region of the brain is a significant contributor to age-related memory loss. This form of memory loss is reversible. The 2013 report offers the strongest evidence to date that age-related memory loss and AD are distinct conditions.[33]

The specter of managing neurodegenerative diseases for which there are currently few or no effective therapies has been a major driver in President Barack Obama's announcement in 2013 to fund the Brain Activity Map initiative. This is a multiyear research effort that might cost $300 million per year or about $3 billion over the first decade in federal support. The goals are breathtakingly ambitious and include developing technologies to understand and initiate new treatments for Alzheimer's and Parkinson's diseases and mental illnesses; advancing knowledge of how the brain's neurons function in large interconnected networks; gaining greater understanding into perception and consciousness; and potentially accelerating advances in artificial intelligence. The Brain Activity Map initiative represents the emergence of a new school of thought on the workings of the brain in biological terms based on insights developed from a half century of work on the science of the mind (cognitive sciences) and science of the brain (neurobiology). This would be the latest in federally supported "big science." But unlike the Soviet space race or the Human Genome Project, the Brain Activity Map initiative is not straightforward, and it is unclear what is actually achievable because of the inherent uncertainties in the complexity of the brain and mind. We do not even know what questions should be asked.[34]

For neurodegenerative diseases, aging is the elephant in the room. It is an immutable risk factor. Those with Alzheimer's are generally older than sixty, and, with every subsequent five years the likelihood of Alzheimer's doubles. Almost half of the population over eighty-five has Alzheimer's. Aging as it relates to chronic disease occurrence and progression is poorly understood. Loss of neurons is part of the normal degenerative process in aging, but just when that normal process becomes aberrant, leading to accelerated degeneration, is difficult to know.

In the next chapter, we explore aging as a risk factor in chronic degenerative diseases. Is aging a risk factor that simply correlates with disease, or is it causal, whereby aging processes contribute to disease pathogenesis?

10

Desperately Seeking Methuselah

Death is an inexorable consequence of complexity. Subtle and not-so-subtle changes and imperfections at every level of biological organization lead to diseases and disorders associated with aging and impose limits on the human life span. Today, the average life span of Americans is 75–80 years. It was about half that at the beginning of the twentieth century, when pneumonia, tuberculosis, and other infectious diseases often robbed people of decades of life. Controlling microbial infections has resulted in the emergence of chronic diseases such as congestive heart failure, cancer, and neurodegenerative diseases.

Since the mid-twentieth century, the progressive graying of the American population stems largely from improved management of cardiovascular diseases. Individuals who would have succumbed to heart disease are now at risk for cancer and neurodegenerative disorders as they age. The death rate from cancer, adjusted for size and age of the population, has declined only 5 percent between 1950 and 2005, but, for heart disease, death rates fell by more than 60 percent in the same time period. The disappointing cancer results may be more apparent than real. Individuals surviving heart attacks become the cancer patients.

Aging is the common risk factor linking most chronic degenerative diseases. This chapter explores how complexity theory informs the problem of aging. Can the processes of aging be retarded or stopped? Can the human life span be increased indefinitely? By addressing design weaknesses, can we make a better human?

Aging is arguably the most familiar yet least understood aspect of the human experience. We first see aging by what it does to our grandparents and parents, and then we experience aging ourselves. Although aging can be defined as progressive functional decline with increasing mortality over time, the process is not uniform and cannot be so simply characterized: to borrow a phrase from US Supreme Court Justice Potter Stewart, "I know it when I see it."[1]

Solving all the chronic disease problems like cancer, heart disease, diabetes, and neurodegenerative diseases will not prevent aging. From a complexity perspective, aging is a spontaneous inevitability: cells and other system components simply fail. Aging is not a result of components wearing out in the sense that a mechanical device wears out over time because of friction and other mechanical forces. Aging is the accumulation of unrepaired damage over time that eventually compromises normal function.

Aging and age-related diseases share common pathways (Figure 10.1). Metabolic and other cellular processes in support of normal growth and development

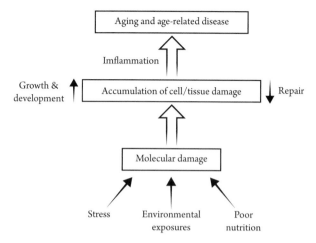

Figure 10.1 Aging and human disease. Chronic human diseases like cancer and heart disease share common pathways with aging. Molecular lesions lead to accumulation of damage in cells and tissues. Damaged cells release inflammatory cytokines. The resulting inflammation is central to the aging and chronic disease process. The level of cell and tissue damage is governed by the capacity for cell and tissue repair. *Source:* The figure is modified from Figure 3 in Kirkwood TBL. Understanding the odd science of aging. *Cell* 2006;120:437–447, with permission from Elsevier.

generate toxic byproducts, resulting in molecular damage. Unrepaired lesions in DNA and proteins lead to the accumulation of damage at the cellular and tissue level. Interleukins and other mediators of the inflammatory response elaborated from damaged cells produce and sustain a local inflammatory environment that results in age-related diseases.

Age-related diseases like heart disease and cancer reflect long-term failure of multicellular systems. More people are living past the age of sixty around the world and are at risk for degenerative diseases. Failure of complex systems is rarely due to a single proximal cause. Comparison of health statistics across countries is informative in revealing the multiplex causality of aging and chronic diseases. Americans have higher rates of most chronic diseases than their same-age counterparts in England in spite of the much lower healthcare costs in that country. Differences at young ages are as large as the differences at older ages for most conditions, including obesity, diabetes, asthma, heart attack, and stroke. Differences cannot be easily explained and involve a number of medical and social factors that interact in complex ways. The American health disadvantage compared with the English arises at early ages, and differences in body weight distributions do not play a clear role, suggesting that disease pathogenesis may be different in the two countries. Behavioral factors alone, including cigarette smoking and diet, are unlikely to be responsible for the generalized pattern of health disadvantages in the United States across health conditions, gender, and age. Social factors, including weakness of America's social safety nets, the magnitude of social inequalities, and the severity of poverty, are also important contributors to poorer life expectancy in the United States.[2] The key explanation for better health outcomes in the UK however might be in the difference in healthcare coverage. The UK has a universal single payer healthcare system. There are millions of uninsured Americans who get only emergency healthcare.

Almost every aspect of an organism's phenotype undergoes age modification with phenomenological complexity (Figure 10.1). Aging-related changes in humans follow dynamic regularities but are, nevertheless, unpredictable. The body's optimal physiological state changes with time. Systems and processes that operate at high efficiency when we are young still function but less efficiently when we age, resistance to stress and loss of adaptive capacity being key examples. The consequences translate into reduced quality of life (difficulty concentrating or engaging in physical activities) and increased disease risk.[3]

The complexity of aging is reflected in the large number of ideas and theories to explain molecular and cellular causes. Over three hundred theories have been proffered to explain mechanisms of aging.[4] None of these theories is entirely satisfactory, but, collectively, they offer a picture of a poorly understood process of complexity that engages every level of biological organization—from cells to tissues to the entire organism.

Recent advances in aging research have greatly clarified the aging process, and three main theories have emerged. Peter Medawar's *mutation accumulation theory* posits that aging is due to random mutations of late-acting genes. These genes show their effects only late in life and, unlike most detrimental mutations, would not be efficiently weeded out by natural selection. Accordingly, these mutations would accumulate over intergenerational time and perhaps cause all the decline and damage usually associated with aging. However, this theory is not fully consistent with what is now known about the regulation of gene expression. Genes are usually expressed in specific tissues at specific times during normal growth and development. The same gene may be turned on in one tissue and turned off in another at different times during the life of the organism. Genetic diseases occur when genes are not suitably expressed at the appropriate time. It is unclear, under Medawar's theory, why certain genes are functional or are expressed differentially only late in life (after the reproductive years). The theory suggests that aging is genetically programmed. There is a key heritable component in human longevity, and large numbers of genes affecting longevity have been identified, but there is little evidence to support genetic programming in aging. In contrast, organismal development beginning in utero is under tight genetic regulation.[5]

A natural extension of the mutation theory is George C. Williams's *theory of antagonistic pleiotropy*. Williams explains aging through pleiotropic genes that have different effects at different ages of the organism. In the antagonistic pleiotropy theory, one of these effects is beneficial, and another is detrimental. In essence, some genes are beneficial early in life but are costly later in life. For example, a robust immune system early in life would protect the organism from infections that could kill it before reaching full reproductive potential. However, later in life, immune function leads to inflammatory processes that promote chronic degenerative states such as cancer and heart disease. Antagonistic pleiotropy suggests aging is an inevitable result of normal physiology. The idea that genetic trade-offs are the cause of aging is an intriguing hypothesis, but there is little supportive evidence. Although many genes associated with aging have been identified, none seems to be associated with benefits apparent early in life.[6]

Thomas Kirkwood's *disposable soma theory* views aging as a systems biology problem. The theory centers on the idea that aging is a consequence of balancing resources between growth/development and somatic maintenance and presumes that the body must prioritize available energy for specific functions. Energy utilization is a zero-sum game because energy resources are finite. The gradual deterioration of the body with age results from the compromise in allocating energy to maintenance and repair functions.[7] Unrepaired cell and tissue damage leads to aging and age-related diseases (Figure 10.1).

The capacity of the body to shift resources as needed is well established. During the flight-or-fight response, blood is preferentially shunted to the heart and skeletal muscles. The disposable soma theory predicts that shortages of food supplies should compromise health and life span. But there is some evidence that a restricted caloric diet actually does the opposite by extending life span. This inconsistency may be more apparent than real. Calorie restriction has broad organismal effects. Limiting calories means the amount of (metabolic) damage to cells and tissues should be reduced, but the energy requirements for maintenance and repair might remain the same.[8]

Seeds of Aging

The seeds of aging are in the cells of life. Old cells can be distinguished from young cells by the accumulation of unrepaired molecular damage. Tissue function is compromised when a threshold number of cells has been damaged. Almost all tissues, including the brain, have some reserve capacity so that, even if some cells are killed or rendered dysfunctional or nonfunctional, normal physiology continues. At some point, however, a loss of tissue and organ function will occur when a critical number of cells are rendered nonfunctional.

One of the earliest observations of cell aging comes from in vitro cell-culture studies showing that mammalian cells are capable of dividing only a limited number of times. Leonard Hayflick defined cell aging (senescence) as the finite replicative life span of human fibroblasts grown in tissue culture.[9] This "Hayflick limit" reflects progressive telomere shortening and eventual chromosomal malfunction due to repeated DNA replication in the absence of telomeres (which are repeated DNA sequences at the ends of chromosomes that serve a protective function). Cancer cells, unlike normal mammalian cells, are capable of dividing indefinitely because of the presence of telomerase, an enzyme that prevents telomere shortening.

It is now known that senescence is a cellular response to an array of constitutive and environmental insults. Senescence can be induced by DNA damage, dysfunctional telomeres, disrupted chromatin, strong mitogenic signals such as those caused by certain oncogenes, and enlarged morphology. Senescent cells influence their local environment by secreting many factors that alter the behavior of neighboring cells and stimulate the immune system. These factors promote inflammation and growth of premalignant cells that may account for age-related decline and reduced tissue repair.

DNA damage is a key senescence trigger. A large body of evidence argues that DNA damage and mutations accumulate with age. Cells harboring mutations at defined loci have been shown to increase with age in humans. Reactive oxygen species, including superoxide ions, hydroxyl radicals, and hydrogen peroxide, are important sources of damage to DNA. Unrepaired DNA lesions can activate the cell cycle checkpoint machinery, leading to senescence or apoptosis and subsequent cellular attrition and tissue dysfunction.[10]

Senescence contributes to four major biological processes. Two are beneficial—tumor suppression and tissue repair. Two are harmful—aging and tumor promotion.[11] Cell senescence plays an important protective role in organisms with renewable tissues, such as bone marrow, skin, and the small intestine. Aging cells can permanently withdraw from the cell cycle, thus preserving the normal proliferation kinetics of the tissues if there is adequate replacement of lost cells. Bone marrow, for example, is a cell-renewal system and the source of red blood cells, white blood cells, and platelets. Unchecked damage to the proliferative elements in the marrow leads to uncontrolled growth characteristic of leukemia.

Cellular senescence appears to act as an important anticancer mechanism early in life by preventing uncontrolled cell growth. Cancer and aging are coupled because of common biochemical pathways involving the *P53* and *RB* tumor suppressor genes. These genes normally suppress cancer formation by killing cells or arresting growth. When these genes are mutated, loss of regulatory control of cell proliferation ensues with increased susceptibility to cancer. As the body ages, the population of senescent cells increases and creates age-related complications. Senescent cells acquire phenotypic changes that might promote cancer by activation of inflammatory cytokines. Senescent cells secrete proteins that alter the tissue microenvironment, impacting tissue structure and function. The accumulation of senescent cells may compromise tissue renewal and repair. Senescence response is an example of antagonistic pleiotropy—promoting early life survival by curtailing cancer development but limiting longevity as senescent cells accumulate.[12]

Senescence is one of several possible cellular states. Cells either have the potential to divide or are nondividing. By undergoing senescence, cells move from a state of potential or active proliferation to a postmitotic condition. Senescence is limited to dividing cells and is essentially irreversible growth arrest. In senescence, cells are alive but cease to move through the cell cycle. Senescent cells can be distinguished from terminally differentiated cells by morphology and signaling events. Differentiation (the acquisition of specialized structures and functions) is usually initiated by physiological cues and does not commonly involve tumor-suppression networks. Senescent cells, on the other hand, result from oncogenic stimuli that inactivate tumor-suppression pathways. Quiescent cells such as liver cells reside in a resting phase but can be induced to reenter the cell cycle if exposed to an appropriate physiological stimulus.

It is unclear how an actively dividing cell that has sustained DNA damage chooses between aging and death. Senescence or aging is a random process. Cells destined to undergo senescence cannot be identified, but the number of aging cells increases with time. The rate at which damage is accumulated is dictated by energy investments in cell maintenance and repair. Apoptosis (death), on the other hand, appears to be deterministic. The cell will self-destruct once a threshold level of DNA damage has been reached. Perhaps senescence occurs when a subthreshold level of damage has been reached. Senescence looks to be the more costly alternative in the long run. Senescent cells secrete damaging factors that affect neighboring cells and promote chronic disease. Apoptosis, on the other hand, kills damaged cells that are then removed from the body. Proliferation of nearby normal cells leads to replacement of lost cells in tissues with cell-renewal capacity.[13]

Senescent cells have been identified in tissues undergoing age-related pathologies, including atherosclerosis in blood vessels and glomerulosclerosis in the kidney. But until recently it has been unclear whether these cells simply reflect the aging process or play a causative role in aging. In studies, senescent cells that have been selectively removed have been associated with the delay of chronic disease. The toxic secretions of senescent cells stimulate the immune system and cause low-grade inflammatory responses. In tissues such as fat and skeletal muscle, removal of senescent cells delayed the onset of age-related pathologies. Furthermore, late-life clearance of aging cells has been shown to attenuate progression of already established age-related disorders. Cellular senescence appears to be causally implicated, and the removal of senescent cells can prevent or delay tissue dysfunction and extend health span.[14]

In a complexity context, senescent cells represent a form of component failure. The population of senescent cells increases with age. The resultant local disruption and microenvironmental changes have a domino effect, leading to tissue and functional disruption. The Weibull failure model is a good fit to the age-specific mortality rates for several cancers. The Weibull model assumes disease is a consequence of the failure of system components and is consistent with our current understanding of cancer progression.[15]

Worn-Out Bodies

Aging is a failure of the organism to keep going. The disposable soma theory argues that aging is a consequence of constraints in body maintenance resulting in a buildup of damage. Optimizing trade-offs between aging and chronic diseases rests on balancing loss of cells (that is, apoptosis) and preserving damaged cells (that is, senescence). The rate of aging appears to be tissue specific and depends on the capacity for repair and tissue cell renewal and on rates of energy utilization and immune function. The aging process is unique to the individual because of the multitude of inputs in the aging algorithm. Two modulators of life span—metabolism and immune response—are critically important. Susceptibility to chronic degenerative diseases is associated with loss of the immune function. Metabolic activity decreases with age.[16]

Immune System Failure

As the body ages the immune system gradually deteriorates and loses the ability to fight disease and ward off infection. Immunosenescence is a natural physiological process and includes an array of vital activities, including degradation of the host's capacity to respond to infections, diminished development and retention of long-term immune memory (including the one generated by vaccination), alteration of immune cell turnover, and an imbalance between innate and adaptive immunity, potentially causing enhanced and persistent inflammatory responses. Immunosenescence is a major contributory factor to the increased frequency of morbidity and mortality among the elderly from various aging-related diseases (Figure 10.2).[17]

The evidence linking immune dysfunction and heightened disease risk is substantial. Primary immunodeficiency results from rare diseases caused by inherited mutations that directly compromise the immune system. These diseases are associated with increased risks of some cancers. The most frequently encountered cancers are lymphomas often triggered by Epstein-Barr virus infections that progress unchecked because of an ineffective immune system. Secondary (acquired) immunodeficiency results from various stressors including aging, malnutrition, and certain therapeutic interventions. Many diseases, including cancers of the bone marrow and lymphatic system, directly or indirectly cause immunosuppression. Certain chronic infections, notably acquired immunodeficiency syndrome (AIDS) caused by the human immunodeficiency virus (HIV), are linked to cancer and opportunistic infections. HIV suppresses the immune system by infecting and killing a critical population of immune cells called T helper cells that are important in cellular immunity.[18]

Medical therapeutics like drugs that suppress the immune system in transplant patients provide compelling evidence for the role of immune surveillance in disease control. Immunosuppressive drugs are two-edged swords. These drugs are vital for successful organ and tissue transplantation by suppressing the immune system to avoid donor-tissue rejection. But this same immunosuppressive activity increases the risks of serious disease normally held in check by the immune system. Therapeutic immunosuppression causes a marked increase in the incidence of nonmelanoma skin cancer and some viral-induced cancers. Cancers of the lung, colon, rectum, bladder, and prostate, but not breast, are also increased by immunosuppression, suggesting that many nonviral cancers are normally kept in check by immune surveillance.[19]

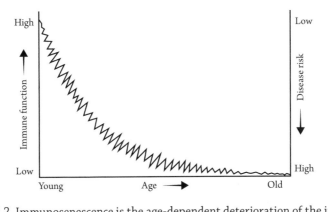

Figure 10.2 Immunosenescence is the age-dependent deterioration of the immune system. As the immune system becomes less competent, certain disease risks increase with age. The functional relationship between age, the immune function, and disease risk is not fully understood, but it is most likely nonlinear.

Slowed Metabolism

Energy flow (thermodynamics) is a fundamental process underlying aging. Chemical composition of the body changes regularly with age. Physiological and biochemical functions progressively decline. The ability to respond adaptively to environmental change is reduced, so our vulnerability to certain diseases increases. Many processes, including the body's metabolism, slow down.

The second law of thermodynamics imposes functional limits on living systems. The human body is only 10–20 percent efficient as an engine, an efficiency comparable to most automobile engines. This low efficiency is a consequence of the small difference between core body temperature (the hot sink) and ambient or environmental temperature (the cold sink). Marathon runners prefer to run in cold weather for this reason—waste heat can be dissipated more efficiently in the cold. The low energy-processing efficiency of the human body is consistent with the second law, which requires most of the processed energy be returned to the environment as waste since for any real, irreversible process entropy must increase. The human body generates about 120 watts of power, of which 100 watts are dissipated as waste heat; the remaining 20 watts power all biological processes.[20]

Paradoxically, there is some evidence that reducing calorie intake may improve health and extend life span. Calorie restriction (CR) diets are typically 60–70 percent of what animals would consume if left to their own devices. Benefits of CR have been observed in a variety of organisms, but the effect is not universal or consistently observed. Long-term effects of CR in Rhesus monkeys show conflicting results. The CR effect is poorly understood, but, if the effect is real, the key appears to be the number of available calories in the diet.[21] The ratio of protein to carbohydrate in the diet has been reported to have a dramatic effect on life span but this probably reflects differences in the availability of calories. In general calories from carbohydrate sources are more readily available as a source of energy. Thermodynamically a calorie is a calorie and it should make no difference what the source as long as calories from different sources are equally available metabolically.

CR animals have been reported to be more resistant to external stresses and appear to forestall or prevent many late-onset diseases, including cancer. CR involves a panoply of sometimes conflicting effects, including reduction in oxidative damage, increased metabolic efficiency, increased genomic stability, increased apoptosis, decreased apoptosis, lowered glycolysis, lower insulin, decreased body temperature, and activated neurohormones. CR and its consequences are clearly complex. Undernutrition (without malnutrition) reduces body mass, creating a high surface area to volume ratio that results in greater heat loss. The higher metabolic efficiency and observed lower body temperatures seen in CR settings support this view. The key question is whether CR benefits are a passive result of lower calorie intake and lower body-mass index or the consequence of an active regulatory program that recognizes food scarcity. The identification of the *SIR2* gene suggests that CR may be a regulated process that involves silencing genes.[22]

Immunosenescence and metabolism are closely linked. The immune system is extremely costly to operate in terms of both energy requirements and protein synthesis. The immune system is constantly generating new cells; about every two weeks, the entire mass of white blood cells is replaced (the life span of most white blood cells is approximately fourteen days). B cells, a type of white blood cell, produce antibodies at an astounding rate of about two hundred antibody molecules per second per B cell. The immune system is made up of an incredible number of different cell types that act in a complex but highly coordinated fashion. The only system in the living world more complex is the human brain. The total metabolic cost of the immune system is probably inestimable because of its complexity, but there is little argument the cost is high. Fever is a generalized immune response because high temperature is not tolerated as well by the infectious agent as by the body. For every one degree Celsius increase in body temperature due to fever, there is a 15 percent increase in metabolic rate. This febrile response is costly, but survival is worth the price. The loss of immune function with age is tied in part to decreased metabolism, and increased risk of disease means that metabolic resources are redirected toward a return to health.[23]

Aging is a complex process involving a large number of genes and multiple cellular pathways. It is unclear how determinants of aging, including caloric intake, stress, endocrine profile, and immune function, impact the aging trajectory. But, clearly, the process is not linear. Aging parameters are interdependent; small changes in one parameter influence others. Aging processes are evident at every level of biological complexity—DNA, proteins, cells, tissues, organisms. As a scalable phenomenon, changes in lower levels of organization lead to emergent properties at higher organizational strata.

It is difficult to uncouple aging from chronic diseases. It is unclear whether aging genes actually retard aging or boost longevity by averting or delaying chronic diseases.

Our understanding of aging in the last two or three decades has increased exponentially. Whether the problem of aging will ever be solved is anyone's guess. If George Williams's theory of antagonistic pleiotropy is right, then any effort to eradicate or modify the aging process must include modification of biological processes that underpin normal physiology. In complex systems, tinkering in one part of the system often has large, unanticipated, and untoward consequences in other parts of the system.[24]

Cheating Death

If heart diseases, cancer, and neurodegenerative diseases can be prevented or delayed, it seems logical that life span would be significantly extended because these diseases occur late in life and are the primary causes of death in old age. But the public health impact of preventing age-related diseases has turned out to be surprisingly small. If the heart-disease burden in the United States were eliminated, the average life expectancy would rise by only about three years. Curing all cancers would add about the same number of years. Risks of cancer and heart disease are highest in older populations. Although these diseases can occur at any time during life, they are manifestations primarily of aging, and preventing these diseases does not slow the aging process.[25]

Boosting longevity means adding years in later life, and that means solving the aging problem. We live in a remarkable era of long life spans. More and more people are living relatively healthy lives into their nineties and hundreds, a consequence of the tremendous gains earned from medical victories over infectious diseases and other advances in medicine and public health. However, pushing that life span higher still will be increasingly difficult.

A number of longevity genes have been identified that influence life span. These genes are highly conserved and have been found in several primitive species as well as in humans. Interference with the gene signaling pathways suggests substantial plasticity of life span that has been discovered via genetic studies of model organisms including the nematode worm *Caenorhabditis elegans*, the fruit fly *Drosophila melanogaster*, and laboratory mice. Mutations in the *IGF1* pathway (a set of genes that responds to signals from the environment or within the animal) can produce significant increases in the life span of *C. elegans*. The *IGF1* pathway regulates insulin signaling and insulin-like growth factor. *mTOR* is another longevity gene with broad regulatory control of cell and organismal growth. The *mTOR* pathway integrates nutrient and hormonal signals, and regulates diverse cellular processes. In addition to influencing life span, *mTOR* has been linked to several human diseases including cancer, diabetes, obesity, cardiovascular diseases, and neurological disorders. In cancer, dysregulation of *mTOR* signaling occurs in diverse human tumors, and suggests *mTOR* inhibitors as a therapeutic strategy. These findings demonstrate the importance of growth control in the pathology of major diseases and overall human health. Whether *IGF1*, *mTOR*, and other longevity genes can be manipulated to increase human life span is conjecture. Although inactivation of longevity genes like *IGF1* and *mTOR* have resulted in life span extension in some model organisms, there has been little work so far to explore life extension in humans or any other mammal.[26]

A key question in gerontology is whether humans have a fixed life span limit. Has the graying of the US population been a steady upward trend over time, or has it slowed in recent years? Are we approaching a theoretical limit on the human life span? As the average life span increases, the probability grows that at least some people will live to a very old age. Recent analyses of maximum life spans of Swedish populations refute the notion that the human life span is fixed and unchanging over time. The entire distribution of ages at death has been shifting upward for more than a century, although the maximum has increased much more slowly than the average.[27]

The remarkable gains made by medical sciences and public health in the last 150 years have almost doubled the American life span. These achievements had nothing to do with solving the aging problem. Instead, ensuring a safe food and water supply, managing waste, and identifying and protecting against microbial agents solved the infectious disease problem and added decades to the average life span (Figure 10.3).

Any serious attempt to extend the human life span must address aging itself. Stopping or even dramatically slowing the aging process appears to be an intractable problem. Any effort to modify normal biology is likely to have significant costs that outweigh benefits of extended life span. It is a Faustian bargain to trade off the quality of life for added years, but that has not stopped some scientists like Aubrey de Grey from making claims that it can be done. De Grey thinks that humans can live

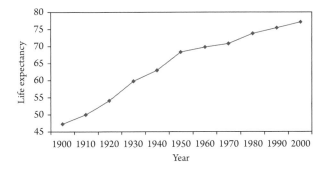

Figure 10.3 Life expectancy in years at birth in the United States, 1900–2000. Life expectancy is the average number of years persons can expect to live, assuming that, in the future, they experience the current age-specific mortality rates in the population. *Source:* US Bureau of the Census.

for hundreds of years, but there is little credible evidence to suggest cheating death is possible. Most proposals, including de Grey's, are based on ill-founded speculation about the aging process and the benefits of living to 150 years and beyond.[28]

Building Better Humans?

The quest for immortality and bodily and spiritual perfection has been a preoccupation of humankind since the beginnings of civilization. Steve Jobs, the über-creative technovisionary, argued that death is life's change agent. The specter of death means that you do not waste your life living another person's choices or aspirations.[29]

If immortality is unattainable, then what do people hope for? When divinities or higher powers are called or invoked, most people wish for good health, happiness, and prosperity, and protection from disease, pain, suffering, and premature death. A collective goal of biomedicine is to improve on what is already there—maintain or even improve our quality of life as we age. Fiction writers have dealt with versions of this issue, portraying various dystopias with genetically engineered humans. Margaret Atwood's *Oryx and Crake* includes the Children of Crake, genetically engineered by Crake to be peaceful, polite, and happy and feel no jealousy. The Crakers were created to address the "problems" of humans, to make them better than current humans. The Crakers have been created to be perfectly suited to their environment. The plausibility of picking "good" traits and eradicating "bad" ones, like the fictional characters in Atwood's book, is already occurring at some levels.[30]

The human body is not perfect. Although it is designed to last for decades, structural and functional failures take a toll. As the body ages, it is subject to degenerative diseases and other pathologies that diminish quality of life. The average age of humans particularly in the developed world is rising at a dramatic rate as life expectancy climbs and birth rate decreases. The number of people worldwide sixty-five years and older is likely to more than double in the period 2003–2030, from 420 million to 973 million.[31] Biomedicine has enjoyed considerable success in treating heart disease and cancer. The five-year relative survival rate for all cancers diagnosed between 1999 and 2006 is 68 percent, up from 50 percent in 1975–1977. The improved outcomes reflect progress in early diagnosis and better therapies.[32] Cancer survivors now live long enough to die of something else.

Certain poorly designed features of the body guarantee the occurrence of chronic, degenerative diseases.[33] An important consequence of ameliorating these defects is the delayed onset or reduced severity of these diseases, leading to a higher quality of life in advanced age. Particularly troublesome are two kinds of cells in the body that generally stop replicating past the stage of growth and development—neurons and muscle fibers. These postmitotic cells have lost the capacity to divide as a consequence of acquiring a high degree of specialization. Age-related damage to these cells cannot be repaired. The only approach to altering pathogenesis due to normal cell loss is early diagnosis and efforts to delay further cell loss and therapeutic measures to replace lost cells.

Here are some possible approaches to the human design problem.

Better Housekeeping

Proteins are synthesized continuously in the cell in support of a wide range of structural and physiological requirements. The synthesis of proteins involves stringing together amino acids in a specific order as determined by the DNA code and folding of the resultant polypeptide into a functional protein. Protein folding is a remarkably complex process that is poorly understood. Misfolding of proteins is implicated in a broad spectrum of diseases, most notably in the nervous system. Neurofibrillary tangles (NFTs) play a central role in neurodegeneration and are the key molecular defects in Alzheimer's disease and other neurodegenerative disorders. The proteins implicated in these different pathologies and the clinical manifestations of the diseases differ, but the molecular mechanism of protein misfolding and the structural intermediates and endpoint of the protein aggregation are remarkably similar. Even though the initiation, aggregation, and spread of defective proteins, particularly in the brain, are not well understood, there is recent evidence suggesting that damaged proteins "spread" through the brain like an infection.

The problems of neurodegenerative disease might be completely manageable if neurogenesis in the brain worked better, replacing spent neurons before they begin to cause problems for themselves and nearby cells. Age-dependent loss of cognitive functioning is a now-defining feature of our time. In the United States, Alzheimer's disease alone affects 10 percent of those sixty-five years of age and older, and the risk doubles for every five additional years. Loss of nerve cells in the brain also affects other neurological processes, including motor functioning. Normal motor functioning depends on intact innervations, and muscle loss in the body could be avoided with excess motor neurons.

A better system to fold proteins and destroy defective, unwanted proteins would reduce the propensity for aggregation and the pathogenic consequences of NFTs. Perfect or near-perfect synthesis, maintenance, and repair of every biomolecule in the body would significantly reduce or eliminate the risk for most age-related diseases. But this is probably unrealistic. The best we can hope for is early detection of disease and slowing the process down.[34]

Of course, even if it worked, this approach is not appropriate for the acute neurological damage that results from head trauma or stroke. A replacement model based on the regeneration of lost or damaged neurons is the better way to go in managing acute injury. In theory, if cells die, a population of adult neural stem cells would quickly replace them. Stem-cell replacement therapy is an active area of research, but restoring regenerative capacity in the clinical setting must await a more complete understanding and control of nerve-cell-population growth dynamics. Tinkering with regenerative potential to make more cells and replace cells that degenerate could spiral out of control and lead to cancer.

Radical Solutions

Normal metabolism generates free radicals that are considered a significant cause of cell damage. Radicals are highly reactive chemical species that can damage DNA and other critical macromolecules. Free radicals are generated primarily in mitochondria, the power houses of the cell where much of metabolism occurs. The accumulation over time of unrepaired free-radical damage has been linked to cancer and other diseases and to the aging process itself. Free radicals cause damage by oxidizing biologically important molecules.

Control of free radicals is a systemwide problem, since metabolism occurs everywhere. The body generates its own free-radical scavengers to minimize oxidative damage. Vitamin E and other antioxidants in the diet also modify damage by neutralizing free radicals before they can damage critical cell targets. Powerful free-radical scavengers such as amifostine have been synthesized for use in cancer therapy to control damage to normal tissue from free-radical-generating chemotherapy and radiotherapy.[35]

In theory, if a gene could be engineered into mitochondrial DNA that protects the cell from free-radical damage, the rate of aging might be slowed, and cancer and other radical-mediated degenerative disease risks reduced or delayed. But interfering with free radicals has potentially serious downsides. Free radicals play an important role in regulation of many biological processes, including vascular tone and blood pressure, metabolism of various biological compounds, enzyme activation, and mediation of cell signaling. Disrupting these important processes could cause more problems than it would solve.

Inflammatory Control

Inflammation is a natural biological process central to the functioning of the nonspecific immune system, the first line of defense against microbial infection and injurious agents. Without the ability to launch an inflammatory response, wounds and infections would never heal. Chronic inflammation is characterized by the simultaneous destruction and healing of tissue. The inflammatory process leads to the local release of cytokines—protein-signaling molecules produced by monocytes, macrophages, lymphocytes, and other cells. Inflammation and the production of cytokines are highly regulated processes and, when thrown out of balance, lead to chronic diseases, including atherosclerosis, rheumatoid arthritis, and cancer. Controlling these age-related diseases is contingent on balancing the progressive dysfunction associated with the inflammatory process and repair and replacement provided by normal cell proliferation.

Better regulation of chronic inflammation without compromising normal immune functioning might lead to delays in age-related chronic disease. Managing disease risks would require that anti-inflammatory controls be instituted early in life and continue indefinitely. It is well known that the chronic inflammation associated with heart disease begins decades before the clinical horizon is reached.[36]

There is compelling evidence that anti-inflammatory drugs reduce heart disease risks. Several large-scale clinical trials demonstrate that cholesterol-lowering therapy with statin drugs reduces coronary event rates in both primary and secondary prevention. These drugs work by inhibiting the synthesis of low-density lipoprotein cholesterol by interference with HMG CoA reductase, a key enzyme in the synthesis pathway in the liver. Hyperlipidemia is a major risk factor for atherosclerosis. The observed benefit of statin therapy, however, cannot be fully explained by the lowering of blood lipids. Evidence from clinical trials and basic science studies suggest that statins also have anti-inflammatory properties that may provide additional clinical efficacy.[37]

It is unclear, however, whether statin's anti-inflammatory benefits extend to other diseases. Pharmacologically, statins might reduce cancer risk via reductions in local inflammation, neovascular formation, and cell proliferation. Some reports suggest that statins reduce the risk of colon, breast, lung, and prostate cancers; but overall evidence is inconsistent. In one meta-analysis including 6,662 incident cancers and 2,407 cancer deaths, statins did not reduce the incidence of cancer or cancer deaths.[38]

The differential protection against heart disease and cancer suggests that a one-size-fits-all approach to disease control is not likely to work. Although many chronic diseases share inflammation as a component of pathogenesis, the role of inflammation appears to be disease specific. Developing drugs that target disease-specific inflammatory processes, instead of current nondiscriminating management of inflammation, has emerged as an important therapeutic strategy.

Making Sense of Aging

Sensory losses are one of the hallmarks of the aging process. A large proportion of the population over the age of sixty-five years has age-related sensory losses that impair overall health, self-sufficiency, and quality of life. The senses become less reliable, with the most dramatic changes affecting vision and hearing. Roughly 30 percent of adults over age sixty-five experience some hearing loss caused by aging, occupational or recreational noise, genetic factors, and certain diseases and trauma. Visual impairments unrelated to conditions that can be treated by corrective lenses are equally common in older populations. As sensory loss becomes more severe, cognitive functioning worsens. Diminished vision and hearing have profound consequences, including social isolation, interference with face-to-face communication, more difficulty using the telephone or cell phone, and loss of interest in what once were pleasurable activities.

Loss of the chemical senses (taste and smell) occurs gradually over time and may not be noticeable. Nevertheless, sensory deficits have serious repercussions; they play a major role in maintaining a healthy nutritional status because chemical senses are key to food enjoyment. Impaired gustation and olfaction not only plays havoc with nutrition but also contributes to social isolation because food serves as a major social function. An individual with a poor sense of smell may not be able to smell smoke. Spoiled food might not be recognized. A diminished sense of taste may mean more salt and sugar in foods and beverages to enhance eating pleasure, but overseasoning food may be unhealthy. Dietary choices may be altered to compensate for diminished or altered sensory perceptions.[39]

Aging produces changes in both the signal receptor (including the eye, middle ear, and taste buds) and the postreceptor neural networks. Historically, sensory deficits have been managed by amplification or modification of sensory signals. Eye-glass prescriptions that correct for visual aberrations have been around for centuries. Modern hearing aids amplify sound in the diminished frequency ranges. Use of spices and salt and sugar enhance the flavor (smell and taste) experiences of food. Short of completely replacing defective receptors, the best that can be done is to enhance available perception and to use a "more-sense" approach to improve the overall sensory experience. For example, making foods more colorful, enhancing flavors through use of sauces, using colorful environments, music, and other sounds (for example, crackling) can compensate for sensory deficits in taste and smell and improve the nutritional experience to a certain extent.[40]

Beyond amplifying and modifying sensory signals, there have been significant advances in signal-receptor technologies. Cochlear implants can facilitate hearing in some profoundly deaf patients. However, understanding the nature of neural processing—specifically, how sensory data are processed in the brain—continues to be a significant challenge. Research and development in technology-enhanced sensory systems currently focus on disease treatment. Improvements in age-related sensory deficits will likely require the same types of technologies but used at a different scale.

Aging and sensory loss appear to be mutually reinforcing. As aging progresses, sensory losses tend to increase, and the growing unreliability of the senses may accelerate the aging process. Sensory-perception systems play a major role in informing the body about its environment and, in so doing, may trigger physiologic decisions that alter longevity. Senses, particularly taste and smell, dictate our diet and the foods we choose to eat. Shifting dietary profiles to compensate for sensory losses by adding more sugar in the diet may have health consequences. Those decisions may influence the rate at which we age.

Aging as Complexity

Technologies are emerging that extend survival by delaying death from chronic fatal diseases. But there is a limit to what can be accomplished; conquering chronic disease does not solve the aging problem. Modifying the aging process—slowing it down or delaying it—is unchartered territory with significant risks because the biological processes involved in aging have considerable overlap with normal biochemistry and physiology.

Aging starts sometime around the onset of reproductive maturity when senescence processes begin. After that, aging marches on inexorably. How we age and how we die are inherently unpredictable. Advanced age is the main risk factor for most chronic diseases and functional deficits in humans, but the fundamental mechanisms that drive aging remain largely unknown, impeding the development of interventions that might delay or prevent age-related disorders and maximize healthy life spans. Cellular senescence, which halts the proliferation of damaged or dysfunctional cells, is an important mechanism to constrain the malignant progression of tumor cells. Senescent cells accumulate in various tissues and organs with aging and have been hypothesized to disrupt tissue structure and function because of the substances they secrete.[41]

However, aging is more than senescence. Like any biological process, aging exhibits scalable and emergent properties that inextricably link superior and more complex layers of biology with the less complex elemental layers below. Will identification and removal of senescent cells in aging tissue reverse or retard the aging process?[42] Is that the solution to aging, or is aging itself an emergent process that cannot be fully understood or controlled by manipulating cells?

Aging, like all other aspects of human biology, medicine, and disease, is best understood in the context of complexity. Evolution is one dimension of the complexity of life; complex systems must have the capacity to evolve in response to chronic environmental change. They also must have adaptive capabilities to deal with acute environmental stresses. Homeostasis is another dimension of complexity that provides the necessary internal stability to do that. As discussed in the next and final chapter, complexity is the unifying theory in biology. It is the common thread that links Darwinian evolution, cell theory, and homeostasis.

11

Emergence Medicine

At the core of life are fundamental contradictions. Basic biological processes, including simple diffusion and nerve impulse conduction, follow well-known laws of physics and are predictable. But contingent, higher-order processes, including cognition and cardiac function, are highly complex, and system behavior is unpredictable. Multicellular organisms exchange matter and energy with their external environment to satisfy thermodynamic requirements, but the internal environment is isolated from the external environment to satisfy homeostasis constraints. At large timescales, physiological functions in a healthy individual look unchanging over time, but the underlying processes exhibit dynamic behavior at smaller timescales. The immune system enhances survival at young ages by vigorously fighting off infections but may lead to chronic diseases later in life by promoting inflammation. Biological systems are incredibly resilient but are also very fragile.

System complexity links these paradoxes. In fact, complexity itself is paradoxical. The more answers we get about complex systems, the more questions come up. In complex systems the ability to make predictions means the future is already known. In theory, human behavior ought to be predictable if the initial conditions associated with higher cognitive functioning are known. In the stock market, future stock prices ought to be predictable if the initial conditions governing complex business behaviors are fully known.[1]

Although detailed behavior of complex systems cannot be fully understood or predicted at a microscopic level, a certain degree of predictability is possible macroscopically. Change in heart rate over time is a good example. Minute-by-minute variations in heart rate appear to be chaotic (see Figure 4.2); but, when measurements are taken over longer time intervals, say, on a daily basis, heart rate is predictable and follows a regular pattern.

Living systems couple deterministic processes with higher-order chaotic behavior. Homeostatic control mechanisms stabilize system performance and, at the same time, allow the system to adapt rapidly to changing environmental conditions.[2] The human body easily toggles between a stable, vegetative state and adaptive, excited states. But living on the edge is a precarious situation. With one small push, stability is lost, and uncontrolled behavior ensues. In cancer, one bad cell is the seed for small localized tissue perturbations that ultimately result in systemwide havoc. Human degenerative diseases are states of dysregulation leading to behavior run amok.

The reductionist approach has dominated biomedical research, yielding significant insights into the mechanisms of relatively simple biological phenomena and the pathogenesis of many human diseases. Investigating component parts as a way of comprehending the whole has been a driving force in the history of science. But the complex nature of living organisms severely limits this approach. The power of elementalism is significantly constrained when components behave interdependently. As a consequence, fully understanding the system requires a combination of reductionist and holistic approaches.

Our understanding of complex biological phenomena such as cognitive functions and cancer is far from comprehensive. Biological processes involve dynamic interactions among multiple genes and a complex interrelationship between genotype and phenotype. Because a biological system is not simply an assembly of all its parts, properties of the system cannot be fully understood without an integrative view of the whole system.

This final chapter advocates a complexity approach to enrich our understanding of human biology and human disease. A complexity perspective provides powerful insights missing in the traditional reductionist view. Chronic degenerative diseases are characterized by complex behaviors that present clinical challenges not encountered in the management of classical microbial diseases. Complexity science is the unifying principle for all biology and medicine and offers interesting and somewhat surprising strategies to deal with contemporary health issues.

Emergence

The secret to understanding biological complexity and complexity of disease is the transition from elementalism to emergence. How emergent behavior comes about is poorly understood, but it appears to be contingent on the number of component connections relative to the number of system components. Emergence is a type of gestaltism, the school of thought that the whole is greater than the sum of the parts. What we observe in the real world is the complex nature of life.[3]

Emergence derives from the self-organization of complex systems. Complex systems, endowed with the capacity for spontaneous order, the foundation for stability and adaptability, are organized into functional strata. Emergence is a stratum property that is contingent on the structure and function of lower strata. Language and other higher cortical functions are emergent properties derived from lower-strata neural networks. To understand language, at least in part, requires knowledge of the neural connections in the various language, auditory, and speech centers of the brain. But an isolated examination of these neural networks neither predicts nor explains language.

The human body may be viewed as a system composed of complex interconnected strata. In the simplest model, the body functions as a large population of cells organized into tissues that are further organized into organs and organ systems. Interstrata communications are facilitated by the nervous system, endocrine system, and cardiovascular system. The ability of the body to maintain steady-state conditions (that is, homeostasis) is a delicate balancing exercise involving many physiological factors influencing intrastrata and interstrata cooperation.

Noninfectious diseases involve multiple strata leading to the loss of steady-state conditions and perturbations of homeostatic parameters. Coronary artery disease is a good example because disease pathogenesis progresses in discrete stages. Coronary artery disease, like most chronic degenerative diseases, is initiated at the cellular level. But the manifestation of signs and symptoms means that higher-level strata (tissues and organs) are involved. The clinical horizon is reached only after significant disease progression that may extend a decade or more. The pathogenesis of coronary artery disease displays a high degree of scalability, progressing from minute changes within the endothelial cell layer of the arterial wall to the development of the atherosclerotic lesion to plaque formation and, finally, to circulatory changes leading to multiple organ and organ system complications. Disease strata even extend beyond the patient. Chronic disease affects the patient's family and social network in profound ways.

The progression of disease from one stratum to the next (that is, disease scalability) marks ever-increasing complexity as pathogenesis progresses. Atherosclerotic plaque formation, the basic pathological lesion underlying coronary artery disease, starts as chronic, unrepaired damage to the blood vessel wall. Localized inflammatory processes in the presence of cholesterol and lipids lead to the development of fatty streaks that by themselves have little physiological consequence. Progression to atherosclerotic plaque formation is not inevitable; plaque formation is dependent on a number of factors, including chronic inflammatory responses and high levels of low-density lipoprotein cholesterol. Each stage in the development of the atherosclerotic lesion is dependent on and more complex than the previous stage. Statins are a powerful class of drugs that can halt or retard arterial plaque formation by reducing levels of low-density lipoprotein cholesterols.[4]

In pathology, emergence means that the manifestation of disease at one scale cannot predict disease characteristics at higher scales. By starting with the smallest changes, coronary artery disease progresses in many stages over a long period of time. Disease progression cannot be easily predicted. Plaque trajectories are marked by periods of rapid development and quiescence.

The appearance of the mature plaque marks the transition from a local pathology to a systemwide pathology. Depending on size and location, the arterial plaque can rupture, releasing a thrombus that causes a stroke, heart attack, or death. Even if the plaque is stable, the reduced blood flow to the heart affects other organ systems like the kidneys and brain. What occurs in a blood vessel in the heart now begins to affect the entire organism. While the manifestations at a cellular level can only be seen at the local level, the manifestations occurring systemwide are more profound.

Signs and symptoms represent emergent properties of disease. Angina pectoris, or chest pain, is a cardinal symptom of heart disease, arising directly from the obstruction of blood flow in the coronary arteries. The resulting cardiac ischemia induces states of oxygen deficiency. When this occurs, aerobic metabolism and oxidative phosphorylation in the cardiac cell mitochondria are inhibited. Accordingly, high-energy phosphates, including adenosine triphosphate (ATP), cannot be regenerated, resulting in the local accumulation of large quantities of adenosine, which cause pain by stimulating nerve endings in the heart. Pain shows a sensitive dependence on initial conditions, suggesting a complicated, nonlinear relationship between myocardial ischemia and pain.[5]

Disease progression as a condition of complexity is also evident in cancer when viewed as an ecological process involving competition between cells for common resources. In the simplest case, cancer cells represent one species and the surrounding normal cells another. Competition means that cellular interactions are harmful. A two-species competition model is deterministic if it is also assumed that the population of competing cells will increase in the absence of competition unless the population is already at its carrying capacity (that is, at the maximum population size that the environment can sustain indefinitely). Under these conditions, definitive statements can be made about the growth and decline of the competing species.

The elementary two-species system is reflective of the earliest stages of tumor development in which the tumor cell population may be considered homogeneous. As the tumor grows and progresses, heterogeneity occurs because of additional mutations in some tumor cells but not others. Heterogeneity effectively introduces into the system new tumor cell subpopulations (species) with different growth rates and interaction characteristics. Such systems can be described by multiple coupled nonlinear equations; these equations can have chaotic solutions and are, consequently, very sensitive to initial conditions. Unless the initial conditions of the cancer are known exactly, tumor growth trajectories are highly uncertain and unpredictable.[6]

Complex diseases cannot be fully understood by focusing on cellular and molecular events that mark the early stages of pathogenesis. To do so hampers a full understanding of how the disease affects the entire organism. While reductionism breaks disease down into its simplest parts and provides important information about pathogenesis and perhaps insights into treatment, the complex nature of chronic degenerative diseases means that understanding of the disease cannot be gleaned from just this information.

Dimensions of Complexity

At an abstract level, complex systems share interesting features. The following dimensions of complexity are found to one degree or another in all complex systems, even as diverse as the World Wide Web and insect colonies.[7]

First, all complex systems use *information*. The concept of information is elastic and difficult to define. In information theory, the term can refer to uncertainty or entropy. Information can mean the electronic signals that are shared between computers on the Internet. In living systems, information is encoded in the genetic material and serves as the blueprint for cell structure and function. Energy in the form of ingested nutrients is another type of information. The neurotransmitters used to link neurons in the brain are yet another kind of information. Price is a form of information that drives economic systems. However information is defined, it is the driver of the complex system.

Second, complex systems have mechanisms to *process information*. In the case of living systems, energy (in the form of foods) is processed through metabolism.

Information coded in the linear arrangement of nitrogenous bases in the DNA is transcribed and translated into structural and functional proteins via protein synthesis. Tornados use energy channels to break down (or process) thermal energy gradients.

Next, *functional dynamic* properties allow complex systems to maintain a stable state and at the same time adapt to changing environmental conditions. Functional dynamics in living systems is accomplished through homeostasis. Without a stable internal environment, information processing could not proceed efficiently. Other types of complex systems impose regulatory controls that constrain the system.

Finally, all complex systems have the capacity to change through *adaptation or evolution*. In biological systems, this is accomplished through genetic diversity and natural selection that improves the chances for survival or success under environmental pressures.

Energy flow density is a useful way to look at information and information processing in complex systems. In this case, energy is the metric for information. Energy flow density is the time rate of free energy flowing through a system per unit mass measured as joules per second per gram (joules s^{-1} g^{-1}). The Earth's oceans and atmosphere have roughly a hundred times the energy flow density of a typical star or galaxy. Photosynthetic plants achieve an energy flow density roughly a thousand times greater than a star. The human body through daily food consumption has an energy flow density about twenty thousand times more than that of a typical star. The human brain consumes about 20 percent of the available energy intake but constitutes only about 2 percent of body weight and has an energy flow density 150,000 times that of a typical star.[8]

Complex systems in nature are open systems. They cannot exist unless information (that is, energy) can be extracted from the environment. Processing the information is an internal function of the system that requires a stable internal environment. The second law of thermodynamics requires that the imported information be degraded and then returned to the environment. Waste in any complex system may be defined as unusable (low-quality) information returned to the environment. The quantity of exported waste (in all its forms) must exceed the amount of usable (high-quality) information imported by the system. The complex system builds order and self-organizes by breaking down high-quality information imported from the environment.

Evolution Versus Functional Dynamics

The problem of morning sickness during pregnancy illustrates the difficulties in uncoupling dimensions of complexity. About 50 percent of women have nausea and vomiting in early pregnancy and an additional 25 percent have nausea alone.[9] The evolutionary dimension posits that nausea and vomiting are protective mechanisms—toxic substances taken by the mother must be expelled since the embryo may be harmed by exposure. Evolutionary adaptation may explain the temporary aversion to certain tastes and smells pregnant women experience, although sensory alterations may also be due to hormonal fluctuations. The Darwinian viewpoint argues that suppressing the emetic response by use of medications endangers the fetus by increasing exposure to toxins. Changing diet to avoid toxins would obviate the need for medications and reduce toxin exposure. The goal of dietary modifications is to avoid foods, odors, and dietary supplements that trigger nausea. Unfortunately, data from randomized trials are lacking to compare different types of diets for the management of nausea and vomiting in pregnancy.

The dynamical dimension focuses on the continual changes that complex systems undergo in structure and behavior. During pregnancy, the body is subject to significant hormonal changes in support of the developing embryo-fetus. Nausea and vomiting are believed to be associated with high levels of human chorionic gonadotropin (hCG) and estrogen during pregnancy. Antiemetics are available to treat nausea and vomiting, but nonpharmacologic approaches, including multivitamin therapy containing vitamin B, are effective for many patients. There are no good data to support the belief that nausea and vomiting are caused by psychological factors. Clinical application of Darwinian medicine by dietary management may lead to undertreatment of women whose quality of life is compromised by hormone-related nausea and vomiting during pregnancy.

The cause of nausea and vomiting in pregnancy is not fully understood, but the stimulus does not appear to be linked with the fetus. Observations that pregnancies without a fetus (a hydatidiform mole) are associated with clinically significant nausea and vomiting suggest that the stimulus is produced in the placenta. The clinical course of nausea and vomiting during pregnancy correlates closely with hCG levels. This tropic hormone stimulates estrogen production from the ovary; estrogen is known to increase nausea and vomiting. Women with twins or hydatidiform moles, who have higher hCG levels than do other pregnant women, are at higher risk for these complications.[10]

Since the 1990s, a small group of biologists and clinicians interested in evolution have been promoting the importance of an evolutionary perspective in clinical medicine. Traditional Western medicine is about understanding disease and disease mechanisms as they presently exist. The focus is on *proximal* causation and their anatomic and physiologic consequences. The evolutionary viewpoint, however, claims that proximal explanations are incomplete. A broader perspective addresses *ultimate* causation and provides important insights into disease diagnosis, therapy, and prevention. Darwinian medicine asks why humans in modern times remain vulnerable to diseases like heart disease and cancer, with promises to lead to better diagnostic tests and therapies. The evolutionary view in medicine looks for the cause of disease based on a patient's signs, symptoms, and medical history by considering interactions among the patient's ancestry, genotypic, and epigenetic variation; the evolutionary history of pathogens to which the patient has been exposed; and the environmental circumstances in which the patient and pathogens meet.[11]

Darwinian medicine is largely theoretical. It takes as its point of departure the oft-repeated saying by geneticist Theodosius Dobzhansky that nothing in biology makes sense except in the light of evolution.[12] But in the realm of clinical medicine, Dobzhansky's claim is neither right nor relevant. The point of departure for clinical medicine is homeostasis. The hypothesis that dynamic functionality of the human body is contingent on constancy of the internal environment is the cornerstone of physiology and clinical medicine.

Evolution has been remarkably successful in explaining otherwise puzzling features of the living world. Darwinian medicine (specifically, genetic analyses) can help sort out who may be susceptible to disease and who may be responsive (or conversely not responsive) to specific treatments. But it remains unclear how evolutionary explanations can inform clinical medicine in devising new diagnostic tests or therapies for disease or public health strategies for disease prevention. Evolutionary explanations have been suggested for human diseases in several diverse categories, including evolved defenses, conflicts with other organisms, novel environments, trade-offs, and design flaws.[13] The discussion of morning sickness is an example where evolution and functional dynamics lead to different solutions to a clinical problem. From an evolutionary perspective, dietary modifications to avoid toxins and the emetic response are preferred to antiemetic drugs. Clinical medicine, on the other hand, views nausea in pregnancy as independent of diet and sees no reason that antiemetic drugs cannot be used to control nausea and vomiting as long as the drugs are not toxic to the fetus.[14]

There is considerable interest in the evolutionary biology community to incorporate principles of evolution in the medical school curriculum. Curriculum revision of any kind means one or more traditional medical topics must be removed or modified to release time for new curriculum topics. Clearly, Darwinian principles are important in developing an overall understanding of life as a natural phenomenon of deep complexity, but, in the clinical context, a broader perspective is needed. The medical curriculum should introduce concepts of complexity science of which evolutionary principles are a part. Specifically, functional dynamics and constraints dictated by homeostasis are central to understanding normal human physiology and disease. What is missing in the national conversation is the role of complexity in human biology and disease. Evolutionary biologists do not talk very much about complexity science, yet it is fundamental to understanding the role of evolution in contemporary medicine. Much of the discussion about evolution in clinical medicine (for example, morning sickness) fails to distinguish between functional dynamics and evolution in complex systems. Curriculum revision in medicine should focus on the broader problems of complexity science that includes a Darwinism ideology.[15]

Beyond Comprehension?

More than a century ago, Henri Poincaré remarked that certain natural systems defied prediction. The long-term behavior of complex, nonlinear systems cannot be reduced to simple mathematical formulae or analyzed by the known laws of physics. Poincaré's stunning revelation meant that comprehending such systems would require a wholly new analytical approach, one that remaps longstanding disciplinary boundaries. Complexity is seen in a diverse set of natural systems, including the sophisticated group behavior of social insects, the unexpected intricacies of the genome, the dynamics of population growth, the self-organized structure of the

World Wide Web, chronic human diseases, economic sciences (including the stock market), and climate change. In spite of considerable advances made since Poincaré's time, it is clear that the vision science offers about natural complex systems will always be incomplete and consequently imperfect.[16]

Is a general theory of complexity feasible given the diversity of complex systems in nature? Are there common denominators that bridge the spectrum of complex natural systems? Can a universal framework be constructed that explains complexity in its broadest sense? We usually think of a scientific theory in mathematically descriptive terms. The holy grail of science continues to be the elucidation of theories as mathematical expressions that explain and predict natural phenomena. However, complex systems defy mathematical description; there are no series of equations that accurately predict climate or the stock market or human behavior. This does not mean that a useful theory is beyond reach, but, if a general theory emerges, it will be expressed qualitatively rather than quantitatively. The search for understanding life's complexity is in its infancy. Indeed, a complete description of complexity is beyond the limits of our knowledge; at this point, there are substantial knowledge gaps that we are not even aware of because we do not know what questions to ask. But an expression of the uncertainties about what we can and cannot know is an important step forward.

The nature of complexity requires that we move forward cautiously. While some complex systems consisting of large networks of simple components interacting by uncomplicated rules can be represented mathematically with simple reiterative formulae, it is another story to think that all complex systems can be modeled in that way.[17] Irreducible complexity defies simple mathematical treatment. But that has not stopped climatologists and other scientists and engineers from modeling complex system behaviors; from these endeavors, we have learned that applying quantitative mathematical models to complex natural processes cannot produce accurate answers. This is the so-called useless arithmetic problem.[18] Complex systems are so highly interconnected that they often have counterintuitive cause-effect results. A tiny almost imperceptible measurement error in an input variable results in gross inaccuracies in model outputs. Life cannot be fully understood by applying mathematical models to biological processes. Mathematical treatment may not be possible in understanding how the brain works. The creativity of the mind is beyond even the most complicated and sophisticated mathematical and numerical analyses.

In biology and medicine, solving complexity is a multidimensional problem involving computational sciences, engineering, physics, chemistry, and biology. At a minimum, complexity in the biological world is a massively interconnected system of networks with numerous overlapping regulatory control loops with innumerable input variables and parameters. Small perturbations anywhere in the system lead to widely variable, unpredictable, and unintended results elsewhere in the system. Alzheimer's disease (AD) and cancer are chronic degenerative diseases that behave in just this way, as was discussed in previous chapters. Living at the edge of chaos means that complex biological systems can be both very resilient and incredibly fragile. You can never know when you might go over the edge!

Physics, chemistry, neurobiology, or computational sciences cannot alone provide solutions to the complexity puzzle. How can emergent properties be measured and understood and what about the surprising creativity and unexpected behaviors observed in complex systems? These seemingly intractable pieces of the complexity problem should not deter us from applying the tools we now have to unravel complexity. Applying computational and analytical methods to nonlinear dynamical clinical data might lead to important insights into disease progression and treatment for complex diseases like heart disease and cancer. While reducing the body to a collection of interconnected networks leans toward reductionism, it can identify key nodes and edges that are critical in specific disease states. If these nodes and edges can be treated with drugs, it is a path forward to prevention and therapy strategies.

Part of the difficulty in developing a general theory of complexity is the lack of a clear definition of "complexity." Without a generally agreed-on definition, it is hard to see how a set of principles and theories can evolve. In chapter 4, general characteristics of complexity are discussed, but the term is never clearly defined. Complex systems are often viewed as large networks of simple interacting elements that, following simple rules, produce emergent and complex behavior. But this simplistic view and other suggested definitions and metrics hardly explain the properties and behaviors of the diverse complex systems found in nature.[19] Complexity sciences, particularly in the biomedical realm, are in their infancy. A fully matured discipline will have achieved understanding of generalized principles of complex behavior, emergence, and other key properties of complex systems. We might even answer Erwin Schrödinger's question *What Is Life?* Still, whether a theory will ultimately emerge is anyone's guess. If there is a general theory of complexity, it is likely to be more descriptive and qualitative than mathematical. Certainly, the characteristics of life discussed in chapter 1, including information storage and retrieval and energy flow and metabolism, are starts to developing a complexity theory of life. The elusiveness of a deep theory of complexity does not mean that complexity is beyond our grasp because it is inherently difficult to understand. To reach an understanding requires innovative and creative ways of thinking about the world.

Complexity limits what can be accomplished quantitatively. Phase transitions and emergent properties cannot be easily described or explained using computational and quantitative methods. However, model building offers a potentially fruitful approach to understanding the behavior of complex systems. Models describe relationships among system components. Qualitative solutions to complex problems seek to describe the general form of the functional relationships between input and output variables. Running various scenarios through such models leads to outcomes that can be evaluated to determine which ones are most probable and reliable. Multiple models can identify aspects of a problem or solution that any single model cannot. Bad predictions can be avoided by steering clear of bad models and using evidence-based procedures. Whether a model is robust or not depends on how well the model predicts actual outcomes. Calibration, or the matching of predicted outcomes with actual outcomes, is the gold standard for model development. But models are never foolproof. As a model of a complex system becomes more complete, it becomes less understandable; as a model grows more realistic, it also becomes just as difficult to understand as the real-world processes it represents. This paradox helps explain why complete models of the human brain and thinking processes have not been created and will undoubtedly remain difficult for years to come. Model building involves a necessary trade-off among generality, realism, and precision.[20]

For example, cancer is one of the most commonly modeled human diseases. Carcinogenesis is a complex, multistep, multipath process. Models of carcinogenesis are typically based on the principle that cellular adaptation requires genetic and/or epigenetic changes that generate new phenotypes. Recent advances in cancer modeling reveal that carcinogenesis requires tumor populations to surmount six distinct environmental proliferation barriers that arise in the adaptive landscapes of normal and premalignant populations—apoptosis, inadequate growth promotion, senescence, hypoxia, acidosis, ischemia. In the simplest models, barriers are considered to be independent and broken down one by one in a linear sequence to achieve tumor growth and spread. More complicated scenarios that lead to the complex and unpredictable behavior of cancer view barriers as interdependent. Alterations in a single multifunctional protein such as RAS may initially serve to overcome one barrier but then may accelerate the subsequent pace of adaptation by lowering other barriers. Growth and spread of cancer can be accomplished using a number of different strategies and combinations of strategies, including changes in specific sequences of barriers.[21]

A Unified Theory of Biology

Complexity is the unifying theory accounting for all key principles in biology—Darwinian evolution, cell theory, and homeostasis. Nothing makes sense in biology except in the light of complexity. Biology lacks a fundamental theoretical framework like theoretical physics that can be described by mathematical laws with predictive power. Physics-like laws for biology are unlikely because of the inherent complexity in biological systems. Creativity and complexity by their very nature preclude prescriptive behavior.

A unified theory of biology needs to explain how dimensions of complexity relate to one another. A central theory of biology should establish a conceptual framework to address unanswered questions in human biology, disease, and medicine. The link between information and evolution is well established through Neo-Darwinism (the modern synthesis) that couples Darwinian evolution with genetics (that is, information coded in the DNA). Until genetics and DNA mutations were folded in, evolution from a mechanistic perspective was necessarily incomplete.

The link between evolution and functional dynamics provides important insights regarding regulation of biological processes and their impacts on functional efficiency. Biological evolution has resulted in a complete separation of the internal cell environment from the external environment.[22] Homeostasis sustains this environmental separation. The evolutionary progression (from small marine organisms to humans) toward isolationism suggests that physiological efficiency at the cellular and systems level is contingent on total internal regulatory control.

The property of degeneracy in complex systems (discussed in chapter 5) is another example where functional dynamics and evolution (natural selection) are bridged. Degeneracy, the capacity of structurally different elements to perform the same function, is a ubiquitous property of complexity at all biological scales. Degeneracy is a requirement for natural selection because natural selection can only operate in a population of genetically dissimilar organisms. This suggests that multiple genes contribute in an overlapping fashion to the construction of each phenotypic feature undergoing selection. For example, loss-of-function mutations in yeast often have little or no detectable functional effect. This observed robustness can better be accounted for by interactions among a network of unrelated genes rather than by the existence of duplicated genes with similar, merely redundant functions.[23]

One of the central problems in all of biology is the relationship between genotype (the information and information-processing dimensions of complexity) and phenotype (the functional dynamics dimension of complexity). How does the genetic information contained in DNA ultimately translate to functional and structural outcomes? How is the genotype-phenotype dynamic perturbed in disease? The Human Genome Project gave us a full description of human DNA base pair by base pair, but that is only the first step in understanding phenotypic expression. Personalized or precision medicine and genetic mapping of human diseases promised to lead to individualized treatments of disease, but that has not been realized because the genotype-phenotype relationship is very complex and poorly understood. Part of the problem is that the genome is not the only determinant of gene expression. The environment also plays a key role by regulating gene expression and silencing genes. Epigenetics, the science of switching genes on and off, provides important insights into the relationship between genetic information and processing and regulatory control dimensions of complexity.[24]

The genotype-phenotype dynamic means causal influences run both up and down the hierarchy of structure and function of biological systems (that is, from system states to dynamical rules and from dynamical rules to system states). The classic example of bottom-up causation is DNA-directed synthesis of proteins that control specific tissue and organismic functions. Top-down causation like epigenetics involves the system as a whole exerting causal control over a gene or other subsystem. The dynamical rules that govern bottom-up and top-down causation are rooted in feedback-control systems that serve to stabilize the systems but at the same time allow for dynamical changes as environmental conditions dictate. Feedback control is observed in both living and nonliving systems, but what distinguishes life from nonlife is top-down information flow—the influence of systemwide information on component behaviors.

Predictions

A unified theory of biology falls short of the predictive power of classical physics because complexity precludes a sufficiently robust understanding of biological processes. The centerpiece of complex systems is their emergent properties and inherent unpredictability. Although complex systems cannot be fully comprehended because of nonlinear behaviors and inherent uncertainties, a complexity perspective offers important insights into human physiology and disease management.

First, complex diseases are not fixable once they are underway. As diseases progress, their complexity also progresses, and this means that higher-order strata are involved. Finding disease early is an important goal of medicine, particularly for degenerative diseases, because early diagnosis leads to treatments that stall disease progression and save lives. However, managing advanced disease is often a real challenge and usually not successful. Many cancers, including breast cancer, colon cancer, and prostate cancer, are essentially curable (with a five-year survival rate greater than 90 percent) if caught and treated at early stages; these same diseases have abysmal survival statistics (typically less than a 20 percent five-year survival rate) when metastasis has taken hold. The war on cancer has shifted from an all-out assault on all cancers to treatment challenges of advanced diseases. To date, little progress has been made in solving cancers of the lung, ovary, pancreas, and stomach. These diseases are already advanced at initial diagnosis and are very difficult to treat.[25] Chronic degenerative diseases are multidimensional, and a combination of treatments works better than a single approach. The cure can be as complex as the disease itself. Prescribing a pill and nothing else to people with clinical depression who question their existence is unlikely to heal them of their overwhelming sorrow.

Second, chronic disease is a stochastic phenomenon: it is characterized by randomness. Who gets cancer or the late onset, sporadic form of AD is unknowable, and when a person gets the disease, the trajectory is unknowable. Genetic and lifestyle factors increase the risk of a disease, but the presence of these host or environmental factors does not mean a person is guaranteed to get any particular disease; on the flip side, the absence of host and environmental factors also cannot be interpreted to mean a person will not get a disease. Typically, clinicians use statistics like five-year survival and median survival time as a measure of survival, but these are simply measures of central tendency and cannot be used to predict disease course in an individual. As we saw in chapter 8, glioblastoma multiforme, an aggressive primary brain cancer, has a mean survival time of about fifteen months. All that means is that, in a population of persons with the disease, half will die within fifteen months and half will survive more than fifteen months after diagnosis. How long a particular patient survives is anyone's guess.[26]

Third, removing all known risk factors does not eliminate chronic diseases, suggesting there is an irreducible risk.[27] Disease prevention should focus on what we know are important risk factors, such as smoking and diet in cancer and cardiovascular diseases. Causality is an intractable problem for chronic degenerative diseases. AD, cancer, heart disease, and other chronic degenerative diseases have long time horizons that separate the disease-causing agent from the disease. For the most part, chronic diseases develop independently of the cause, and the clinical features of the disease cannot be used to determine disease etiology.

There is an irreducible background of disease for which causes cannot be identified. The consequences for public health are considerable. The probability of getting cancer from a small dose of a cancer-causing agent is highly uncertain. It is impossible to distinguish a disease that occurs spontaneously from one caused by environmental exposure. The public health policy implications are significant because large sums are allocated to reduce already very small levels of environmental pollutants linked with disease risk that cannot be reliably measured.[28]

Fourth, screening tests to detect disease at its earliest stages are not beneficial for everyone. Even the best screening tests available have high false-positive rates when used in populations with low disease prevalence. High false-positive rates mean that positive tests lead to additional tests, biopsies, higher medical costs, and patient and family anxiety, all unnecessary. Part of the problem is that biochemical tests like PSA for prostate cancer and CA-125 protein for ovarian cancer were developed using a reductionist approach to early detection—identifying substances associated with diseased cells without considering the complexity of the disease itself. This approach marginalized the significance of the false-positive problem because the focus of research and development is identifying and characterizing biomarkers of disease. The importance of the nonspecific nature of these tests surfaced only when the technology was introduced in the marketplace. Had research and development been launched from a patient and societal perspective—the complexity view—important questions would have been asked at the beginning about who might and might not benefit from the test. The lesson learned from the reductionist approach is screening technologies have limited utility. Screening tests should be limited to patient populations for which there is evidence of increased risk of disease. The question is how frequently and how far ahead of symptoms screening tests should be performed.

The enthusiasm for screening appears to be on the wane. Recent studies suggest PSA tests do not save lives and ovarian-cancer screening of the general female population does not reduce mortality. Mammography is a useful screening test to find early breast cancer, but not in thirty- or forty-year-old women. However, women at high risk (those who are positive for certain cancer genes or who have a mother or sister who was diagnosed with breast cancer) may benefit from their first mammogram at age forty, with repeat studies at least once every other year. Obstacles to the ideal use of screening technologies are mostly due to complexity and other inherent biological barriers of many diseases. Screening tests identify pseudodisease with detectable lesions that are never destined to grow and require medical intervention. Uncertainties in disease trajectories are an inherent problem of complexity. The future is in developing biological markers, including genetic tests for specific pathologies to identify high-risk subpopulations that would benefit from screening and early diagnosis. Screening of high-risk populations reduces the false-positive rate because disease prevalence is higher.

Fifth, the explosion in medical technology cannot be sustained at present rates because of the inherent irreducible complexity of biological systems. Inherent system uncertainties become increasingly problematic as technologies probe deeper and deeper into complex systems. Biological complexity constrains what we can know about the human body and human disease. Imaging and other technologies have provided medicine with an incredible amount of information for the diagnosis, treatment, and prevention of disease, but there is a limit to what we can know, and technology will be less and less useful. As technologies become increasingly more sophisticated, we should expect less return on technological efficiency as the complexity-driven asymptotic limits on what we can know are

approached. And as we have seen with cancer-screening tests, technological inno-
vation leads to unintended consequences, excessive costs, and reduced return on
investment.[29]

There are arguments that we should not rely so much on technology. If you feel
ok, maybe you are ok. Interestingly, the limited value of early disease detection in
long-term health is supported by extensive evidence that well-being described on a
patient questionnaire predicts long-term survival more effectively than laboratory
and clinical tests or other high-technology data. A 2012 Danish study analyzing the
findings of fourteen scientifically designed clinical trials of routine checkups that
followed patients for more than twenty years found no reduction in risk of death
or serious illness in the group who had medical checkups compared to the group of
patients who did not.[30] As Sir William Osler argued more than a century ago, "Listen
to your patient; he will tell you the diagnosis."

Final Thoughts

There is one final contradiction. This last paradox has nothing to do with disease
complexity per se. Instead, it is concerned with the management of complex disease.
When it comes to chronic disease management, responsibility should fall on the
individual, not the healthcare professional. The burden should be shifted from the
healthcare community to the individual to practice good health habits, rather than
rely on the healthcare professional to find disease that may not be there.

The last twenty years have shown a remarkable shift in disease patterns worldwide. Many developing areas of the world have overcome infectious and communicable diseases as public health threats. The challenge now for worldwide medicine and
public health is managing the increased incidence of chronic degenerative diseases
like cancer and heart diseases. The decline in deaths from malnutrition and infectious diseases like measles and tuberculosis has resulted in more of the world's population living into old age and dying from chronic degenerative diseases. In 2010,
eight million people died of cancer worldwide, compared to about 5.8 million in
1990. This shift in disease patterns reflects improved public health practices in the
developing world, including better access to medical services, food, and sanitation.[31]

Today's public health challenges are considerable. Deaths from infectious diseases are still a significant problem in many parts of the underdeveloped world.
Adult mortality poses equally difficult challenges for the world's public health system because personal behavior affects chronic disease risks. Tobacco use continues
to be a rising threat worldwide; curtailing cigarette consumption could save millions
of lives every year. It is considerably more difficult to get people to change behaviors than to administer a vaccine that protects children from infectious diseases like
measles.

The current medical model emphasizes descriptions and management of health
and disease as tests, rather than individual subjective assessments. Clinical laboratory tests are more informative in acute and emergency situations where changes
in quantitative clinical test results are often ahead of subjective assessments. But
in the case of chronic disease management, healthcare by the individual is the best

medicine. Diet, exercise, not smoking, and dozens of personal decisions made on a daily basis are far more important in long-term health than early detection of disease. In the long term, the patient's personal assessment is probably as good a barometer of health status as any medical test.

Understanding health and disease requires knowledge of how the design and function of the human body make us what we are. Medical science needs a broader perspective on disease than the conventional viewpoint that things ought to be fixable if we can just find the right magic bullet. Contemporary medicine focuses on deterministic processes in health and disease, but we need an approach that targets disease as a systems problem with features of complexity. Complexity and emergence in biological systems suggest that some diseases simply cannot be fixed or stopped; admitting the limits of diagnostic and therapeutic medicine in managing chronic degenerative diseases should fuel the growing trend toward preventive medicine.[32] As we have emphasized throughout this book, disease prevention is always preferable to therapy and cure. Disease prevention is essentially manipulating emergence. Chronic disease healthcare of the future is, in reality, emergence medicine.

GLOSSARY

Acid-base buffer	Dilute aqueous solution of a conjugate acid-base pair that prevents significant changes in pH when a small quantity of a strong acid or strong base is added
Action potential	Rapid, transient change in the membrane potential of excitable cells; in the nervous system serves as the signal transported along nerve axons
ADH	Antidiuretic hormone; a hormone produced by the hypothalamus and stored and released by the posterior pituitary gland, which promotes water retention by the kidney
AIDS	Acquired immunodeficiency syndrome; a disease of the human immune system caused by the human immunodeficiency virus (HIV)
Allostasis	Physiological process that maintains stability (homeostasis) when organisms actively adjust to stress and other conditions
Alzheimer's disease	Most common form of dementia; disease worsens with progression, leading to death; there is no cure
Amifostine	Drug used to protect against harmful effects of chemotherapy and radiation
Amyloid protein	Insoluble fibrous proteins found in several tissues and associated most commonly with Alzheimer's disease, but also other diseases, including atherosclerosis and type 2 diabetes
Amyloidosis	Process of extracellular deposition and accumulation of amyloid protein. The buildup of amyloid protein leads to plaque in the brain—a marker for Alzheimer's disease
Analgesic	Pain reliever
Angina pectoris	Chest pain often associated with coronary artery disease
Angiogenesis	Growth of new blood vessels from preexisting vessels

Angiography	Medical imaging procedure to visualize blood vessels, particularly in the heart
Antagonistic pleiotropy	Some traits controlled by a gene are beneficial to the organism, and other traits controlled by the same gene are harmful
Antiemetic	Medication to prevent or stop nausea and vomiting
Apoptosis	Cell death resulting from a series of genetically programmed events
APP	Amyloid precursor protein; membrane-bound protein found in nerve and other tissues and from which amyloid proteins are derived; Alzheimer's disease is associated with beta-amyloid
Aquaporin	Water channel protein in the cell membrane that facilitates movement of water by osmosis
Aqueous	Type of chemical solution in which water is the solvent; in living systems all biological processes occur in dilute aqueous solutions
Arrhythmia	Abnormal electrical activity in the heart that leads to irregular heart beat
Asymptotic	Pertaining to limiting value of a dependent variable when the independent variable approaches zero or infinity
Atherosclerosis	Deposition of fat-like substances in the walls of arteries, causing vessel narrowing
ATP	Adenosine triphosphate; key source of free energy that drives biological processes
Atrial septal defect	Opening in the wall (septum) separating the left and right atria, leading to abnormal blood flow between the left heart and the right heart
Axon	Long extension of the neuron that generates and propagates nerve signals (action potentials) to target cells or other nerve cells
B cell	Type of lymphocyte in the blood involved in the immune response
BCR-ABL oncogene	Chromosomal abnormality involving the fusion of parts of chromosomes 9 and 22 encoding a kinase protein that causes unregulated cell growth; the protein is associated with certain types of leukemia, notably chronic myelogenous leukemia
Beta-amyloid	Fragment of amyloid precursor protein that form the plaques in brain tissue typically seen in Alzheimer's disease
Bifurcation	Process whereby a stable steady-state system spontaneously breaks its symmetry when entering a nonlinear mode beyond some energy threshold, resulting in two new possible dynamic steady states; the system selects one of the states depending on system history and environmental conditions

Biomarker	Indicator of a biological state; an objective measure of a normal or pathologic process that may be used to diagnose disease or measure response to a therapeutic intervention
Blood doping	Use of products like erythropoietin to enhance oxygen transport to muscles
Brain plasticity	Modifications in neural networks due to changes in behavior, the environment, or neural processes; changes due to brain injury or disease
Brownian motion	Random movement of particles suspended in a fluid
CABG	Coronary artery bypass graft; cardiac surgical procedure using artery and vein grafts from other parts of the body to bypass blocked coronary arteries
Cachexia	The loss of fat and skeletal muscle mass; a significant factor in the poor performance status and high mortality rate of cancer patients
Cancer	Set of more than one hundred different diseases characterized by uncontrolled growth and spread of abnormal cells
Capacitance	Ability of an object to store electric charge; plasma membrane of the cell has capacitance because it can be electrically charged
Carcinogen	Biological, chemical, or physical agent that causes cancer
Carcinogenesis	Origin, production, or development of cancer
Cardiomyocyte	Muscle cell found in the walls of the ventricles of the heart; responsible for the heart's pumping action
Catheterization	Placement of a thin, flexible tube (catheter) in a body cavity, blood vessel, or duct to treat diseases or to perform medical procedures; cardiac catheterization involves inserting a catheter in the coronary arteries
Causal factor	In public health refers to agents that cause disease; removal of the causal agents eliminates or reduces disease incidence depending on what other casual factors may be present; see "Risk factor"
Chaos	A property of some complex systems characterized by sensitivity to initial conditions; small changes in inputs result in large, disproportionate outputs in the system, leading to unpredictable behavior
Chemotherapy	Treatment of cancer with cell-killing drugs or other drugs that interfere with growth and spread of cancer; treatment may be administered to cure the patient, to prolong life, or to maintain quality of life by reducing the severity of signs and symptoms
Cheyne-Stokes respiration	Irregular or arrhythmic breathing pattern observed in patients with certain brain lesions and patients in coma

Closed system	System isolated from its surroundings such that there is no exchange of energy or mass with the environment
Codon	Fundamental unit of genetic information; a three DNA base sequence that specifies a particular amino acid
Comorbidity	Presence of other diseases or disorders in addition to the primary disease
Complexity	Property of certain systems characterized by components acting interdependently such that behavior of the entire system cannot be accounted for or predicted by the properties of individual components
Complexity paradox	The more we know about human biology and disease, the less we seem to understand
Condition	Characteristic of a system that dictates the dynamics of change of system states over time; equilibrium is a condition of a system
Cori cycle	Metabolic pathway in which lactic acid produced by glycolysis is converted into glucose in the liver; also called lactic acid cycle
Coronary angiogram	Medical imaging procedure using X-rays and radio-opaque dyes to visualize the coronary arteries in the heart; definitive diagnostic test for coronary artery disease
Cytology	Study of cell structure, function, and biochemistry
Cytolysis	Bursting of cell due to excess water uptake because of osmotic imbalance between the intracellular and extracellular environment; plants and bacteria do not undergo cytolysis because of the presence of a cell wall
DCIS	Ductal carcinoma in situ; collection of abnormal cells in the lining of the milk ducts that have not invaded nearby breast tissues; whether DCIS leads to invasive cancer in a particular case is unclear
Degenerative disease	Deterioration of tissue or organ function or structure over time due disease to cell loss or damaged cells; Alzheimer's disease and cancer are examples
Dementia	Group of diseases associated with serious loss of cognitive ability; Alzheimer's disease is the most common form of dementia
Depolarization	Change in the excitable cell membrane potential that makes it less negative; if the depolarization exceeds a voltage threshold in nerve cells an action potential may result
Deterministic chaos	Future behavior of chaotic systems is fully determined by initial conditions, but the deterministic nature of these systems does not make them predictable; see "Chaos"

Determinism	Philosophy stating that all events are determined by preexisting causes
Diabetes type 2	Metabolic disorder characterized by high blood glucose levels due to insulin resistance or insulin insufficiency
Differentiation	The process whereby cells acquire specialized structures and functions
Disease	Functional or structural condition of the body judged to be abnormal; associated with specific signs and symptoms
Dissipative structure	System operating far from thermodynamic equilibrium that efficiently dissipates the heat energy generated to sustain it; dissipative structures have the capacity to change to higher levels of orderliness (self-organization) to become more efficient; see "Bifurcation"
DNA	Deoxyribonucleic acid; the macromolecule in the cell that encodes the genetic instructions for development and functioning of all living organisms
Dyslipidemia	Abnormal levels of lipids (cholesterol and fat) in the blood plasma
Edema	Tissue swelling caused by accumulation of fluid
Edges	In biological networks refers to the interactions occurring between nodes; see "Nodes"
Elementalism	An approach that focuses on individual components as a way of understanding complex systems
Emergence	Properties of a complex system that cannot be predicted or understood by examining system components
Endothelium	Thin layer of epithelial cells that line the interior walls of blood vessels
Energy flow density	Time rate of flow of energy per unit mass; measured in joules per second per kilogram
Enterotoxin	Toxin produced by a microorganism that targets the intestines
Entropy	Measure of disorder in thermodynamic systems; nature tends toward maximum disorder (zero entropy); highly ordered systems have high negative entropy
Epidemiology	An observational science of the study of the distribution and causes of disease in defined populations
Epigenetics	Changes in gene expression or cellular phenotype caused by mechanisms other than alterations in the sequence of DNA bases
Epithelial cells	Form sheet of cells that line or cover tissues and organs; makes up tubules and covers the surface of the body; one of the four major types of cells in the body

Equilibrium	In thermodynamics refers to the condition when there is no net flow of energy or matter and no driving forces in the system; in living systems external sources of energy are necessary to maintain the system far from equilibrium
Erythropoietin	Hormone secreted by the adult kidney that acts on bone marrow cells to stimulate red blood cell production
Etiology	Causes of disease
Excitable cell	Cells that can be stimulated to create a small electric current; include neurons and muscle cells
Extracellular fluid	Aqueous fluid that surrounds cells and makes up the blood plasma
Facilitated diffusion	Passive movement of a solute molecule down its concentration gradient through a membrane via a specific carrier protein
False-negative rate	Percentage of subjects with disease who test negative for the disease
False-positive rate	Percentage of subjects without disease who test positive for the disease
Fibroblast	Connective tissue cell that synthesizes the extracellular matrix and collagen
Fractal	An object or quantity that displays self-similarity or repeating patterns on all scales
Free energy	Portion of available energy available to do work; remaining energy is waste energy
Free radical	Highly reactive chemical species because of the presence of an unpaired electron; e.g., hydroxyl free radical
FTO gene	Gene that produces the fat mass and obesity-associated protein; certain protein variants are correlated with obesity in humans
Functional dynamics	Functional changes occurring over time in living systems at the cellular, tissue, organs, and organismal level
Gene	Molecular unit of heredity; unit of inheritance associated with a defined region of DNA
Gene silencing	Switching off of a gene; a process of gene regulation by epigenetic mechanisms
Genetic drift	Changes in gene frequencies from generation to generation as a result of random processes
Genetic mutation	Change in the genetic material associated with changes in the linear sequence of bases in the DNA
Genomics	The entirety of an organism's hereditary information and its interactions

Genotoxic	Biological, chemical, or physical agent that damages cellular DNA, thereby causing mutations
Gerontology	Study of the biological, medical, psychological, and social aspects of aging
Glioblastoma	An aggressive cancer arising from glial cells in the brain
Goldman equation	Total equilibrium potential across a cell membrane is determined by the intracellular and extracellular concentrations of all electrolytes present
Gradient	Describes in which direction and at what rate a physical or chemical quantity including pressure, temperature, and concentration changes at a particular location in the system; gradients are the driving force for many biological processes
Half-life	Time required for a quantity to fall to half its value as measured at the beginning of the time interval; measure of how long a drug remains in the blood
Hayflick limit	The number of times a normal cell population will divide until cell division stops; cancer cells have no Hayflick limit
hCG	Human chorionic gonadotropin; hormone produced during pregnancy; stimulates secretion of estrogen and progesterone
HDL cholesterol	High-density lipoprotein cholesterol; high levels associated with reduced heart disease risk; sometimes referred to as "good" cholesterol; see "LDL cholesterol."
Hemodynamics	Branch of physiology dealing with the forces involved in the circulation of the blood
Hillock	Portion of the nerve cell body connected to the axon
HIV	Human immunodeficiency virus; causal factor for acquired immunodeficiency syndrome (AIDS)
HMG-CoA reductase	3-hydroxy-3-methyl coenzyme A reductase; statin drugs lower low-density lipoprotein cholesterol levels by inhibiting HMG-CoA reductase in the liver
Homeostasis	Constancy of the body's internal environment including body temperature, pH, and various electrolytes and biologically important molecules
Homocysteine	A homolog of the amino acid cysteine; elevated levels have been associated with certain forms of heart disease
Host factor	Genetic, immunologic, physiologic, and other individual traits that affect susceptibility to disease
Hydatidiform mole	Intrauterine mass formed by degeneration of products of conception

Hyperlipidemia	Abnormally high concentration of fats or lipids in the blood
Hyperpolarization	Change in the excitable cell membrane potential that makes it more negative; inhibits action potentials in nerve cells
Hypertension	Physiologic state characterized by high blood pressure
Hypotension	Physiologic state characterized by low blood pressure
Hypoxia	Physiologic state of oxygen deficiency
Iatrogenic effect	Physical or mental condition caused by medical intervention itself
Immunosenescence	Gradual deterioration of the immune system due to natural aging
Immunosuppression	Diminished immune function due to disease or treatment
Inflammation	Pain, heat, swelling, and tenderness in tissues in response to infection or injury; generalized immune response that is part of healing process
Interleukins	Group of multifunctional cytokines; produced by T cells and other types of immune cells to regulate the immune response
Internal energy	State of a system that represents total energy contained in the system
Interstitial fluid	Water-based environment surrounding cells
Ion	Atom or molecule with a net negative or positive charge; anions (e.g., Cl^-) are negative ions and have more electrons orbiting the nucleus than protons in the nucleus; cations (e.g., K^+, Na^+) are positively charged ions and have fewer electrons orbiting the nucleus than protons in the nucleus
Ischemia	Inadequate blood supply to tissues, particularly the heart
Isothermal	In thermodynamic systems heat exchange that does not involve a change in temperature
LDL cholesterol	Low-density lipoprotein cholesterol; high levels are associated with increased heart disease risk, sometimes called "bad" cholesterol. See "HDL cholesterol."
Lesion	Localized, abnormal structural change
LNT theory	linear no-threshold theory; used to predict numbers of cancers in populations exposed to low doses of radiation carcinogen; under LNT cancer risk is assumed to be a linear function of dose without a dose threshold
Lipogenesis	metabolic formation of fat occurring inside the cell
Lipophilic	Ability of a solute molecule to dissolve in lipids, oils, and other nonpolar solvents; nonpolar solutes generally have high lipophilicity

Lumen	Inside space of a tubular structure such as an artery or intestine
Lymphocyte	Type of white blood cell important in immune function; includes B cells, T cells, and natural-killer cells
Macrophage	Tissue-based cell that is important in nonspecific and specific immunity
Membrane conductance	Ability of cell membrane to allow substances to cross; cells can change conductance properties by opening or closing specific ion channels in the membrane
Membrane potential	Voltage difference between the inside and outside of the cell
Metabolic syndrome	Combination of medical disorders leading to increased risk of cardiovascular disease and diabetes; insulin resistance and obesity are recognized factors
Metastable states	Long-lived states of a system that are less stable than the ground (most stable) state of the system
Metastasis	Cancer spreading from site of origin to other sites in the body
Mitogen	Substance that stimulates cell division
Mitosis	Cell division; the daughter cells have identical genetic information as the parent cell
Modularity	Degree to which a system's components may be separated into distinct functional areas; e.g., brain modules for vision, language
Morphology	Branch of biology dealing with form and structure of organisms
mRNA	Messenger ribonucleic acid; involved in synthesis of proteins in cells
Myocyte	Muscle cell
Na^+-K^+ pump	An intermembrane protein complex that pumps K^+ into the cell and Na^+ out of the cell by using ATP as an energy source
Nanotechnology	Manipulation of matter at the atomic or molecular level
Natural selection	Mechanism of evolution; gradual, nonrandom process by which biological traits become more or less common in a population
Negative feedback	In control systems reduces fluctuations and returns output to or toward the set point; confers output stability; contrast with "Positive feedback"
Neo-Darwinism	Comprehensive theory of evolution joining population biology and genetics with Darwin's theory of evolution by natural selection; also referred to as the Modern Synthesis
Neoplasm	Abnormal mass of tissue as a result of uncontrolled proliferation of abnormal cells; cancer

Nernst equation	Calculates the membrane potential due to the concentration gradient of a single type of ion across the permeable membrane
Neurodegenerative disease	Loss of structure or function of neurons and neuronal networks due to cell loss or damaged cells; Alzheimer's disease and brain cancer are examples
Neurofibrillary tangles	Aggregates of hyperphosphorylated tau protein in the brain; biomarker for Alzheimer's disease
Nocebo effect	Inert substance that produces an undesirable effect
Node of Ranvier	Gap in the myelin sheath along the nerve axon where the action potential is regenerated
Nodes	In biological networks refers to proteins, metabolites, genes, and cells
Nootropic	Medication that masks cognitive deficiencies by enhancing other cognitive and memory processes
Normotensive	Normal blood pressure; 120 mm Hg systolic pressure and 80 mm Hg diastolic pressure
Occlusion	An obstruction or closure of a body passage
Oncogene	a type of cancer gene that is a mutated form of the normal proto-oncogene whose function is control of cell growth and division
Oncogenic	Causing the formation of a cancer
Open system	System that can exchange mass and energy with its surroundings
Organic disease	Any disease in which there is a physical change in the structure or function of an organ or tissue
Osmosis	Movement of water across a semipermeable membrane from a region of low solute concentration to a region of high solute concentration; the membrane is impermeable to the movement of solute molecules
Oxidative phosphorylation	Metabolic process that generates ATP in the mitochondria of cells
Palliative therapy	Therapy that removes or reduces the signs and symptoms of a disease but does not cure the disease
Parasympathetic	Part of autonomic nervous system; controls digestion and other nervous system activities while at rest; complementary to the sympathetic system
Pathogenesis	Mechanisms resulting in the development of disease
Pathology	Study of disease and disease processes
Pathophysiology	Disordered physiological processes associated with disease/injury; functional changes associated with or resulting from disease or injury

Perfusion	Flow of blood through a tissue or organ to supply nutrients and oxygen and remove waste
Permeability	Property of cell membrane that allows atoms or molecules to cross membrane; a membrane is semipermeable when it is permeable to some solute molecules but not others
PET	Positron emission tomography; a medical imaging procedure that produces three-dimensional images of functional processes in the body; imaging is based on detection of gamma rays created by positron-emitting radionuclides
Pharmacokinetics	Branch of pharmacology concerned with the way drugs are taken into, move around, and are eliminated from the body
Phenotype	An organisms' observable characteristics or traits
Placebo effect	Inert substance that produces a desirable effect
Plasticity	Capacity of healthy brain tissue to assume functions of damaged areas
Pleiotropy	One gene controls for more than one phenotypic trait in an organism
Polarity	Polar molecules such as water or sucrose have an unequal sharing of electrical charges in their chemical bonds; nonpolar molecules such as lipids have equal sharing of electrons in chemical bonds; polar solutes dissolve in polar solvents but not nonpolar solvents.
Polydipsia	Excessive thirst
Polymorphism	Existence of two or more clearly different phenotypes in the same population of a species
Polyuria	Excessive urine output
Positive feedback	In control systems serves to amplify system output and increases the deviation from the set point; contrast with "Negative feedback"
Positive predictive value	For diagnostic and screening tests refers to the probability that a person with a positive test actually has the disease
Potential energy	Energy that can be converted to electrical, heat, or mechanical energy to do work
Presenilin	Class of transmembrane proteins that regulate certain intracellular calcium ion levels; mutations in the genes that encode presenilin proteins in the brain are linked to familial early-onset Alzheimer's disease
Proliferation	Capacity of cells to divide
Promyelocyte	A precursor cell in the granulocyte series that produces certain types of white blood cells
Prophylaxis	Preventive care; medical intervention that prevents disease

Proteinuria	Protein in the urine; normally, there should be no protein in urine
Proteomics	The study of proteins, their structures, and their functions
Proto-oncogene	Normal gene that regulates cell proliferation and differentiation; mutated forms of proto-oncogenes called oncogenes lead to cancer
PSA	Prostate specific antigen; a protein normally secreted by the prostate gland; elevated levels in the blood may signal cancer
Pseudodisease	Small lesions that are not destined to develop into disease requiring treatment; e.g., DCIS in the female breast
Pulmonary edema	Excessive fluid in the lungs
Quiescent cells	Dormant cells that do not cycle through the cell cycle
Radiation therapy	Use of high-energy radiation to treat cancer; often combined with surgery and chemotherapy
Reductionism	View that studying component parts of a system explains the system; a complex system is the sum of its parts
Redundancy	More than one component or network of components performs the same function in a complex system; the genetic code is redundant because more than one codon may code for the same amino acid
Resting membrane potential	Membrane potential of a cell at rest; cell interior is negative to the exterior due to the slow leakage of potassium ions out of the cell
Risk factor	Factor that is correlated with disease incidence but not a cause of the disease; e.g., age is a risk factor for cancer
Robustness	Property that permits a complex system to maintain its functions despite internal and external perturbations; can involve activation of other components of the system when another element is disabled
Saltatory conduction	Jumping movement of action potentials along axons from one node of Ranvier to the next
Senescence	Accumulation of detrimental changes in cells and tissues with passage of time; the process of aging
Sensitivity	In diagnostic tests the percentage of people with disease who test positive for the disease; true-positive rate of the test
Sign	Objective assessment of disease usually detected by a physician on physical examination or by clinical test
Solute	Atoms or molecules dissolved in a solvent creating a solution; in living systems solutes include ions, small molecules, and large proteins

Solvent	Substance that dissolves solutes; in living systems the solvent is water
Specificity	In diagnostic and screening tests the percentage of healthy persons who test negative for the disease; true negative rate of the test
SSRIs	Selective serotonin reuptake inhibitors; a class of antidepressants that act to increase serotonin levels
Statins	Class of drugs that lower blood cholesterol levels by inhibiting liver enzyme HMG-CoA reductase, which is important in production of low-density lipoprotein cholesterol; used in the treatment of coronary artery disease
Steady state	Properties of a system that do not change over time; in living systems, maintenance of the steady state requires input of energy
Stem cell	An unspecialized cell with the capacity for self-renewal and differentiation; embryonic stem cells have the capacity to become any tissue in the body; adult stem cells can generate only certain types of tissues
Stochastic	A process characterized by random behavior governed by probabilities
Stroma	Connective, supportive framework of tissues and organs
Superposition	A principle in quantum theory that an electron or other particle exists simultaneously in a number of states; when the particle is measured, only one of the states is observed.
Sympathetic nervous system	Part of the autonomic nervous system; maintains homeostasis; mediates flight-or-fight response; works in opposition to the parasympathetic nervous system
Symptom	Subjective experience of the patient as reported to the physician
Synergy	The effect of combined agents is greater than the sum of effects of the individual agents
System	Set of interacting elements forming an integrative whole; whether a system is simple or complex is determined in part by the nature and interdependence of system components, including the relative numbers of network nodes and edges
Tamoxifen	An estrogen anatagonist that blocks estrogen receptors; prescribed for the treatment and prevention of hormone receptor positive breast cancer
Tau protein	Proteins that stabilize microtubules in the cell; biochemical changes in tau proteins result in neurofibrillary tangles in nerve cells leading to Alzheimer's and other neurodegenerative diseases

Telomeres	Region of repetitive DNA at the ends of chromosomes that serve a protective function; telomere dysfunction is associated with aging and cancer
Therapy	Medical intervention that seeks to cure disease or reduce signs and symptoms of disease
Thrombus	Blood clot that can impede blood flow in the heart or in a blood vessel
Tumorigenesis	Development of a tumor
Tumor-suppressor gene	Class of cancer genes that causes loss of proliferative control of cells
Turgor pressure	Osmotic pressure exerted against cell walls that gives plants the ability to stand upright
Vascular resistance	Resistance to flow of blood in peripheral arteries
Vasomotor nerves	Motor nerves that cause dilation or contraction of blood vessels
Villi	Small, finger-like projections in the intestine that greatly increase absorptive area for nutrients
Vitalism	Doctrine ascribing the functions of a living organism to a vital principle distinct from chemical and physical forces
Voltage-gated membrane channel	Channel protein that opens or closes in response to a change in the local membrane potential
Waste energy	Portion of available energy that cannot be used to do work; e.g., waste heat

NOTES

Preface

1. Not all complex systems behave unpredictably. A timepiece is complex, but timekeeping is predictable. Living systems, however, are complex in both structure and function. Functional complexity is nonlinear, and chaotic behavior leads to emergent properties.
2. The sentence is borrowed from Theodosius Dobzhansky, who claimed in 1964, "nothing in biology makes sense except in the light of evolution." This volume argues evolution is a dimension of complexity.

Chapter 1

1. Laplace P-S. *A Philosophical Essay on Probabilities*, translated into English from the original French 6th ed. by Truscott FW and Emory FL. New York: Wiley; 1902:4.
2. Poincaré H. *Science and Method*. London: Nelson; 1908:68.
3. The idea for the racing analogy comes from Nate Silver's discussion of chaos theory and weather predictions. Silver N. *The Signal and the Noise*. New York: Penguin Press; 2012.
4. Descartes R. *Discourse on Method and Meditations*, translated by Lafleur LJ. New York: The Liberal Arts Press; 1960.
5. Some theological views take a different perspective and hold that humans occupy the center of the Universe and are made in God's image. The rationalization of scientific and religious views about the place of humans on Earth and in the Universe has been the subject of much scholarship for centuries. However, this topic is beyond the scope of this book.
6. What makes humans unique among mammalian species does not necessarily define what makes us human. See Gazzaniga MS. *Human: The Science Behind What Makes Us Unique*. New York: HarperCollins; 2008.
7. Two other key characteristics of life are important at the population and species level but are not critical to the functioning and survival of the individual. In a population context, individual organisms must be able to reproduce their own kind to sustain population growth and species survival. Evolution is characteristic of populations and, through the processes of genetic mutation and natural selection, results in subtle changes in organisms to maximize lifetime reproductive success as environmental conditions change. Thus, reproduction and Darwinian evolution operate at the population level. Survival of an individual organism does not require that the organism be reproductively intact or respond to evolutionary pressures.
8. Important differences exist between prokaryotic cells (e.g., bacteria) and eukaryotic cells (e.g., human cells). Unlike prokaryotes, eukaryotic cells have a cell nucleus and a highly compartmentalized cytoplasm that serves to separate specialized cell functions. Nevertheless, key biological processes, including protein synthesis and glucose metabolism, are similar.
9. Gibson DG, et al. Creation of a bacterial cell controlled by a chemically synthesized genome. *Science* 2010;329:52–56.

10. Changeux, JP. *Neuronal Man*. Princeton, NJ: Princeton University Press; 1985. Changes in the genome (mutations) lead to either death or severe dysfunction; very few viable mutations are passed on from generation to generation that would result in visible structural changes. This means that human beings today are the same as human beings five hundred years ago (genetic determinism assures invariance of structure).

11. Viruses are simpler but are not considered to be living in the sense that bacteria and higher-order cells and multicellular organisms are. Viruses can only replicate their genetic machinery by infecting living cells and using those cells as a platform for replication. Out of the cell, viruses are inert organic entities that are made up of RNA or DNA encased in a protein coat.

12. Death in the context of the decay of steady-state to equilibrium conditions is consistent with the legal and medical definitions of death—an individual who has sustained either (1) irreversible cessation of circulatory and respiratory functions or (2) irreversible cessation of all functions of the entire brain, including the brain stem. See Uniform Definition of Death Act of 1980, which was approved by the American Medical Association in 1980 and by the American Bar Association in 1981.

13. The energy flow density is calculated by dividing the energy flow through the organ by the organ weight and assumes a 70-kg man and average daily caloric intake of 2,000 kcal. The organ weight correction is necessary because energy flow (joules/second) is dependent on organ size. The resting state is defined as a cardiac output of 5 L per minute; during exercise, cardiac output is assumed to increase to 25 L per minute.

14. The term *homeostasis* was first coined by Harvard physiologist Walter B. Cannon in 1932. See Cannon WB. *The Wisdom of the Body*. New York: W.W. Norton; 1932. The idea that multicellular organisms have an internal environment isolated from the external environment was first introduced by Claude Bernard in the nineteenth century.

15. Cell renewal systems include the skin, small intestine, and bone marrow. Other tissues, notably the brain and skeletal muscle, have no renewal capacity.

16. Germ cells in the female ovary and male testis divide by meiosis, a process resulting in the introduction of genetic variability in the gametes (egg and sperm). This genetic variability is responsible for phenotypic differences observable in siblings from the same father and mother.

17. Schrödinger E. *What Is Life?* Cambridge: Cambridge University Press; 1944.

18. Davies P. *The Cosmic Blueprint*. Philadelphia: Templeton Foundation Press; 1988.

Chapter 2

1. Theories are different from laws. In the philosophical sense, "theory" is used to suggest there is room for reasonable doubt, whereas "law" suggests that there is ample supportive evidence and that the law may be accepted without further debate. For a further discussion of laws of nature, seeCartwright NB. *How the Laws of Physics Lie*. Oxford: Clarendon Press; 1983;Davies P. *The Mind of God*. New York: Simon and Schuster; 1992;Mitchell S. *Unsimple Truths: Science, Complexity and Policy*. Chicago: University of Chicago Press; 2009.

2. The era of modern physics was launched at the beginning of the twentieth century with Albert Einstein's theories of relativity and the introduction of quantum theory.

3. For a detailed discussion of determinism and the classical laws of physics, see Davies P. *The Cosmic Blueprint*. Philadelphia: Templeton Foundation Press; 1988; and Prigogine I. *The End of Certainty: Time, Chaos and the New Laws of Nature*. New York: Free Press; 1996.

4. Davies, *The Cosmic Blueprint*.

5. The diminution in blood pressure in a given patient cannot be predicted very well because of individual variations in drug sensitivities. Control of blood pressure solely by adjusting blood volume further assumes absence of significant comorbidities. Antidiuretic drugs do not work in every patient with high blood pressure for a number of reasons. Some patients do not respond well to these drugs. In other patients, the high blood pressure is due to medical reasons unrelated to water retention and high blood volume. Management of hypertension can be challenging and often requires a multiple drug strategy.

6. The human brain has a computational capacity of about 1,015 operations per second, based on the number of synapses in the human brain and nerve impulse firing rate. Although no desktop computer can approach this capability, massive parallel computers are now approaching human brain capacity. SeeMoravec N. When will computer hardware match the human brain? *Journal of Evolution and Technology* 1998;1:1–12.

7. The zeroeth law establishes the concept of temperature, and the third law establishes a barrier that prevents reaching a temperature of absolute zero. An excellent primer on the four laws of thermodynamics is provided in Atkins P. *Four Laws That Drive the Universe.* New York: Oxford University Press; 2007.

8. The extracellular and intracellular environments actually contain many different types of ions and molecules, but only sodium ions are considered here to facilitate discussion of diffusion.

9. Eddington AS. *The Nature of the Physical World.* Cambridge: Cambridge University Press; 1928; Snow CP. *The Two Cultures: And a Second Look.* Cambridge: Cambridge University Press; 1959; Davies, *The Mind of God.*

10. Schrödinger, E. *What Is Life? The Physical Aspect of the Living Cell.* Cambridge: Cambridge University Press; 1944. The structure of DNA as the heritable material in cells and the deciphering of the genetic code were essentially completed by the early 1960s.

11. For further discussions on the arrow of time, see Davies, *Cosmic Blueprint*; Prigogine, *The End of Certainty*; Schneider ED, Sagan D. *Into the Cool: Energy Flow, Thermodynamics, and Life.* Chicago: University of Chicago Press; 2005.

12. Norbert Weiner refers to the second law of thermodynamics in discussing establishment of enclaves of systems and order in a moral and chaotic universe. These enclaves will not remain there indefinitely by any momentum of their own. In a similar vein the order established in living systems cannot be sustained indefinitely without import of energy. Wiener N. *I Am a Mathematician: The Later Life of a Prodigy.* Cambridge, MA: MIT Press; 1964.

13. For further discussions on the validity of physical laws and how laws may fail in their predictions, see Cartwright, *How the Laws of Physics Lie*; and Mitchell, *Unsimple Truths.*

14. System conditions include whether the object is moving through air or a vacuum. If the object is moving through air, frictional forces need to be accounted for. The initial velocity of the object is also a system condition. If the object is moving at a velocity very close to the speed of light, Newton's second law is invalid because of relativistic considerations that result in an increase in the mass of the object.

15. Groopman JE. *How Doctors Think.* Boston: Houghton Mifflin; 2007.

16. In his essay "Is Everything Determined?" Stephen Hawking discusses the problem of free will and the difficulties in predicting human behavior. Physical laws cannot predict behavior because the equations cannot be solved. Even if they could be solved, the act of making a prediction disturbs the system. Hawking S. *Black Holes and Baby Universes and Other Essays.* New York: Bantam Books; 1994.

17. McKane AJ, Nagy JD, Newman TJ, Stefanini MO. Amplified biochemical oscillations in cellular systems. *Journal of Statistical Physics* 2007;128:165–191.

Chapter 3

1. Almost immediately following Tchaikovsky's demise, the cause of death was questioned. While his death has traditionally been attributed to cholera, some scholars have theorized he committed suicide or was poisoned. See Poznansky A. *Tchaikovsky's Last Days: A Documentary Study.* Oxford: Clarendon Press; 1996.

2. Cholera remains among the most feared diarrheal diseases because it can lead to dehydration and death within hours following infection. The disease has an incubation period of only 24–48 hours. Symptoms of cholera begin with painless, watery diarrhea that may often be followed by vomiting. Only two hundred cases have been reported in the United States since 1973, and most cases have occurred among those traveling to the United States from cholera-affected communities or who have eaten food from affected communities. While the

disease is no longer an issue in countries where minimum hygiene and food and water safety standards are met, it remains a threat in almost every developing country. Cholera is most prevalent, but not limited to, areas such as the Middle East, Africa, and Southeast Asia. In 2010, about 310,000 cases were identified worldwide. Only 10 percent of people infected with *Vibrio cholerae* have life-threatening signs and symptoms. Most infected persons experience only mild diarrhea and vomiting. In the 10 percent of cases with life-threatening disease, excessive dehydration due to diarrhea can lead to low blood pressure, reduced blood perfusion to major organs, cardiac fibrillation, and possibly death. Fluid and electrolyte replacement and antibiotics are first-line therapies for cholera. For further details about cholera, seeBroeck D, Horvath C, et al. Vibrio cholerae: cholera toxin. *International Journal of Biochemistry and Cell Biology* 2007;39:1771–1775;Debasish S, Karim M, et al. Single-dose Azithromycin for the treatment of cholera in adults. *New England Journal of Medicine* 2006;354:2452–2462;Zuckerman J, Rombo L, Fisch A. The true burden and risk of cholera: implications for prevention and control. *Lancet Infectious Diseases* 2007;7:521–530;World Health Organization. *World Health Statistics—2012*. Geneva: WHO Press; 2012.

3. Bullock TH, Orkand R, Grinnell A. *Introduction to Nervous Systems*. New York: W. H. Freeman; 1977.

4. James Clerk Maxwell formulated the theory of electromagnetism associated with the movement of electric charges. An electric current is generated by the motion of any charged atom or molecule.

5. The cell membrane is complex and contains phospholipids that easily allow nonpolar molecules through, but not polar molecules. Phospholipids are long-chain fatty acids with a water-soluble phosphate group capping one end. For technical information on how membranes are penetrated, see Sadava D, Hillis DM, Heller C, Berenbaum MR. *Life: The Science of Biology*. 9th ed. Sunderland, MA: Sinauer Associates/Freeman; 2011:105–145.

6. Fick's law of diffusion summarizes our intuitive understanding of diffusion and can be used to describe diffusion across a cell membrane barrier. Fick's law states the rate of diffusion is directly proportional to the concentration gradient and membrane permeability. In Figure 3.1, the slope of the straight line is a measure of membrane permeability—the steeper the slope the more permeable is the membrane and the faster diffusion occurs. Diffusion is fundamentally a process based on random, microscopic movements of molecules (sometimes referred to as Brownian motion). Since solute molecules are more energetic at higher temperatures, when temperature and solubility characteristics remain constant, the concentration gradient is the major determinant of diffusion rate. Berg HC. *Random Walks in Biology*. Princeton, NJ: Princeton University Press; 1993.

7. Energizing pumps is metabolically expensive. The human brain accounts for 20 percent of resting oxygen consumption, and 50 percent of the ATP produced by brain cells is used to run sodium and other pumps that exchange sodium, potassium, and other ions across cell membranes necessary to generate electrical activity in the brain. Laughlin SB, de Ruyter van Steveninck RR, Anderson JC. The metabolic cost of neural information. *Nature Neuroscience* 1998;1:36–41.

8. Dependence on the number of solute molecules rather than on the chemical and physical characteristics of the solute molecules is a colligative property of solutions. Colligative properties are observed in dilute solutions and include osmotic pressure, boiling point elevation, freezing point depression, and vapor pressure.

9. Van't Hoff's law (derived from the ideal gas laws) predicts osmotic pressure at a given temperature and solute concentration. To apply this law, it is assumed aqueous solutions are very dilute, and van't Hoff's law predicts osmotic pressures almost exactly. If more concentrated solutions are involved, correction factors can be applied to improve van't Hoff predictions. Lachish U. Osmosis and thermodynamics. *American Journal of Physics* 2007;75:997–998.

10. Tonicity refers to the solute concentration of the extracellular environment relative to that of the intracellular environment. A solution is hypertonic if the solute concentration is higher outside than inside the cell. The solution is hypotonic if the solute concentration is lower than inside the cell. An isotonic or balanced solution has the same solute concentration

outside as the inside of the cell. Cell volume and water content are critical to cell function. SeeRitz P, Salle A, Simard G, et al. Effects of changes in water compartments on physiology and metabolism. *European Journal of Clinical Nutrition* 2003;57(Suppl 2): S2–S5.

11. Renal physiology is complex. For a complete discussion of how the kidneys balance water and electrolytes, see Sadava et al., *Life*, or other college-level introductory biology texts. Diabetes insipidus is pathophysiologically unrelated to the more common diabetes mellitus. The diseases have the same name because of the common signs and symptoms of excessive urination (polyuria) and excessive thirst (polydipsia).

12. Alon U. *An Introduction to Systems Biology: Design Principles of Biological Circuits.* Boca Raton, FL: Chapman & Hall/CRC Press; 2007.

13. The Goldman equation considers all permeable ions in calculating the membrane potential based on the electrochemical gradient contributions of each ion. The Nernst equation is a special case and calculates the equilibrium potential for a single permeable ion based on the electrochemical gradient across the cell membrane. The electrochemical gradient is the combination of the chemical gradient due to the difference in chemical concentration across the cell membrane and the electrical gradient due to the imbalance in charge across the cell membrane. Currents in cell membranes are different from electric currents found in electronic devices like cell phones or toaster ovens. In cells, the current is due to the movement of various charge-carrying ionic species. Current in electronic devices results from the movement of electrons.

14. The membrane resting potential is not constant but oscillates slowly about a central value that is determined by the Goldman equation.

15. Capacitors consist of a nonconducting material sandwiched between two conducting materials. In the cell membrane, the phospholipid is electrically nonconducting and separates the intracellular fluid from the extracellular fluid, which are both conducting. Energy is stored in the electrostatic field set up by the separation of charges.

16. The action potential is generated by a coordinated opening and closing of potassium and sodium channels. The action potential is another deterministic process. The rapid influx of sodium depolarized the membrane. The maximum voltage achieved is approximated by the equilibrium potential for sodium as predicted by the Goldman equation. In some instances, calcium ions take the place of sodium ions in generating action potential.

17. MacKinnon R. Potassium channels. *Federation of European Biochemical Societies Letters* 2003;555:62–65.

18. Heavner JE. Local anesthetics. *Current Opinion in Anaesthesiology* 2007;20:336–342.

19. Huxley AF, Stämpfli R. Evidence for saltatory conduction in peripheral myelinated nerve fibres. *J Physiol.* 1949;108:315–339. For a general discussion of neurophysiology, see Sadava et al., *Life*.

20. Approximately two million people worldwide have multiple sclerosis (MS). There are twice as many cases in women as in men, for reasons that are not completely understood. Multiple sclerosis is the leading cause of nontraumatic neurologic disability in young adults in the United States and Europe. The hallmark of the acute MS lesion, inflammatory demyelination, has been largely accepted as evidence of a macrophage-mediated attack on normal myelin. The autoimmune attack causes distinct lesions in the central nervous system. The causes of the disease are not fully understood but are believed to include genetic and environmental factors, such as exposure to Epstein Barr virus, vitamin D deficiency, and metabolic causes. There is no cure for MS, but therapies are available to retard disease progression and reduce severity of symptoms. SeeDutta R, Trapp BD. Pathogenesis of axonal and neuronal damage in multiple sclerosis. *Neurology* 2007;68(22, Suppl. 3):S22–S31.

21. Electrical synapses are much faster than synapses that involve neurotransmitters and are found in reflex pathways that must be very fast. Unlike neurotransmitter-based synapses, there is no signal gain, and the signal gets weaker as it moves across the synaptic gap. Neurotransmitter synapses, the more common type, are more complex and vary their signal strengths. Kandel ER, Schwartz JH, Jessell TM. *Principles of Neural Science.* 4th ed. New York: McGraw-Hill; 2000.

22. Neurotransmitters must be cleared from the synaptic cleft quickly. Otherwise, depolarization or hyperpolarization occurs continuously. Neurotransmitter levels are controlled by reuptake mechanisms, diffusion out of the synaptic cleft, or enzymatic degradation. Changeux JP. *Neuronal Man*. Princeton, NJ: Princeton University Press; 1985; Changeux JP. Chemical signaling in the brain. *Scientific American* 1993;269(5):58–62.

23. Correcting neurological and behavioral abnormalities by adjusting levels of neurotransmitters in the brain is challenging. Conceptually, it is difficult to appreciate how simple neurochemical adjustments can lead to predictable outcomes in complex systems. Patients do not respond in the same way, and treatment efficacy may be dependent on severity of disease. It is not surprising, therefore, that the efficacy of SSRIs is disputed. In one recent report that analyzed a number of previously published clinical studies, benefits of antidepressant medications could not be clearly demonstrated in patients with mild or moderate symptoms; therapeutic benefits, however, appear substantial in patients with severe depression. Fournier JC, DeRubeis RJ, Hollon SD, et al. Antidepressant drug effects and depression severity. *Journal of the American Medical Association* 2010;303(1):47–53.

24. Skeletal muscle contraction and relaxation are complex processes. Hundreds of thousands of muscle fibers bundle together to make up skeletal muscle. Each muscle is made up of long bundles of myofibrils that are tightly packed together in a parallel fashion. Myofibrils are contractile units in a highly ordered arrangement of longitudinal myofilaments composed of actin and myosin. Together, they produce movement by contraction through the sliding filament model. In the relaxed muscle, actin and myosin do not overlap each other. But when a nerve impulse stimulates the muscle, contraction occurs by pulling these proteins next to each other. Because this occurs in every myofibril, the entire muscle will shorten, allowing it to move the bones to which it is attached. For a current review of muscle physiology, see Davies KE, Nowak KJ. Molecular mechanisms of muscular dystrophies: old and new players. *Nature Reviews Molecular Cell Biology* 2006;7:762–773.

25. Newton's first law of motion, the law of inertia, states that a body at rest remains at rest unless acted upon by an external force, while a body in motion remains so unless acted upon by an external force. An arm resting at someone's side will remain there unless the person voluntarily contracts and relaxes muscles in the arm to raise the arm. The arm moves because the force generated by the movement of muscles exceeds the arm's inertia or tendency to remain at rest. Newton's second law is the law of acceleration and relates acceleration to force. The second law is commonly expressed as *force equals mass times acceleration*. The second law can be interpreted to mean it takes a lesser force to move a lighter body. If two bodies with different masses are subject to the same force, the lighter body will move first. Newton's first law is a special case of the second law. A body moving at constant velocity (zero acceleration) exerts no force and will remain in motion at constant velocity until a force acts on the body. But in our everyday experiences, masses moving at constant velocity do not stay in motion forever as predicted by Newton's first law. Every moving object will tend to slow down and stop because of external forces like friction and gravitation. To keep a mass moving requires application of an external force to overcome the natural forces that tend to slow down and stop the body. A boxer who knocks out his opponent with a left hook invokes the second law (although he probably does not know it!). The left arm and boxing glove accelerate rapidly as the punch is thrown. When the boxing glove contacts the opponent's jaw, there is a rapid deceleration of the arm and glove, and the resulting force is transferred to the opponent's jaw, resulting in a knockout. Newton's third law is the law of action and reaction. A body will remain stationary as long as forces acting on the body in one direction are countered by equal forces acting on the body in the opposite direction. A 2-kg object held by a person with the arm fully extended will remain stationary as long as the upward force exerted by the person's arm exactly counters the weight. When these opposing forces are in equilibrium, the object remains stationary. But in time, the arms fatigue, and the object drops to the floor because the upward force cannot counter the gravitational downward force.

26. The ECF compartment represents all the water outside cells. Most of total body water is found inside cells. The ECF accounts for about 33 percent of total body water; intracellular water accounts for 67 percent. See Sadava et al., *Life*.

27. Capillaries in the brain do not have pores. The tight capillary walls are part of the blood-brain barrier that protects the brain from exposure to toxins.

28. For detailed discussions of hydrostatic pressure and osmotic pressure in the capillary bed, see, for instance, Jenkins GW, Kemnitz CP, Tortora GJ. *Anatomy and Physiology: From Science to Life*. New York: Wiley; 2007; Sadava et al., *Life*.

29. As discussed in chapter 2, most of the energy generated by the body is dissipated as waste heat. Of the 125 watts generated by the body at rest, only about 25 watts are used by the body to do useful work. The remaining 100 watts is dissipated as heat equivalent to the output of an ordinary light bulb. The human body is equivalent to a mechanical engine operating at 20 percent efficiency. The brain generates more power than any other organ. The 20 watts of power is extraordinary given that the brain is only 2 percent of total body mass.

30. Blood volume also contributes to peripheral vascular resistance. To maintain blood flow, blood pressure is increased to compensate for increased system resistance. An important class of medications to reduce high blood pressure reduces the water content of the blood. Diuretics act on the kidney to reduce blood volume by enhancing water loss.

31. McCall RP. *Physics of the Human Body*. Baltimore: Johns Hopkins University Press; 2010. The blood also contains white blood cells and platelets, but these cell types represent a tiny fraction of total blood cellularity.

32. Alyeska Pipeline Service Co. *Facts: Trans Alaska Pipeline System '09* (PDF). Alyeska Pipeline Service Co., 2009. Available at http://alyeska-pipe.com/TAPS/PipelineFacts.

33. Nickerson CA, Ott CM, Mister SJ, et al. Microgravity as a novel environmental signal affecting Salmonella enterica serovar Typhimurium virulence. *Infection and Immunity* 2000;68:3147–3152; Newman SA. Physico-genetic determinants in the evolution of development. *Science* 2012;338:217–219.

34. Martin M. Does homeostatic pressure explain tumor growth? *Journal of the National Cancer Institute* 2009;101:914–915.

Chapter 4

1. Some lower life forms have the capacity to reverse the aging process. Tiny jellyfish age in reverse by growing younger and younger until the earliest stages of development are reached, and then the life cycle begins anew. The "immortal" jellyfish can transform itself from any stage in its development. This transformation potential is not observed in higher life forms, including humans, and is unparalleled in the animal kingdom.Piraino S, et al. Reversing the life cycle: medusae transforming into polyps and cell transdifferentiation in *Turritopsis nutricula* (Cnidaria, Hydrozoa). *Biological Bulletin* 1996;190:302–312.

2. The biosphere is a cornucopia of complexity that demonstrates an arrow of time. Organic evolution has led to the emergence of increasingly complex life forms from simple bacteria to multicellular organisms. Complexity is one-directional, forward. There is no evidence of reverse evolution whereby simple life comes from more complex life. Neo-Darwinism is an important theory in biology that has been remarkably successful in explaining the evolution of species in the past through processes of mutation-driven genetic variation and natural selection, but Darwinian theory is historical, not predictive. The theory cannot explain the increase in biological complexity evident in the biosphere. For further discussions of the arrow of time metaphor, see Davies P. *The Cosmic Blueprint*. Philadelphia: Templeton Foundation Press; 1988; Progogine I. *The End of Certainty: Time, Chaos and the New Laws of Nature*. New York: The Free Press; 1996; Chaisson EJ. *Cosmic Evolution: The Rise of Complexity in Nature*. Cambridge, MA: Harvard University Press; 2001.

3. Complex behaviors can occur in simple systems as well as complex ones. A simple pendulum can exhibit unpredictable and complex behaviors when the pendulum swings in a very large arc. The key to complex behavior is not the macrostructure or function of the system but whether the system exhibits nonlinear dynamical behavior.

4. Equilibrium, near-equilibrium, and far-from equilibrium conditions are discussed in detail in Davies, *Cosmic Blueprint*;Kaufman S. *At Home in the Universe*. New York: Oxford University Press; 1995; Progogine, *End of Certainty*; Schneider ED, Sagan D. *Into the Cool: Energy Flow, Thermodynamics, and Life*. Chicago: University of Chicago Press; 2005.

5. In this discussion, we focus on properties of complexity relevant to human biology. Other interesting properties of complexity are seen elsewhere in nature. Insect colonies like ants, bees, or termites provide a spectacular demonstration of the interplay between co-operation and competition. For a tour of the diversity of complex systems, seeMitchell M. *Complexity: A Guided Tour*. New York: Oxford University Press; 2009. The comment attributable to Gell-Mann was taken from Schneider and Sagan, *Into the Cool*, 23.

6. Life feeds on negative entropy and is "order from order." See Schrödinger E. *What Is Life?* Cambridge: Cambridge University Press; 1944.

7. For more on system complexity and information content, see Davies, *Cosmic Blueprint*.

8. The butterfly effect is attributable to E. Lorenz. For an excellent overview of chaos and applications in medicine and physiology, see Gleick J. *Chaos: Making a New Science*. New York: Penguin Books; 1987.

9. Glass L and Mackey MC. *From Clocks to Chaos: The Rhythms of Life*. Princeton NJ: Princeton University Press; 1988:36–56.

10. Goldberger AL, et al. Fractal dynamics in physiology: alterations with disease and aging. *Proceedings of the National Academy of Sciences* 2002;99(Suppl. 1):2466–2472.For an excellent introduction to fractals, see Gleick, *Chaos*.

11. Weibel ER. What makes a good lung? *Swiss Medical Weekly* 2009;139:375–386.

12. Rzhetsky A, et al. Probing genetic overlap among complex human phenotypes. *Proceedings of the National Academy of Sciences* 2007; 104:11694–11699.

13. Human cancer is a collection of more than one hundred separate diseases characterized by the abnormal growth and spread of abnormal cells. Control of cell proliferation is lost, in part, because key signaling networks that serve a growth regulatory function have been inactivated. Kleinsmith provides an excellent overview of the molecular biology of cancer. See Kleinsmith LJ. *Principles of Cancer Biology*. San Francisco: Pearson Benjamin Cummings; 2006.

14. *MYC* is a member of a class of cancer genes called oncogenes. Oncogenes are mutated forms of proto-oncogenes that are normal constituents of the human genome controlling cellular growth and proliferation.

15. Ecker JR. ENCODE explained. *Nature* 2012;489:52–53 (four other brief papers describing the ENCODE project immediately follow); The ENCODE Project Consortium. An integrated encyclopedia of DNA elements in the human genome. *Nature* 2012;489:57–74.

16. Glass and Mackey, *From Clock to Chaos*.

17. Uncertainty derives from quantum mechanics and the Heisenberg uncertainty principle. All properties of a system cannot be completely known. Werner Heisenberg developed the uncertainty principle based on studies of particle motion. A particle can be completely described by its position and momentum, but if the particle's momentum is known exactly, its position can only be estimated. Conversely, complete knowledge of position means the particle's momentum cannot be known exactly. A fundamental tenet of quantum mechanics is that measuring a property of a physical system always disturbs it.

18. Causal mechanisms are well understood for some complex diseases (for example, solar UV-induced skin cancer) but poorly understood for others (for example, brain cancers and Alzheimer's disease). Spontaneous disease rates are highly variable. More than 90 percent of female breast cancer and prostate cancer have no known causal factors. About 10 percent of lung cancer occurs spontaneously; see American Cancer Society. *Cancer Facts and Figures—2012*. Atlanta, GA: American Cancer Society; 2012. DNA damage is an important common element in natural and environmental cancer. DNA damage occurs spontaneously, and the frequency of damage is increased with environmental exposure. DNA damage in radiation carcinogenesis has been particularly well studied. See Billen D. Spontaneous DNA damage and its significance for the "negligible dose" controversy in radiation protection. *Radiation Research* 1990;124:242–245.

19. For further reading on chaos, linear dynamics, and complexity in medicine, see Glass and Mackey, *From Clock to Chaos*; West BJ. *Fractal Physiology and Chaos in Medicine*. Singapore: World Scientific Publishing; 1990; Goldberger AL. Non-linear dynamics for clinicians: chaos theory, fractals, and complexity at the bedside. *Lancet* 1996;347:1312–1314; Goldberger et al., Fractal dynamics in physiology; Lipsitz LA, Goldberger AL. Loss of

"complexity" and aging: potential applications of fractals and chaos theory in senescence. *Journal of the American Medical Association* 2002;267:1806–1809.

20. Goldberger AL, et al. What is physiological complexity and how does it change with aging and disease? *Neurobiology of Aging* 2002;23:23–26.

21. The PSA test has been called into question as a screening tool for prostate cancer in the general male population because the test does not reduce prostate cancer mortality and has a high false-positive rate, necessitating additional tests and procedures in some patients. See Welch HG. *Should I Be Tested for Cancer?* Berkeley: University of California Press; 2004; Chou R, Croswell JM, Dana T, et al. Screening for prostate cancer: a review of the evidence for the U.S. Preventive Services Task Force. *Annals of Internal Medicine* 2011;155:762–771.

Chapter 5

1. The constancy of the internal environment is a unifying principle of physiology: "The fixity of the milieu supposes a perfection of the organism such that the external variations are at each instant compensated for and equilibrated.... The stability of the internal environment is the condition for the free and independent life." Bernard C. *Lectures on the Phenomena of Life Common to Animals and Plants*, translated by Hoff HE, Guillemin R, and Guillemin L. Springfield, IL: Charles C. Thomas Publishers; 1974:190. Original publication: 1878.

2. For good general discussions of complexity and its applications to biology, seeNicolis G, Prigogine I. *Exploring Complexity: An Introduction*. New York: Freeman; 1989;Kauffman S. *At Home in the Universe: The Search for the Laws of Self-Organization and Complexity*. New York: Oxford University Press; 1995.

3. The range of normal for each test in Table 5.1 reflects interindividual variation among measurements in a large group of healthy individuals in the population. The normal range for most physiological parameters varies considerably because of differences in age, gender, ethnicity, and location. Koeppen BM, Stantop BA. *Renal Physiology*. 4th ed. Philadelphia: Elsevier; 2007:183.

4. Posttherapy changes in PSA have been associated with improved survival in patients. However, the relationship between PSA levels and response to treatment has not been firmly established owing to the fact the disease is complex and not all treatment effects are attributable to declining PSA levels. See Fleming MT, Morris MJ, Heller G, et al. Post-therapy changes in PSA as an outcome measure in prostate cancer clinical trials. *Nature Clinical Practice Oncology* 2006;3:658–667.

5. Claude Bernard and Walter Cannon were two of the major players in the early development of physiology as a basic medical science, in particular, the development of the concept of homeostasis. The text discussions of Bernard and Cannon were taken from the following sources: Cannon WB. *The Wisdom of the Body*. New York: Norton; 1932; Cross CJ, Albury WR. Walter B. Cannon, L. J. Henderson and the organic analogy. *Osiris* 2nd ser;1987;3:165–192; Gross CG. Claude Bernard and the constancy of the internal environment. *Neuroscientist* 1998;4:380–385.

6. Wiener N. *Cybernetics or Control and Communication in the Animal and the Machine*. Cambridge, MA: MIT Press; 1961. Original publication: 1948.

7. McEwen B, Lasley EN. *The End of Stress as We Know It*. Washington, DC: Joseph Henry Press; 2002.

8. Nicolis and Prigogine, *Exploring Complexity*; Macklem PT. Emergent phenomena and the secrets of life. *Journal of Applied Physiology* 2008;104:1844–1846.

9. For a provocative discussion of sensory timing and perception, see Eagleman DM. Brain time. In Brockman M, ed. *What's Next? Dispatches on the Future of Science*. New York: Vintage Books; 2009:155–169.

10. See any introductory college chemistry textbook for a discussion of buffers, equilibrium reactions, and pH. Recall that pH is on a logarithmic scale. The hydrogen ion concentration $[H^+]$ is 10 times higher at pH 6 than at pH 7.

11. Other buffers perform a more minor role in regulating the pH of the blood. The phosphate buffer consists of phosphoric acid (H_3PO_4) in equilibrium with dihydrogen phosphate ion ($H_2PO_4^-$) and H^+. Hemoglobin also acts as a pH buffer in the blood. During exercise, hemoglobin helps control the pH of the blood by binding some of the excess hydrogen ions that are generated in skeletal muscle. At the same time, molecular oxygen is released for use by the muscles.

12. Mackey MC, Glass L. Oscillation and chaos in physiological control systems. *Science* 1977;197:287–289.

13. There are numerous examples of oscillatory behavior in living systems. See for example, Mackey and Glass, Oscillation and chaos; Sturis J, Van Cauter E, Blackman JD, Polonsky KS. Entrainment of pulsatile insulin secretion by oscillatory glucose infusion. *Journal of Clinical Investigation* 1991;87:439–445; McKane AJ, Nagy JD, Newman TJ, Stefanini MO. Amplified biochemical oscillations in cellular systems. *Journal of Statistical Physics* 2007;128:165–191.

14. Changeux JP. *Neuronal Man*. Princeton, NJ: Princeton University Press; 1985:77–83.

15. For detailed discussions of robustness and degeneracy in complex biological systems, see Edelman GM, Gally JA. Degeneracy and complexity in biological systems. *Proceedings of the National Academy of Sciences* 2001;98:13763–13768; Mitchell SD. *Unsimple Truths: Science, Complexity, and Policy*. Chicago: University of Chicago Press; 2009.

16. Neural plasticity is a remarkable but poorly understood process. The loss of one function can be compensated by the gain in another function. A person who becomes blind may acquire a heightened sense of hearing. Gazzaniga MS. *The Ethical Brain*. New York: Dana Press; 2005; Rose S. *The Future of the Brain: The Promise and Perils of Tomorrow's Neuroscience*. New York: Oxford University Press; 2005.

17. McQuaid J, Schleifstein M. *Path of Destruction: The Devastation of New Orleans and the Coming Age of Superstorms*. New York: Little, Brown; 2006.

18. Table 5.2 shows the reserve capacity of selected physiologic systems as reflected by the difference between normal (homeostasis) and disease conditions that severely compromise normal function. Reserve capacity can also be defined in terms of the increased function in the physiologic system under exercise conditions. For example, the human lung has an excess gas exchange capacity of 1.5 during exercise compared to rest. See Weibel ER. What makes a good lung? *Swiss Medical Weekly* 2009;139:375–386.

19. Try this little experiment. Fill a jar with tap water, and place it on the kitchen table. Introduce a small quantity of food dye (a volume much smaller than the water volume), and let the jar sit undisturbed. After a short time, the dye is no longer visible because molecules are uniformly distributed in the water. Random behavior is not a new idea. Henri Poincaré, the French philosopher and mathematician, discussed these ideas at the turn of the twentieth century. See Poincaré. H. *Science and Method*. London: Nelson; 1908.

20. There are other routes of excretion. If the substance is excreted via the salivary glands or large intestines, concentrations in those tissues would have to be considered.

21. The amount of drug in the body is also determined by how the drug is formulated and how rapidly the drug is released into the bloodstream after ingestion.

22. Starfield B. Is US health really the best in the world? *Journal of the American Medical Association* 2000;284(4):483–485.

23. Ariga M. *Passions and Tempers: A History of the Humours*. New York: HarperCollins; 2007; Mukherjee S. *The Emperor of All Maladies: A Biography of Cancer*. New York: Scribner; 2010.

24. Mackey and Glass, Oscillation and chaos.

Chapter 6

1. Alvin Weinberg coined the word *trans-scientific* to describe technical problems that cannot be solved by science alone.Weinberg AM. Science and trans-science. *Minerva* 1972;10:209–222.

2. Vital signs include pulse or heart rate, respiration rate, blood pressure, and body temperature.

3. Half of all pregnancies in the United States result in prenatal or postnatal death or an otherwise less-than-healthy baby. Early pregnancy loss (during the first eight weeks of pregnancy) occurs in 20–30 percent of implantations. Spontaneous abortions (occurring at eight

to twenty weeks of pregnancy) occur in 10–20 percent of clinically recognized pregnancies. Minor developmental defects occur in about 15 percent of live births. Major congenital anomalies occur in 2–3 percent of live births. Chromosomal defects appear to be a major cause of spontaneous abortions and anatomical malformations. See National Research Council, Committee on Developmental Toxicology. *Scientific Frontiers in Developmental Toxicology and Risk Assessment.* Washington, DC: National Academy Press; 2000.

4. Welch HG, Black WC. Using autopsy series to estimate the disease "reservoir" for ductal carcinoma in situ of the breast: how much more breast cancer can we find? *Annals of Internal Medicine* 1997;127(11):1023–1028; Welch HG. *Should I Be Treated for Cancer?* Berkeley: University of California Press; 2004.

5. The *International Statistical Classification of Diseases and Related Health Problems* (ICD) is a medical classification by the World Health Organization and codes for diseases and a wide variety of signs, symptoms, abnormal findings, complaints, social circumstances, and external causes of injury or disease. Under this system, every health condition can be assigned to a category and given a code. Categories can include a set of similar diseases. World Health Organization. *ICD-10: International Statistical Classification of Diseases and Related Health Problems.* 10th rev ed. New York: World Health Organization; 2010.

6. This is particularly true for diseases with microbial etiologies. Only limited resources, even in wealthy countries like the United States, are available for disease-prevention programs. Allocating resources to get the biggest bang for the buck requires an understanding of national disease burdens, causal factors, and their interaction.

7. Patterson KD, Pyle GF. The geography and mortality of the 1918 influenza pandemic. *Bulletin of the History of Medicine* 1991;65(1):4–21.

8. Koch's postulates represent an important milestone in clinical microbiology. Nevertheless, their utility has significant limitations. Not all microbial diseases meet every Koch criterion. The recognized cause of cholera, *Vibrio cholerae,* can be isolated from both sick and healthy people, invalidating postulate (2). Viruses do not cause illness in all infected individuals, a requirement of postulate (1). For example, poliovirus causes paralytic disease in about 1 percent of those infected.

9. American Cancer Society. *Cancer Facts and Figures—2012.* Atlanta: American Cancer Society; 2012.

10. Mandelblatt JS, Cronin KA, Bailey S, et al. Effects of mammography screening under different screening schedules: model estimates of potential benefits and harms. *Annals of Internal Medicine* 2009;151:738–747.

11. Breast cancer is the most common cancer in American women. About 200,000 new cases are diagnosed each year. Approximately 20 percent of patients with breast cancer, or 40,000 women, are expected to die of their disease annually. American Cancer Society, *Cancer Facts and Figures—2012*; Bleyer A, Welch HG. Effect of three decades of screening mammography on breast cancer incidence. *New England Journal of Medicine* 2012;367:1998–2005.

12. Candidate cancer drugs go through three additional phases of clinical evaluation. Phase 2 is used to evaluate the activity of the drug against certain cancers and to establish dose-response. Phase 3 establishes the therapeutic effectiveness of the drug and the benefit-to-risk ratio. Phase 4 involves further development of the drug following marketing approval for the purposes of optimizing clinical utility and exploring activity in other cancer types.Sznol M. Drug development. In DeVita VT, Lawrence TS, Rosenberg SA, eds. *DeVita, Hellman and Rosenberg's Cancer Principles and Practice of Oncology.* 8th ed. Philadelphia: Lippincott Williams & Wilkins; 2008:385–392.

13. Saif MW, Chu E. Antimetabolites In DeVita VT, et al. *DeVita, Hellman and Rosenberg's Cancer Principles and Practice of Oncology*, 427–437.

14. Vioxx is the trade name for rofecoxib. Other nonsteroidal anti-inflammatory drugs, including ibuprofen, do not show elevated heart disease risk. Ray WA, Stein CM, Daugherty JR, et al. COX-2 selective non-steroidal anti-inflammatory drugs and risk of serious heart disease. *Lancet* 2002;360:1071–1073.

15. Lewis G. Some studies of social causes of and cultural response to disease. In: CGN Mascie-Taylor, ed. *The Anthropology of Disease*. Oxford: Oxford University Press; 1993:73–124.

16. Groopman J. *How Doctors Think*. Boston: Houghton Mifflin; 2007:209.

17. Dunlop D, Inch RS. Variations in pharmaceutical and medical practice in Europe. *British Medical Journal* 1972;3:749–752; Gillik MR. Medicine as ecoculture. *Annals of Internal Medicine* 2009;151:577–580.

18. Nessim S, Smith DS. Survivorship: obstacles and opportunities. In Dollinger M, Rosenbaum EH, Temparo M, Mulvihill SJ, eds. *Everyone's Guide to Cancer Therapy: How Cancer Is Diagnosed, Treated and Managed Day to Day*. Kansas City, MO: Andrews McMeel Publishing; 2002.

19. Payer L. *Medicine and Culture: Varieties of Treatment in the US, England, West Germany and France*. New York: Henry Holt; 1996; Gillik, Medicine as ecoculture.

20. Perceptions of disease risk differ culturally and socially. In Fiji, fat bodies signify social connections, financial resources, and, thus, "health." In the United States, obesity is viewed as a clear sign of unhealthy living. Public health messages link obesity to cancer, diabetes, heart disease, and early mortality. Differences in national culture provide important perspectives on the dynamic relationship between health and disease. Within the structure of the National Health Service, British doctors attempt to do less. They take fewer X-rays and prescribe fewer drugs than in the United States. Accordingly, the British patient is less likely to be labeled as sick and require treatment. In Britain, society's traditional and conventional wisdom is that "if you feel well, you are well." In the United States, a wellness model of healthcare management is promoted by many healthcare insurers, and, as a consequence, the "well-person" examination is encouraged. American physicians are more thorough in the search for disease. See Marsh GN, Wallace RB, Whewell JB. Anglo-American contrasts in general practice. *British Journal of Medicine* 1976;1:1321–1325; Loustaunau MO, Sobo EJ. *The Cultural Context of Health, Illness, and Medicine*. Westport, CT: Bergin & Garvey; 1997.

21. Payer, *Medicine and Culture*, 103.

22. For a general review of medical enhancement, see Mehlman MJ. *The Price of Perfection: Individualism and Society in the Era of Biomedical Enhancement*. Baltimore: Johns Hopkins University Press; 2009.

23. Berbatis CG, Sunderland VB, Bulsara M. Licit psychostimulant consumption in Australia, 1984–2000: international and jurisdictional comparison. *Medical Journal of Australia* 2002;177:539–543; McCabe SE, Knight JR, Teter CJ, Wechsler H. Non-medical use of prescription stimulants among American college students: prevalence and correlates from a national survey. *Addiction* 2005;99:96–106; International Narcotics Control Board. *Psychotropic Substances*. New York: United Nations; 2009.

24. Coronary atherosclerosis begins at a young age. About one in six teenagers already have atherosclerotic plaque in their coronary arteries based on in vivo intravascular ultrasound. See Tuzcu EM, Kapadia SR, Tutar E, et al. High prevalence of coronary atherosclerosis in asymptomatic teenagers and young adults: evidence from intravascular ultrasound. *Circulation* 2002;103(22):2705–2710.

Chapter 7

1. A stress echocardiogram is a study using ultrasound to visualize the heart during controlled exercise conditions. The imaging study can reveal abnormal heart muscle motion during exercise that may be suggestive of coronary artery blockage. If certain arteries are blocked or severely occluded, cardiac muscle movement in the area of the heart that is vascularized by the diseased artery would show abnormal motion.

2. Roger VL, Go AS, Lloyd-Jones DM, et al. Executive summary: heart disease and stroke statistics—2011 update. A report from the American Heart Association. *Circulation* 2011;123:459–463; Roger VL, Go AS, Lloyd-Jones DM, et al. Heart disease and stroke statistics—2011 update. A report from the American Heart Association. *Circulation* 2011;123:e18–e209.

3. Reaven GM. Role of insulin resistance in human disease. *Diabetes* 1988;37:1595–1607; Gale EAM, Alberti KGMM, Zimmet PZ. Should we dump the metabolic syndrome? No. *BMJ* 2008;336:640–641.

4. Grundy SM, Cleeman JI, Daniels SR, et al. Diagnosis and management of the metabolic syndrome: an American Heart Association/National Heart, Lung, and Blood Institute Scientific statement. *Cardiology in Review* 2005;13:322–327.

5. Less than 1 percent of cancers in the United States are seen in pediatric patients (ages 0–14 years). Childhood cancers include leukemia (cancer of the bone marrow) and tumors of the bone, kidney, and nervous system. American Cancer Society. *Cancer Facts and Figures—2012*. Atlanta: American Cancer Society; 2012.

6. The BMI is a measure of a person's fatness or thinness and is a proxy for the amount of body fat. It is calculated by dividing body weight (in kilograms) by the square of the height (in meters). Normal BMI ranges from 18 to 25 kg/m². A BMI below 18 is considered underweight; BMI between 25 and 30 is overweight. To determine your BMI in kg/m², divide your weight (in pounds) by the square of your height (in feet) and multiply the quotient by 4.88 (a dimensional conversion factor).

7. Ravusin E, Swinburn BA. Pathophysiology of obesity. *Lancet* 1992;340:404–408; Flegal KM, Carroll MD, Ogden CL, Johnson CL. Prevalence and trends in obesity among U.S. adults, 1999–2000. *Journal of the American Medical Association* 2002;288(14):1723–1727; Ogden CL, Flegal KM, Carroll MD, Johnson CL. Prevalence and trends in obesity among U.S. children and adolescents, 1999–2000. *Journal of the American Medical Association* 2002;288(14):1728–1732.

8. Ravusin and Swinburn, Pathophysiology of obesity; Swinburn BA, et al. The global obesity pandemic: shaped by global drivers and local environments. *Lancet* 2011;378:804–814; Gortmaker SL, Swinburn BA, Levy D, et al. Changing the future of obesity: science, policy, and action. *Lancet* 2011;378:838–847.

9. Frayling TM, Timpson NJ, Weedon MN, et al. A common variant in the *FTO* gene is associated with body mass index and predisposes to childhood and adult obesity. *Science* 2007;316:889–894; Gerken T, Girard CA, Tung YC, et al. The obesity-associated FTO gene encodes a 2-oxoglutarate-dependent nucleic acid demethylase. *Science* 2007;318:1469–1472.

10. Hall KD, Sacks G, Chandramohan D, et al. Quantification of the effect of energy imbalance on body weight. *Lancet* 2011;378:826–837.

11. Ebbeling CB, Swain JF, Feldman FA, et al. Effects of dietary composition on energy expenditure during weight-loss maintenance. *Journal of the American Medical Association* 2012;307:2627–2634.

12. Insulin serves as an anabolic hormone stimulating cells to take up energy-rich glucose in times of excess. Catabolic hormones, such as glucagon and adrenaline, counteract the physiological effects of insulin. Under homeostatic conditions, hormones are balanced to meet energy requirements. In type 2 diabetes, the pancreas continues to produce insulin, but the body's cells are unable to use it. Type 1 diabetes is characterized by insufficient production of insulin by the pancreas. Diabetes type 1 is usually diagnosed in children or adolescents. Treatment often involves insulin replacement to control blood glucose.

13. Roger et al., Executive summary; Roger et al., Heart disease and stroke statistics.

14. In a 2008 study, diabetic patients who were otherwise normotensive, nonsmokers, and normolipidemic were at equal risk for cardiovascular disease as those who previously suffered from heart disease. Sari I, Soydinc S, et al. Uncomplicated diabetes mellitus is equivalent for coronary artery disease: new support from novel angiographic myocardial perfusion-myocardial blush. *International Journal of Cardiology* 2008;127:262–265.

15. Seshasai SRK, Kaptoge S, Thompson A, et al. Diabetes mellitus, fasting glucose, and risk of cause-specific death. *New England Journal of Medicine* 2011;364:829–841. It is unclear whether cancer risk is a direct consequence of unregulated blood sugar or of overproduction of insulin or inability of the body to respond to insulin.

16. Cubbon R, Kahn M, Kearney MT. Secondary prevention of cardiovascular disease in type 2 diabetes and prediabetes: a cardiologist's perspective. *Clinical Practice* 2007;62:287–299; Saunders J, Mathewkutty S, Drazner MH, McGuire DK. Cardiomyopathy in type 2 diabetes.

Herz 2008;33:184–190; Lopaschuk GD, et al. Myocardial fatty acid metabolism in health and disease. *Physiological Reviews* 2010;90:207–258.

17. Cubbon et al., Secondary prevention of cardiovascular disease in type 2 diabetes and prediabetes; LeRoith D, Rayfield E. The benefits of tight glycemic control in type 2 diabetes mellitus. *Clinical Cornerstone* 2007;8:S19–S29; Steinmerz A. Lipid-lowering therapy in patients with type 2 diabetes: the case for early intervention. *Diabetes/Metabolism Research and Reviews* 2008;24:286–293.

18. The left anterior descending coronary artery is often referred to as the "widowmaker" because blockages in this artery frequently result in death. The artery is a major source of blood for the left ventricle, the heart's main pumping chamber.

19. Causality has deep philosophical meaning and has been the subject of philosophical study for centuries. What does it mean that state B was "caused" by agent A? In an effort to simplify this discussion, an operational definition of causality is adopted. An agent is causal if changing exposure to the agent results in a change in disease incidence. The simplest functional relationship is a linear, no-threshold dose-response where any dose is assumed to be associated with disease risk and doubling the dose of the agent doubles the risk of disease. Risk factors are also related to disease, but the relationship is not functional. For example, female breast cancer is strongly associated with age. However, age per se does not cause breast cancer. Instead, age is a marker for one or more underlying biological processes that are causal.

20. Causality can be very difficult to establish because correlations are often weak and supporting evidence for causality is limited or absent. There are very few studies in which large numbers of people have been exposed to graded doses of a disease-causing agent and disease incidence and mortality documented through medical surveillance and follow-up. The single largest study of this kind is the Life Span Study of Japanese atomic bomb survivors. The study began in the early 1950s and is ongoing. Hill AB. The environment and disease: association or causation? *Proceedings of the Royal Society of Medicine* 1965;58:295–300; McCormick J. The multifactorial aetiology of coronary heart disease: a dangerous delusion. *Perspectives in Biology and Medicine* 1988;32:103–108.

21. McCormick, Multifactorial aetiology of coronary heart disease; Tseng ZH, Secemsky EA, Dowdy D, et al. Sudden cardiac death in patients with human immunodeficiency virus infection. *Journal of the American College of Cardiology* 2012;59:1891–1896.

22. There are some exceptions. Solar ultraviolet (UV) light and some of the hundreds of chemicals in cigarette smoke are mutagenic and cause cancer and other disorders, including immune suppression and hypertension.

23. Xeroderma pigmentosum is a rare genetic disorder characterized by defective DNA repair and high risk for solar UV light-induced skin cancer. The genetic defect increases susceptibility to skin cancer because solar UV damage to DNA is not repaired. Sun exposure increases the incidence of skin cancer, but, in the absence of solar UV, skin cancer risk is not elevated. Kraemer KH, Slor H. Xeroderma pigmentosum. *Clinical Dermatology* 1985;3:33–69.

24. Stress and other environmental factors can cause permanent tissue damage or physiological alterations such that removal of the offending factor does not eliminate the disease. Cigarette smoke, for example, is an important factor in the development of atherosclerotic plaque formation in coronary artery disease. However, once plaques are formed, smoking cessation does not reverse the process. The value of quitting lies in preventing other plaques from forming.

25. For excellent reviews of the role of epigenetics in human disease, see Domann FE, Futscher BE. Flipping the epigenetic switch. *American Journal of Pathology* 2004;164:1883–1886; Egger G, Liang G, Aparicio A, et al. Epigenetics in human disease and prospects for epigenetic therapy. *Nature* 2004;429:457–463; Skinner MK, Manikkam M, Guerrero-Bosagna C. Epigenetic transgenerational actions of environmental factors in disease etiology. *Trends in Endocrinology and Metabolism* 2004;21:214–222.

26. Pinney SE, Simmons RA. Epigenetic mechanisms in the development of type 2 diabetes. *Trends in Endocrinology and Metabolism* 2004;21:223–229; Egger et al., Epigenetics in human

disease and prospects for epigenetic therapy; Gluckman PD, Hanson MA, Buklijas T, et al. Epigenetic mechanisms that underpin metabolic and cardiovascular diseases. *Nature Reviews Endocrinology* 2009;5:401–408.

27. Skinner et al., Epigenetic transgenerational actions of environmental factors in disease etiology.
28. Gluckman et al., Epigenetic mechanisms that underpin metabolic and cardiovascular diseases.
29. Domann and Futscher, Flipping the epigenetic switch; Egger et al., Epigenetics in human disease and prospects for epigenetic therapy; Gluckman et al., Epigenetic mechanisms that underpin metabolic and cardiovascular diseases; Berger SL, Kouzarides T, Shiekhattar R. An operational definition of epigenetics. *Genes and Development* 2009;23:781–783.
30. Gluckman et al., Epigenetic mechanisms that underpin metabolic and cardiovascular diseases.
31. Pinney and Simmons, Epigenetic mechanisms.
32. Stein Z. *Famine and Human Development: The Dutch Hunger Winter of 1944–1945.* New York: Oxford University Press; 1975.
33. Feinberg AP, Vogelstein B. Hypomethylation distinguishes genes of some human cancers from their normal counterparts. *Nature* 1983;301:89–92; Domann and Futscher, Flipping the epigenetic switch.
34. The robustness of the data shown in Table 7.1 is questionable. Agus reports genetic and environmental contributions for a wide variety of diseases without any supporting evidence. Agus's data are reported here only to illustrate the large variations in genetic and environmental contributions to human disease.
35. Willett WC. Balancing life-style and genomics research for disease prevention. *Science* 2002;296:695–698. About 70 to 90 percent of colon cancer, stroke, coronary heart disease, and type 2 diabetes are potentially preventable by lifestyle modifications.
36. American Cancer Society. *Cancer Facts and Figures—2012.* Atlanta: American Cancer Society; 2012.
37. American Cancer Society. *Cancer Facts and Figures—2012.* The American Cancer Society publishes cancer statistics by cancer site on a regular basis. Ionizing radiation and cigarette smoke are arguably the two most thoroughly studied human carcinogens. Extensive epidemiological studies indicate that the nature of the smoking–radiation interaction in lung cancer is very complex. The nonlinear nature of the interaction appears to be dependent on the dose of radiation and smoking intensity. See National Research Council. *Health Effects of Exposure to Radon.* BEIR VI report. Washington, DC: National Academy Press; 1999; Furukawa K, Preston DL, Lonn S, et al. Radiation and smoking effects on lung cancer incidence among atomic bomb survivors. *Radiation Research* 2010;174:72–82.
38. Chorzempa, A. Type 2 diabetes mellitus and its effect on vascular disease. *Journal of Cardiovascular Nursing* 2006;21:485–492; Cubbon et al., Secondary prevention of cardiovascular disease in type 2 diabetes and prediabetes; Gerich JE. Type 2 diabetes mellitus is associated with multiple cardiometabolic risk factors. *Clinical Cornerstone* 2007;8:53–68; Grubbs R, Sica DA. Taking the pressure off type 2 diabetes mellitus: implementing hypertension guidelines. *Progress in Cardiovascular Nursing* 2007;22:159–165; LeRoith and Rayfield, Benefits of tight glycemic control in type 2 diabetes mellitus.
39. McCormick, Multifactorial aetiology of coronary heart disease.
40. A 2009 report from the Institute of Medicine examined eleven studies and concluded that heart attack reduction caused by smoking bans ranged from 6 percent to 47 percent, based on health outcomes measured by admission records of local hospitals. Institute of Medicine. *Secondhand Smoke Exposure and Cardiovascular Effects: Making Sense of the Evidence.* Washington, DC: National Academies Press; 2009.
41. Mitchell SD. *Unsimple Truths: Science, Complexity, and Policy.* Chicago: University of Chicago Press; 2009:74.
42. Tuzcu EM, Kapadia SR, Tutar E, et al. High prevalence of coronary atherosclerosis in asymptomatic teenagers and young adults: evidence from intravascular ultrasound. *Circulation*

2002;103(22):2705–2710; Anselmino M, Gohlke H, Mellbin L, Ryden L. Cardiovascular prevention in patients with diabetes and prediabetes. *Herz* 2008;33:170–177; Steinmerz, Lipid-lowering therapy in patients with type 2 diabetes.

43. IARC Monograph Working Group. Non-Ionizing Radiation, Part II: Radiofrequency Electromagnetic Fields [includes mobile telephones]. *IARC Monographs* 102. Lyon, France: International Agency for Research on Cancer; 2011.

44. Reasner CA. Reducing cardiovascular complications of type 2 diabetes by targeting multiple risk factors. *Journal of Cardiovascular Pharmacology* 2008;52:136–144.

45. Collins KM, Dantico M, Shearer NBC, et al. Heart disease awareness among college students. *Journal of Community Health* 2004;29:405–420.

46. American Cancer Society. *Cancer Facts and Figures—2012.*

Chapter 8

1. Malignant gliomas are rare primary brain tumors that are very difficult cancers to treat. They arise from abnormal glial cells that divide uncontrollably. Normal glial cells serve important support functions for neurons in the central nervous system. The disease cannot be cured even when the bulk of the tumor is removed surgically because some tumor cells always remain and can cause regrowth. Standard therapy involves whole-brain irradiation with concomitant and additional chemotherapy with temozolomide, a cancer drug that sensitizes cells to the effects of radiation. Although most patients tolerate the combination therapy well, the combination therapy extends survival in most patients only by a few months to perhaps one to two years. See Stupp R, Hegi ME, Mason WP, et al. Effects of radiotherapy with concomitant and adjuvant temozolomide versus radiotherapy alone on survival in glioblastoma in a randomised phase III study: 5-year analysis of the EORTC-NCIC trial. *Lancet Oncology* 2009;10(5):459–466.

2. Cancer statistics exclude nonmelanoma skin cancers (over one million cases annually in the United States) because they are rarely fatal and are easily removed surgically.American Cancer Society. *Cancer Facts and Figures—2012.* Atlanta: American Cancer Society, Inc.; 2012;World Health Organization. *The World Health Organization's Fight Against Cancer: Strategies That Prevent, Cure and Care.* Geneva: WHO Press; 2007.

3. Jemal A, Siegal R, Xu J, Ward E. Cancer statistics—2010. *CA Cancer Journal for Clinicians* 2010;60:277–300; Leaf C. *The Truth in Small Doses: Why We're Losing the War on Cancer—and How to Win It.* New York: Simon & Schuster; 2013: 17–61.

4. Doll R, Peto R. The causes of cancer: quantitative estimates of avoidable risks of cancer in the United States today. *Journal of the National Cancer Institute* 1981;66(6):1191–1308.

5. Hanahan D, Weinberg RA. The hallmarks of cancer. *Cell* 2000;100:57–70.

6. Hanahan D, Weinberg RA. Hallmarks of cancer: the next generation. *Cell* 2011;144:646–674.

7. Loeb LA. Mutator phenotype may be required for multistage carcinogenesis. *Cancer Research* 1991;51:3075–3079; American Cancer Society, *Cancer Facts and Figures—2012.*

8. The history of cancer from ancient to modern times is fascinating. For an excellent detailed history, see Mukherjee S. *The Emperor of All Maladies: A Biography of Cancer.* New York: Scribner; 2010.

9. Gould SJ. The median isn't the message. *Discover* 1985;6:40–42; American Cancer Society, *Cancer Facts and Figures—2012.* The median is one measure of central tendency. In a population of individuals with this disease half will survive more than fifteen months, and half will survive less. As a measure of central tendency, the median is insensitive to extremes. Some patients may survive only a few months, but others have been known to survive five years or more.

10. Tisdale MJ. Cachexia in cancer patients. *Nature Reviews Cancer* 2002;2:862–871.

11. Many cancers have no known causes. In about 90 percent of women with breast cancer and men with prostate cancer, causal factors cannot be identified. Glioblastoma, the subject of the case study at the beginning of the chapter, has no known causes.

12. Cigarette smoke contains thousands of chemicals, about sixty of which are strongly linked to cancer. Cigarette smoking is responsible for about 30 percent of all cancer deaths annually in the United States; in fact, the leading cause of cancer mortality in both men and women is lung cancer. Cigarette smoking has also been linked to larynx, oral cavity, and esophageal cancer, and, to a lesser extent, to cancers of the bladder, kidney, pancreas, and uterine cervix. See American Cancer Society, *Cancer Facts and Figures—2012*.

13. Management of infectious disease in general requires knowledge of the infectious agent since disease pathogenesis is intimately connected to the offending microbe and treating the disease requires elimination of the microbe. However, in chronic degenerative diseases such as coronary artery disease, neurodegenerative diseases, and cancer, the disease is characterized by prolonged disease development following exposure to the causal agent. Once the disease is clinically evident, eliminating causal factors has no clinical consequence. Causal-agent exposure is uncoupled from the clinical presentation of the disease. Of course, while smoking cessation in a lung cancer patient does nothing for the management of the current disease, it can reduce or eliminate the risk of disease in the future. Lung cancer treatment is the same in smokers and nonsmokers.

14. About 10 percent of cancers occur in children and young adults (under twenty years). Childhood cancers, however, have a different pathogenesis from cancers in adults. See American Cancer Society, *Cancer Facts and Figures—2012*.

15. A component-failure model is not the only explanation of the age-dependent cancer mortality data. Other statistical models, including that for tumor growth, also fit the data satisfactorily. See Frank SA. *Dynamics of Cancer: Incidence, Inheritance and Evolution*. Princeton, NJ: Princeton University Press; 2007.

16. The guardian of the genome, p53 was named "molecule of the year" in 1996. See Alberts B, et al. *Molecular Biology of the Cell*. New York: Garland; 2002:1344–1345.

17. Nicolis G, Prigogine I. *Exploring Complexity*. New York: Freeman; 1989; Kauffman S. *At Home in the Universe*. New York: Oxford University Press; 1995; Prigogine I. *The End of Certainty: Time, Chaos and the New Laws of Nature*. New York: The Free Press; 1997.

18. Foulds L. The experimental study of tumor progression: a review. *Cancer Research* 1954;14(5):327–339.

19. Kleinsmith LJ. *Principles of Cancer Biology*. San Francisco: Pearson Benjamin Cummings; 2006:175–199.

20. Fidler IJ. The pathogenesis of cancer metastasis: the "seed-and-soil" hypothesis revisited. *Nature Reviews Cancer* 2003;3:453–458.

21. Boutwell RK. Some biological aspects of skin carcinogenesis. *Progress in Experimental Tumor Research* 1963;4:207–250.

22. Doll and Peto, Causes of cancer.

23. Godtfredsen NS, Prescott E, Osler M. Effect of smoking reduction on lung cancer risk. *Journal of the American Medical Association* 2005;294:1505–1510.

24. Chlebowski RT, et al. Breast cancer after use of estrogen plus progestin in postmenopausal women. *New England Journal of Medicine* 2009;360(6):573–587.

25. Kleinsmith, *Principles of Cancer Biology*, 214–215.

26. For an overview of cancer as an evolutionary phenomenon, see Greaves M. *Cancer: The Evolutionary Legacy*. Oxford: Oxford University Press; 2002; Merlo LMF, Pepper JW, Reid BJ, Maley CC. Cancer as an evolutionary and ecological process. *Nature Reviews Cancer* 2006;6:924–935.

27. Nowell PC. The clonal evolution of tumor cell populations. *Science* 1976;194:23–28.

28. Merlo et al., Cancer as an evolutionary and ecological process.

29. Kenny PA, Bissell MJ. Tumor reversion: correction of malignant behavior by microenvironmental cues. *International Journal of Cancer* 2003;107:688–695; Fidler, Pathogenesis of cancer metastasis.

30. Hanahan and Weinberg, The hallmarks of cancer; Hanahan and Weinberg, Hallmarks of cancer: the next generation.

31. Kenny and Bissell, Tumor reversion; Fidler, Pathogenesis of cancer metastasis.

32. Merlo et al., Cancer as an evolutionary and ecological process.

33. Mukherjee, *Emperor of All Maladies*, 248.

34. Basso K, et al. Reverse engineering of regulatory networks in human B cells. *Nature Genetics* 2005;37:382–390.

35. Kleinsmith, *Principles of Cancer Biology*, 45–50.

36. An epigenetic trait is a stably heritable phenotype resulting from changes in a chromosome without alterations in the DNA sequence. See Berger SL, Kouzarides T, Shiekhattar R. An operational definition of epigenetics. *Genes and Development* 2009;23:781–783.

37. Kanwal R, Gupta S. Epigenetics and cancer. *Journal of Applied Physiology* 2010;109:598–605.

38. Domann FE, Futscher BE. Flipping the epigenetic switch. *American Journal of Pathology* 2004;164:1883–1886.

39. Welch HG, Black WC. Using autopsy series to estimate the disease "reservoir" for ductal carcinoma in situ of the breast: how much more breast cancer can we find? *Annals of Internal Medicine* 1997;127:1023–1028.

40. Fearon ER, Vogelstein B. A genetic model for colorectal cancer. *Cell* 1990;61:759–767.

41. Donnenberg VS, Donnenberg AD. Multiple drug resistance in cancer revisited: the cancer stem cell hypothesis. *Journal of Clinical Pharmacology* 2005;45:872–877.

42. Merlo et al., Cancer as an evolutionary and ecological process.

43. Prigogine, *End of Certainty*, 57–72.

44. Kenny and Bissell, Tumor reversion; Fidler, pathogenesis of cancer metastasis; Godtfredsen et al., Effect of smoking reduction on lung cancer risk.

45. Merlo et al., Cancer as an evolutionary and ecological process.

46. By "anywhere" is meant both in and outside the body. Cancer cells can grow on walls or countertops. Unlike most normal human cells, they are very easy to culture in a laboratory setting. See Skloot R. *The Immortal Life of Henrietta Lacks*. New York: Crown; 2010.

47. Kauffman, *At Home in the Universe*, 166; Page RE, Mitchell S. Self-organization and the evolution of division of labor. *Apidologie* 1998;29:171–190.

48. Crespi B, Summers K. Evolutionary biology of cancer. *Trends in Ecology and Evolution* 2005;20:545–552.

49. Frank, *Dynamics of Cancer*.

50. Chemotherapy as a primary cancer treatment has been successful in the management of a small number of cancers including childhood leukemia and testicular carcinoma. American Cancer Society, *Cancer Facts and Figures—2012*.

51. Diagnosis of cancer includes staging or assessing the size and spread of disease. Early stage cancers have a higher probability of being controlled than later stage disease. See Kleinsmith, *Principles of Cancer Biology*, 201–207.

52. Druker BJ, Lydon NB. Lessons learned from the development of an abl tyrosine kinase inhibitor for chronic myelogenous leukemia. *Journal of Clinical Investigation* 2000;105:3–7.

53. Gerlinger M, et al. Intratumor heterogeneity and branched evolution revealed by multiregion sequencing. *New England Journal of Medicine* 2012;366:883–892 54.

54. Actual costs are highly variable and depend on site and extent of disease, whether hospitalizations are required, and costs of specific treatments including cancer drugs.

55. Chapter 6 discusses the link between stage of disease and five-year survival. See Table 6.1.

56. Screening (and diagnostic) tests can be defined by the test sensitivity, test specificity, and the predictive value. Test sensitivity is the probability that a patient with the disease tests positive. Test specificity is the probability that a normal individual will have a negative test. Sensitivity and specificity are coupled. Increasing the sensitivity of a test forces the test to be less specific and vice versa. In the text, the positive predictive value is used and refers to the probability that an individual testing positive has a disease. In some tests, the negative predictive value may be important (the probability that a person with a negative test result does not have the disease). Disease prevalence is a key determinant of positive predictive value and is defined as the number of cases of the disease in a defined population at a particular time. The following boundary cases illustrate the importance of disease prevalence: if everyone in the population had the disease, there would be no false-positive results,

and every positive result would be a true positive. In this case, the positive predictive value would be 100 percent. Conversely, if no one in the population had the disease, there would be no true positive results, and every positive result would be a false positive. In this case, the positive predictive value would be 0 percent.

57. Mandelblatt JS, et al. Effects of mammography screening under different screening schedules: model estimates of potential benefits and harms. *Annals of Internal Medicine* 2009;151:738–747; Partridge AH, Winer EP. On mammography—more agreement than disagreement. *New England Journal of Medicine* 2009;361(26):2499–2501.

58. American Cancer Society, *Cancer Facts and Figures—2012*; Moyer VA on behalf of the U.S. Preventive Services Task Force. Screening for ovarian cancer: U.S. Preventive Services Task Force reaffirmation recommendation statement. *Annals of Internal Medicine* 2012;157(12):1–56. The task force recommendations relied heavily on a large mortality study that showed no reduction in ovarian cancer mortality in women screened for ovarian cancer versus women not screened. See Buys SS, Partridge E, Black A, et al. PLCO Project Team. Effect of screening on ovarian cancer mortality: the Prostate, Lung, Colorectal and Ovarian (PLCO) Cancer Screening randomized controlled trial. *Journal of the American Medical Association* 2011;305:2295–2303.

59. Chou R, et al. Screening for prostate cancer: a review of the evidence for the U.S. Preventive Services Task Force. *Annals of Internal Medicine* 2011;155(111):762–771.

60. Mukherjee, *Emperor of All Maladies*, 14–16.

61. Godtfredsen et al., Effect of smoking reduction on lung cancer risk.

62. American Cancer Society, *Cancer Facts and Figures—2012*.

63. Doll and Peto, Causes of cancer.

64. Pearce MS, et al. Radiation exposure from CT scans in childhood and subsequent risk of leukemia and brain tumors: a retrospective cohort study. *Lancet* 2012;380:499–505. Computed tomography (CT) scans in children have been linked to a small increased risk for later developing leukemia and brain cancer. The cancer link was particularly significant when patients were given multiple examinations that increased the patient cumulative dose. Single-exam doses are low and not associated with increased cancer risk. A causal link between X-ray exposure and cancer could not be established because the study was not designed to account for confounding variables.

65. Marchant GE, Mossman KL. *Arbitrary and Capricious: The Precautionary Principle in the European Union Courts*. Washington, DC: AEI Press; 2004.

66. Science alone is insufficient to establish public health policy. Political and social forces also drive the process. In spite of established decades-old scientific evidence linking formaldehyde exposure in the workplace with leukemia, formaldehyde has just recently been categorized as a known human carcinogen by the US government's National Toxicology Program. The reason for the delay is complex but likely includes lobbying by plywood and other formaldehyde industries to hinder classification. Government response to the increased rate of tobacco consumption, particularly among young people in some areas of the United States, illustrates the importance of reinventing effective social messaging to deter smoking. Convincing evidence that smoking is harmful has been well established since the 1950s. Old warning labels, however, have lost their punch, and more aggressive and disturbing social messages now appear in the public domain. Mossman KL. *Radiation Risks in Perspective*. Boca Raton, FL: Taylor & Francis; 2007; National Toxicology Program. *Report on Carcinogens*. 12th ed. Research Triangle Park, NC: US Department of Health and Human Services, Public Health Service, National Toxicology Program; 2011.

67. Colditz GA, et al. Applying what we know to accelerate cancer prevention. *Science Translational Medicine* 2012;4:127rv4; Vogelstein B, et al. Cancer genome landscapes. *Science* 2013;339:546–558.

68. Chemotherapy drugs will still be needed to treat cancers like leukemia and lymphoma that do not start off as a localized tumor, as does breast cancer or prostate cancer. Leukemia and lymphoma are sometimes referred to as liquid tumors and are usually spread regionally. Local treatment by surgery or radiotherapy is not effective in treating disseminated disease.

Chapter 9

1. Alzheimer's disease may be inherited; however, less than 1 percent of Alzheimer's patients have the inherited form of the disease. Autosomal dominant mutations at *APP, PS1, PS2,* and Trisomy 21 have all been linked to Alzheimer's disease. Acosta-Baena N, Sepulveda-Falla D, Lopera-Gómez CM, et al. Pre-dementia clinical stages in presenilin 1 E280A familial early-onset Alzheimer's disease: a retrospective cohort study. *Nature Neurology* 2011;10:213–220.

2. Deutsch, D. *The Beginning of Infinity.* New York: Viking; 2011.

3. The computational power of the brain may be approximated as follows: There are about 10^{11} neurons in the adult brain. Each neuron has roughly 10^3 synaptic connections to other neurons, resulting in a total of 10^{14} synaptic connections. Action potentials (operations per synaptic connection) are generated at a rate of 100 to 200 per second (assuming one action potential takes five milliseconds). The product of these factors gives about 10^{16} operations per second.

4. Analog processing and digital processing are distinguished by the information generated. Digital processes are limited to discrete pieces of information. In digital computing, the values are yes and no or on and off. Other values are not allowed. Analog processing encodes information on a continuum. There is no inherent limit to values that can be assigned. If digital is black and white, analog represents infinite shades of gray. The advantage of digital systems is their greater fidelity because information is locked into discrete values. Signal quality, however, is greater in an analog system because more information can be encoded. Digital technology can mimic analog technology if the resolution is high enough in the digital system (for example, a digital picture can approximate an analog one if the resolution is high enough). Higher resolution is achieved by acquiring more information by increasing exposure time.

5. Changeux, JP. *Neuronal Man.* Princeton, NJ: Princeton University Press; 1985.

6. Penrose R. *The Emperor's New Mind: Concerning Computers, Minds, and the Laws of Physics.* Oxford: Oxford University Press; 1989; Penrose R. *Shadows of the Mind: A Search for the Missing Science of Consciousness.* Oxford: Oxford University Press; 1994.

7. Kiehl KA, Smith AM, Hare RD, et al. Limbic abnormalities in affective processing by criminal psychopaths as revealed by functional magnetic resonance imaging. *Biological Psychiatry* 2001;50:677–684; Harris S. *The Moral Landscape: How Science Can Determine Human Values.* New York: Free Press; 2010.

8. Karns CM, Dow MW, Neville HJ. Altered cross-model processing in the primary auditory cortex of congenitally deaf adults: a visual-somatosensory fMRI study with a double-flash illusion. *Journal of Neuroscience* 2012;32:9626–9638.

9. Shermer M. Why you should be skeptical of brain scans. *Scientific American Mind* 2008;19:66–71.

10. Hauser W, Hansen E, Enck P. Nocebo phenomena in medicine: their relevance in everyday clinical practice. *Deutsches Arzteblatt International* 2012;109:459–465.

11. Oken BS. Placebo effects: clinical aspects and neurobiology. *Brain* 2008;131:2812–2823.

12. Wimo A, Prince M. *World Alzheimer Report 2010: The Global Economic Impact of Dementia.* London: Alzheimer's Disease International; 2010; Herrmann W, Obeide R. Biomarkers of neurodegenerative disease. *Clin Chem Lab Med* 2011;49:343–344; Hurd MD, et al. Monetary costs of dementia in the United States. *New England Journal of Medicine* 2013;368:1326–1334.

13. Thies W, Bleiler L, Alzheimer's Association. Alzheimer's Association report 2011: Alzheimer's disease facts and figures. *Alzheimer's and Dementia* 2011;7:208–244.

14. Mazoteras MV, Abellan van Kan G, Cantet C, et al. Gait and balance impairments in Alzheimer disease patients. *Alzheimer Disease and Associated Disorders* 2010;24:79–84.

15. Acosta-Baena et al., Pre-dementia clinical stages in presenilin 1 E280A familial early-onset Alzheimer's disease.

16. Chin J, Roberson ED, Mucke L. Molecular aspects of memory dysfunction in Alzheimer's disease. In Byrne J, ed., *Learning and Memory: A Comprehensive Reference.* Vol. 4. New York: Elsevier; 2008:245–293.

17. National Institutes of Health. NIH State-of-the-Science conference statement on preventing Alzheimer's disease and cognitive decline. *NIH Consensus and State-of-the-Science Statements* 2010;27(4).

18. Hadley EC, Lakatta EG, Morrison-Bogorad M, et al. The future of aging therapies. *Cell* 2005;120:557–567.
19. Hardy J, Allsop D. Amyloid deposition as the central event in the aetiology of Alzheimer's disease. *Trends in Pharmacological Sciences* 1991;12:383–388.
20. Chin et al., Molecular aspects of memory dysfunction in Alzheimer's disease.
21. Hardy and Allsop, Amyloid deposition as the central event in the aetiology of Alzheimer's disease.
22. Maccioni RB, Farıas G, Morales I, et al. The revitalized tau hypothesis on Alzheimer's diseasae. *Archives of Medical Research* 2010;41:226–231.
23. de la Monte SM, Wands JR. Alzheimer's disease is type 3 diabetes-evidence reviewed. *Journal of Diabetes Science and Technology* 2008; 2(6): 1101–1113.
24. Soto C. In vivo spreading of tau pathology. *Neuron* 2012;73:621–623; de Calignon A, Polydoro M, Suarez-Calvet M., et al. Propagation of tau pathology in a model of early Alzheimer's disease. *Neuron* 2012;73:685–697; Liu L, Drouet V, Wu JW, et al. Trans-synaptic spread of tau pathology in vivo. *PLoS One* 2012;7(2): e31302.
25. Chin et al., Molecular aspects of memory dysfunction in Alzheimer's disease.
26. Lambert JC, Amouyei P. Genetics of Alzheimer's disease: new evidences for an old hypothesis? *Current Opinions in Genetics and Development* 2011;21:295–301.
27. Ringman JM. Setting the stage for prevention of familial Alzheimer's disease. *Nature Neurology* 2011;10:200–201; Acosta-Baena et al., Pre-dementia clinical stages in presenilin 1 E280A familial early-onset Alzheimer's disease.
28. Jonsson T, Atwal JK, Steinberg S, et al. A mutation in *APP* protects against Alzheimer's disease and age-related cognitive decline. *Nature* 2012;488:96–99.
29. Clark CM, Schneider JA, Bedell BJ, et al. Use of Florbetapir-PET for imaging β-amyloid pathology. *Journal of the American Medical Association* 2011;305:275–283.
30. Frisoni GB, Hampel H, O'Brien JT, et al. Revised criteria for Alzheimer's disease: what are the lessons for clinicians? *Lancet Neurology* 2011;10:598–600.
31. Cooke S. Memory enhancement, memory erasure: the future of our past. In Brockman M, ed., *What's Next? Dispatches on the Future of Science.* New York: Vintage Books; 2009:131–143.
32. The risk of Alzheimer's disease doubles every five years after the age of sixty-five. If a treatment postpones onset by five years *without increasing life span*, the number of affected persons would be reduced by half. Brookmeyer R, Gray S, Kawas C. Projections of Alzheimer's disease in the United States and the public health impact of delaying disease onset. *American Journal of Public Health* 1998;88:1337–1342.
33. Pavlopoulos E, et al. Molecular mechanism for age-related memory loss: the histone-binding protein RbAp48. *Science Translational Medicine* 2013; 5(200): 200ra115. doi:10.1126/scitranslmed.3006373
34. Boffey PM. The next frontier is inside your brain. *New York Times.* February 24, 2013: Sunday Review, 10.

Chapter 10

1. Gewirtz P. On "I Know It When I See It." *Yale Law Journal* 1996;105:1023–1047 (the phrase appears in Justice Stewart's concurring opinion in *Jacobellis v. Ohio*, a pornography case decided by the US Supreme Court in 1964).
2. Martinson ML, Teitler JO, Reichman NE. Health across the lifespan in the United States and England. *American Journal of Epidemiology* 2011;173(8):858–865; Avendano M, Ichiro Kawachi I. Invited commentary: the search for explanations of the American health disadvantage relative to the English. *American Journal of Epidemiology* 2011;173(8):866–869; Martinson ML, Teitler JO, Reichman NE. Martinson et al. respond to "Search for Explanations of the American Health Disadvantage." *American Journal of Epidemiology* 2011;173(8):870.
3. Kirkwood TBL. Understanding the odd science of aging. *Cell* 2006;120:437–447.
4. Medvedev ZA. An attempt at a rational classification of theories of aging. *Biological Reviews of the Cambridge Philosophical Society* 1990;65:375–398.

5. Medawar PB. *An Unsolved Problem in Biology*. London: Lewis; 1952; Kirkwood, Understanding the odd science of aging.

6. Williams GC. Pleiotropy, natural selection and the evolution of senescence. *Evolution* 1957;11(4):398–411; Kirkwood, Understanding the odd science of aging.

7. Kirkwood TBL. Evolution of aging. *Nature* 1977;270:301–304; Kirkwood, Understanding the odd science of aging; Vijg J, Campisi J. Puzzles, promises and a cure for ageing. *Nature* 2008;454:1065–1071.

8. Guarente L, Picard F. Calorie restriction—the *SIR2* connection. *Cell* 2005;120:473–482.

9. Hayflick L. The limited in vitro lifetime of human diploid cell strains. *Experimental Cell Research* 1965;37:72–76; Shay JW, Wright WE. Hayflick, his limit, and cellular ageing. *Nature Reviews Molecular and Cell Biology* 2000;1:72–76; Kirkwood, Understanding the odd science of aging.

10. Balaban RS, Nemoto S, Finkel T. Mitochondria, oxidants, and aging. *Cell* 2005;120:483–495; Lombard DB, Chua KF, Mostoslavsky R, et al. DNA repair, genome stability, and aging. *Cell* 2005;120:497–512.

11. Campisi J. Cellular senescence: putting the paradoxes in perspective. *Current Opinion in Genetics and Development* 2011;21:107–112.

12. Kirkwood, Understanding the odd science of aging; Campisi J. Senescent cells, tumor suppression and organismal aging: good citizens, bad neighbors. *Cell* 2005;120:513–522;Baker DJ, et al. Clearance of p16^Ink4a-positive senescent cells delays ageing-associated disorders. *Nature* 2011;479:232–236.

13. Kirkwood argues that, while programmed cell death (apoptosis) makes sense when damaged cells pose a particular threat (for example, cancer), senescence is likely the less costly alternative by inducing permanent cell-cycle arrest. A primary function of senescence is to arrest cycling cells that have been stressed or damaged such that continued division would pose a threat. Kirkwood, Understanding the odd science of aging.

14. Senecent cells can be distinguished from normal by expression of signature proteins. Cells expressing p16Ink4a have senescent properties, and their removal is linked to attenuation of age-related disease. Campisi J. Cellular senescence; Baker et al., Clearance of p16Ink4a-positive senescent cells delays ageing-associated disorders.

15. The Weibull model does not provide an exclusive fit to the data. Other models, including the Gompertzian growth model, can also be fit to the data. As a descriptive model, the Weibull makes no assumptions about underlying processes leading to system failure. Frank SA. *Dynamics of Cancer: Incidence, Inheritance, and Evolution*. Princeton, NJ: Princeton University Press; 2007:136–138.

16. Kirkwood, Understanding the odd science of aging.

17. Cambier J. Immunosenescence: a problem of lymphopoiesis, homeostasis, microenvironment and signaling. *Immunological Reviews* 2005;205(1):5–6.

18. Kleinsmith LJ. *Principles of Cancer Biology*. San Francisco: Pearson Benjamin Cummings; 2006:152–153.

19. Peto J. Cancer epidemiology in the last century and the next decade. *Nature* 2001;411:390–395.

20. The daily energy consumption of the human body is about 2,000 kilocalories per day. This translates into an energy dissipation rate of about 100 joules per second or 100 watts, enough to power a conventional light bulb. The 100 watts actually represents dissipated heat that is not used to do useful work. Almost everyone has at one time or another experienced how uncomfortable it can be in a poorly ventilated room with a large number of people. See Schneider ED, Sagan D. *Into the Cool: Energy Flow, Thermodynamics, and Life*. Chicago: University of Chicago Press; 2005.

21. A 25-year study of Rhesus monkeys begun in 1987 and concluded in 2012 demonstrated that calorie restriction did not lengthen life span compared to monkeys on a normal diet. Causes of death from cancer and heart disease were the same in both underfed and normally fed monkeys. The study conflicts with a 2009 Rhesus monkey study that concluded calorie restriction does extend life span. Study differences cannot be explained easily but might be related to how the causes of death are interpreted. Colman RJ, et al. Caloric restriction delays disease onset and mortality in rhesus monkeys. *Science* 2009;325:201–204; Mattison

JA, Roth GS, Beasley TM, et al. Impact of caloric restriction on health and survival in rhesus monkeys from the NIA study. *Nature* 2012;489:318–321.

22 The *SIR* (silent information regulator) genes mediate effects of CR through endocrine changes (for example, reduced insulin secretion) and increased resistance to the harmful effects of stress. As a consequence, aging slows. Guarente and Picard, Calorie restriction—the *SIR2* connection;Hadley EC, Lakatta EG, Morrison-Bogorad M, et al. The future of aging therapies. *Cell* 2005;120:557–567.

23. Blalock JE, Smith EM. Conceptual development of the immune system as a sixth sense. *Brain, Behavior and Immunity* 2007;21:23–33.

24. Williams, Pleiotropy, natural selection and the evolution of senescence; Editorial. Aging research comes of age. *Cell* 2005;120:435; Kirkwood, Understanding the odd science of aging; Campisi J. Cellular senescence; Stipp D. *The Youth Pill: Scientists at the Brink of an Anti-Aging Revolution*. New York: Current; 2010.

25. Olshansky SJ, Carnes BA, Cassell C. In search of Methuselah: estimating the upper limit to human longevity. *Science* 1990;250:634–640; Olshansky SJ, Carnes BA, Désesquelles A. Prospects for human longevity. *Science* 2001;291:1491–1492; Stipp, *The Youth Pill*.

26. Huang S, Houghton PJ. Targeting mTOR signaling for cancer therapy. *Current Opinion in Pharmacology* 2003;3:371–377;Sarbassov DD, Ali SM, Sbatini DM. Growing roles for the mTOR pathway. *Current Opinion in Cell Biology* 2005;17:596–603; Bonawitz ND, et al. Reduced TOR signaling extends chronological life span via increased respiration and upregulation of mitochondrial gene expression. *Cell Metabolism* 2007;5:265–277; Tsang CK, et al. Targeting mammalian target of rapamycin (mTOR) for health and diseases. *Drug Discovery Today* 2007:12:112–124;Van Heemst D. Insulin, IGF-1 and longevity. *Aging and Disease* 2010;1:147–157.

27. Wilmoth JR, et al. Increase of maximum life-span in Sweden, 1861–1999. *Science* 2000;289:2366–2368.

28. Aubrey de Grey is a biogerontologist who developed the concept of strategies for engineered negligible senescence (SENS) to describe a diverse range of regenerative medical therapies that would repair age-related damage to human tissue for the purposes of maintaining a state of "negligible senescence." As long as SENS therapies were applied, age-related diseases would be postponed. De Grey's work has received considerable attention but has been severely criticized as too speculative given the current state of technology and understanding of the aging process. See de Grey A, Rae M. *Ending Aging: The Rejuvenation Breakthroughs That Could Reverse Human Aging in Our Lifetime*. New York: St. Martin's Press; 2007.

29. Stanford University Commencement address delivered by Steve Jobs, CEO of Apple Computer and of Pixar Animation Studios, on June 12, 2005. Jobs died of pancreatic cancer on October 5, 2011.

30. Atwood M. *Oryx and Crake*. New York: Anchor Books; 2003; McGregor JL. Transhumanism and obligations to future generations. In Tirosh-Samuelson H, Mossman KL, eds. *Building Better Humans? Refocusing the Debate on Transhumanism*. Berne: Peter Lang; 2011:397–416.

31. Centers for Disease Control and Prevention. Public health and aging: trends in aging—United States and worldwide. *Morbidity and Mortality Weekly Report* 2003;52(6):101–106.

32. American Cancer Society. *Cancer Facts and Figures—2012*. Atlanta: American Cancer Society; 2012. Some cancers, like lung and pancreatic cancer, remain difficult to treat. Even when diagnosed at an early stage, the 5-year-survival rates of these cancers are less than 50 percent.

33. There are many design flaws that lead to compromised function in aging bodies. Design flaws in joints, bones, and teeth, to name a few, are not discussed but are, nevertheless, important as sources of decreased quality of life as the body ages.

34. Soto C. In vivo spreading of tau pathology. *Neuron* 2012;73:621–623.

35. Amifostine (trade name Ethyol) is the only drug approved by the FDA for use in radiation therapy. It is used to prevent xerostomia (dry mouth) in patients treated for head and neck cancers. The drug readily floods normal tissues but enters tumor cells more slowly. If amifostine is given within minutes of radiotherapy treatment, there is a differential sparing

of normal tissues compared with tumors. X- and gamma radiation kill cells by generating large numbers of free radicals that cause extensive damage to DNA. The efficacy of clinical radioprotectors is limited by the amount of protection afforded tumors. Amifostine is the result of decades of research by the US Army to develop protective agents that could be given to soldiers during nuclear war, an example of how military research can have clinical benefits. See Hall EJ, Giaccia AJ. *Radiobiology for the Radiologist*. 6th ed. Philadelphia: Lippincott Williams & Wilkins; 2006:131–132.

36. Enos WF, Colmes RH, Beber J. Coronary disease among United States soldiers killed in action in Korea. Preliminary report. *Journal of the American Medical Association* 1953;152:1090–1093.This report documents the presence of significant coronary lesions in soldiers who were battle casualties in Korea. The average age of soldiers included in the report was 22.1 years.

37. Blake GJ, Ridker PM. Are statins anti-inflammatory? *Current Controlled Trials in Cardiovascular Medicine* 2000;1:161–165.

38. Dale KM, et al. Statins and cancer risk: a meta-analysis. *Journal of the American Medical Association* 2006;295(1):74–80.

39. Schiffman SS. Taste and smell losses in normal aging and disease. *Journal of the American Medical Association* 1997;278:1357–1362; Lin FR, et al. Hearing loss and incident dementia. *Archives of Neurology* 2011;68;214–220.

40. Chencharick J, Mossman K. Nutritional consequences of the radiotherapy of head and neck cancer. *Cancer* 1983;51:811–815.

41. Campisi J. Senescent cells, tumor suppression and organismal aging.

42. Baker et al., Clearance of $p16^{Ink4a}$-positive senescent cells delays ageing-associated disorders.

Chapter 11

1. Gleick J. *Chaos: Making a New Science*. New York: Penguin; 1987; Mitchell M. *Complexity: A Guided Tour*. New York: Oxford University Press; 2009.

2. Heart rate changes very rapidly when the body is threatened with serious injury or death. The flight-or-fight response initiates release of adrenaline and stimulates the sympathetic nervous system rapidly to increase cardiovascular performance by raising blood pressure and heart rate.

3. Deutsch D. *The Beginning of Infinity: Explanations That Transform the World*. New York: Viking; 2011:107–124.

4. Young JL, Libby P. Atherosclerosis. In Lilly LS, ed. *Pathophysiology of Heart Disease*. 4th ed. Baltimore: Lippincott Williams & Wilkins; 2007:118–140.

5. Sylven C. Mechanisms of pain in angina pectoris—a critical review of the adenosine hypothesis. *Cardiovascular Drugs and Therapy* 1993;7:745–759. Angina pectoris represents a visceral pain caused by reversible myocardial ischemia. The majority of ischemic attacks are symptomless. When pain is manifested, it appears late during the ischemic event. The pain is complex in its quality and bears little relation to the region of myocardial ischemia.

6. Species competition models have been used in the ecological sciences for many years and describe the growth and decline of species in shared environments. Smale S. On the differential equations of species in competition. *Journal of Mathematical Biology* 1976;3:5–7.

7. Mitchell, *Complexity*, 3–12.

8. Energy flow in stars is orders of magnitude greater than in a human because the star is much more massive. Energy flow density corrects for differences in mass between systems. The concept of energy flow density is also discussed in chapter 1 when comparing energy utilization by selected organs in the human body. Chaisson E. *Cosmic Evolution: The Rise of Complexity in Nature*. Cambridge, MA: Harvard University Press; 2001; Chaisson E. *Epic of Evolution: Seven Ages of the Cosmos*. New York: Columbia University Press; 2006.

9. Lacroix R, Eason E, Melzack R. Nausea and vomiting during pregnancy: a prospective study of its frequency, intensity, and patterns of change. *American Journal of Obstetrics and Gynecology* 2000;182:931–937.

10. Niebyl JR. Nausea and vomiting in pregnancy. *New England Journal of Medicine* 2010;363:1544–1550.

11. Williams GC, Nesse RM. The dawn of Darwinian medicine. *Quarterly Review of Biology* 1991;66:1–22.

12. Dobzhansky T. Biology, molecular and organismic. *American Zoologist* 1964;4:443–452.

13. Nesse RM, Williams GC. *Why We Get Sick: The New Science of Darwinian Medicine.* New York: Times Books; 1994; Nesse RM, Bergstrom CT, Ellison PT, et al. Making evolutionary biology a basic science for medicine. *Proceedings of the National Academy of Sciences* 2010;107(Suppl. 1):1800–1807.

14. A well-known example of antiemetic drug toxicity is the thalidomide tragedy. In 1961, clinical evidence became available that thalidomide, an effective antiemetic drug for the treatment of morning sickness, when taken early in pregnancy, caused an enormous increase in a previously rare syndrome of congenital anomalies involving the limbs. Prior to withdrawal from the market in 1961, about seven thousand affected infants were born to women who had taken this drug. A single dose of the drug was sufficient to produce effects. The usual preclinical animal tests did not detect that thalidomide had teratogenic activity because different animal species metabolize the drug differently. Pregnant mice and rats (the most common test animals) do not generate malformed offspring when given thalidomide. Rabbits produce some malformed offspring, but the defects are different from those seen in affected human infants. An excellent overview of the thalidomide tragedy is provided in The Insight Team of the Sunday Times of London. *Suffer the Children: The Story of Thalidomide.* New York: Viking Press; 1979.

15. Nesse et al., Making evolutionary biology a basic science for medicine.

16. Poincaré H. *Science and Method.* London: Thomas Nelson; 1908; Mitchell, *Complexity.*

17. Wolfram S. *A New Kind of Science.* Champaign, IL: Wolfram Media; 2002.

18. Pilkey OH, Pilkey–Jarvis L. *Useless Arithmetic: Why Environmental Scientists Can't Predict the Future.* New York: Columbia University Press; 2007.

19. Complexity has been defined and measured in terms of system size, entropy, algorithmic information content, logical depth, thermodynamic depth, computational capacity, statistical complexity, fractal dimensions, and degree of hierarchy. Mitchell, *Complexity.*

20. Levin R. The strategy of model building in population biology. *American Scientist* 1966;54:421–431; Silver N. *The Signal and the Noise.* New York: Penguin Press; 2012.

21. Gatenby RA, Gillies RJ. A microenvironmental model of carcinogenesis. *Nature Reviews Cancer* 2008;8:56–61.

22. Gross CG. Claude Bernard and the constancy of the internal environment. *Neuroscientist* 1998;4:380–385.

23. Edelman GM, Gally JA. Degeneracy and complexity in biological systems. *Proceedings of the National Academy of Sciences* 2001;98:13763–13768.

24. Domann FE, Futscher BE. Flipping the epigenetic switch. *American Journal of Pathology* 2004;164:1883–1886.

25. Kleinsmith LJ. *Principles of Cancer Biology.* San Francisco: Pearson Benjamin Cummings; 2006.

26. American Cancer Society. *Cancer Facts and Figures—2012.* Atlanta, GA: American Cancer Society; 2012.

27. Peto J. Cancer epidemiology in the last century and the next decade. *Nature* 2001;411:390–395; Willett WC. Balancing life-style and genomic research for disease prevention. *Science* 2002;296:695–698.

28. Mossman KL. *Radiation Risks in Perspective.* Boca Raton, FL: Taylor & Francis; 2007:109–128.

29. Gleick, *Chaos*; Kelly K. *Out of Control: The New Biology of Machines, Social Systems and the Economic World.* New York: Addison-Wesley; 1994; Castellani B, Hafferty FW. *Sociology and Complex Science: A New Field of Inquiry.* Berlin: Springer Verlag; 2009.

30. Krogsboll L, et al. General health checks in adults for reducing morbidity and mortality from disease: Cochrane systematic review and meta-analysis. *BMJ* 2012;345:e7191.

31. Recent shifts in disease patterns around the world are documented in the *Global Burden of Disease Study 2010*, a comprehensive report of estimates of disease and mortality in more

than 180 countries published in 2012 in a series of papers in *Lancet*, a British medical journal. Lozano R. Global and regional mortality from 235 causes of death for 20 age groups in
1990 and 2010: a systematic analysis for the Global Burden of Disease Study 2010. *Lancet*
2012;380:2095–2128; Murray CJL. Disability-adjusted life years (DALYs) for 291 diseases
and injuries in 21 regions, 1990–2010: a systematic analysis for the Global Burden of
Disease Study 2010. *Lancet* 2012;380:2197–2223; Lim SS. A comparative risk assessment
of burden of disease and injury attributable to 67 risk factors and risk factor clusters in 21
regions, 1990–2010: a systematic analysis for the Global Burden of Disease Study 2010.
Lancet 2012;380:2224–2260.

32. Macklem P. Emergent phenomena and the secrets of life. *Journal of Applied Physiology*
2008;104:1844–1846; Bates JHT. Emergency medicine. *Journal of Applied Physiology*
2008;104:1849.

SELECTED BIBLIOGRAPHY

There is considerable interest in the application of complexity to medicine and public health but few resources to draw on. Most books on complexity deal with applications in climatology, economic sciences, evolution, dynamical systems theory, and computational and information sciences. Although a number of research articles have been published on nonlinear behavior, chaos, and emergent phenomena in living systems (for example, cardiovascular physiology), I am unaware of any book that provides a comprehensive exploration of complexity phenomena in human biology and disease.

Acquiring a basic knowledge of any discipline requires considerable time and effort reading introductory and advanced texts to become familiar with fundamental concepts and theories. Complexity science is especially challenging because it is a "super"-discipline that depends on a working knowledge of more fundamental disciplines like mathematics, computer science, physics, and chemistry. Further, as discussed throughout this book, there is no general or unified theory of complexity to facilitate disciplinary structuring or understanding.

In writing this book, I relied on several texts that provide a broad overview of complexity relevant to the human biology domain. James Gleick's *Chaos: Making a New Science* (New York: Penguin, 1987) is a must-read for anyone interested in complexity phenomena in nature and the role of chaos in complexity. Yet, while Gleick's book focuses on the complex behavior of the atmosphere, oceans, and wildlife populations, only a few examples of chaos in human biology and disease are included, like brain function and the surprising order in the chaos that develops in the beating of the human heart.

In *Complexity: Life at the Edge of Chaos* (Chicago: The University of Chicago Press, 1992), Roger Lewin explores the broad landscape of complexity science. Written in the form of a series of dialogues between the author (a science writer) and many experts (supporters and a few skeptics), the book takes the reader from archaeological remains to rain forests to the Santa Fe Institute, arguably the world's foremost center for the study of complex systems. The only aspect of human biology discussed is the brain and consciousness. Lewin also explores Darwinian evolution as an example of controversy in the complexity field.

Stuart Kauffman's *At Home in the Universe* (New York: Oxford University Press, 1995) is a highly theoretical exploration of self-organization and order in complex systems. Kauffman, one of the leading thinkers in complexity science, contends that complexity itself triggers self-organization and that if enough different molecules pass a certain threshold of complexity they begin to self-organize into a new entity—a living cell. Considerable attention is paid to evolutionary processes.

Melanie Mitchell offers a well-written overview of complexity sciences in her *Complexity: A Guided Tour* (New York: Oxford University Press, 2009). Mitchell discusses a wide range of natural and computational systems to explain how large-scale complex, organized, and adaptive behavior can emerge from simple interactions among components. As a computer scientist, Mitchell focuses on information and computation, but some attention is given to evolutionary theory as an example of biological complexity.

The only book I found that directly addresses complexity science in medicine is Colin Alexander's *Complexity and Medicine: The Elephant in the Waiting Room* (Nottingham, UK: Nottingham University Press, 2010). The author posits medicine's failure to solve many noninfectious diseases to a reluctance to incorporate complexity theory and employ it as a tool for investigating disease. Alexander explores chaos theory and complex self-regulating dynamical systems using diseases of the musculoskeletal system as examples. The focus of the book is etiology of disease.

In addition to these and other background sources, newspaper and magazine articles reporting recent medical advances provided excellent source material. I relied heavily on the *New York Times* (particularly the Tuesday *Science Times* section) for reports on cutting-edge research as examples of principles of complexity in disease pathogenesis, disease diagnosis, and therapy. I used these popular press pieces to identify the original reports in the technical and clinical literature as recorded in the "Notes" section of each chapter.

In the "Notes" to a chapter, the reader will, of course, find the specific references to support claims and statements; many of these are technical articles published in professional journals. Several full-length books in addition to the ones discussed above are, in my opinion, valuable and accessible to all interested readers, and I list them below:

Atkins P. *Four Laws That Drive the Universe*. New York: Oxford University Press; 2007.

Berg HC. *Random Walks in Biology*. Princeton, NJ: Princeton University Press; 1993.

Cannon WB. *The Wisdom of the Body*. New York: Norton; 1932.

Chaisson EJ. *Cosmic Evolution: The Rise of Complexity in Nature*. Cambridge, MA: Harvard University Press; 2001.

Changeux, JP. *Neuronal Man*. Princeton, NJ: Princeton University Press; 1985.

Davies P. *The Cosmic Blueprint*. Philadelphia: Templeton Foundation Press; 1988.

Deutsch, D. *The Beginning of Infinity*. New York: Viking; 2011.

Mitchell S. *Unsimple Truths: Science, Complexity and Policy*. Chicago: University of Chicago Press; 2009.

Prigogine I. *The End of Certainty: Time, Chaos and the New Laws of Nature*. New York: The Free Press; 1996.

Penrose R. *The Emperor's New Mind: Concerning Computers, Minds, and the Laws of Physics*. Oxford: Oxford University Press; 1989.

Schneider ED, Sagan D. *Into the Cool: Energy Flow, Thermodynamics, and Life*. Chicago: University of Chicago Press; 2005.

Schrödinger E. *What Is Life?* Cambridge: Cambridge University Press; 1944.

INDEX

A

Abellan van Kan, G., 242
absorptive tissues, 36
acetylcholine, 44
acid-base buffers, 81, 209, 232
acidosis, 202
Acosta-Baena, N., 242
acoustic neuromas (brain cancer), 131
acquired immunodeficiency syndrome (AIDS),
    183, 209
actin, in skeletal muscle contractions, 45, 228
action potential
    definition of, 209
    nerve cell depolarization for, 40–41, 40f
    nodes of Ranvier and, 43
    oscillation amplitude and, 82–83, 83f
    spatial and temporal frequencies of, 165
adaptive capacity, 4–5, 16, 62
adenosine triphosphate (ATP), 20, 35, 39, 82, 143,
    210
ADH (antidiuretic hormone), 37, 209
ADHD (attention deficit hyperactivity
    disorder), 112
aging, 177–192
    cancer risk increase with, 141, 144
    cellular molecular damage, 180–182
    complexity in, 191–192
    complexity loss and, 67–68
    in degenerative diseases, 117
    as disease risk factor, 121
    free radicals, 189
    immune system failure, 182–183
    inflammatory control, 189–190
    longer life spans, 185–187
    memory loss related to, 176
    metabolism, slowing of, 183–185
    neurodegenerative diseases
        and, 168–176
    protein synthesis, 188–189
    reversal in jellyfish, 229
    as risk factor, 16–17

sensory losses, 190–191
theories of, 179–180
AIDS (acquired immunodeficiency syndrome),
    183, 209
Alberti, K. G. M., 235
Alberts, B., 239
Alexander, C., 250
allostasis, 77, 209
Allsop, D., 243
Alon, U., 227
Alzheimer's disease
    biomarkers for, 106–107
    complexity of, 98–99, 168–175, 171f
    diagnosis of, 103
    inheritability of, 242
    lower cancer risk in, 139
    as neurodegenerative disease, 117
    NFTs (neurofibrillary tangles) in, 187
    overview, 209
    public health impact of, 243
American Bar Association, 224
American Cancer Society, 230, 233, 237
American Heart Association, 234
American Medical Association, 224
American Sign Language, 111
amifostine (radiation therapy drug), 189, 209,
    245–246
Amouyei, P., 243
amyloidosis, in Alzheimer's
    disease, 170, 172, 209
Amyvid (florbetapir) tracer for Alzheimer's
    disease, 174
anaerobic metabolism, in cancer, 143
analgesic drugs, 88t, 209
Anderson, J. C., 226
anesthetics, action of, 42
anger control, 44
angina pectoris, 163, 195, 209, 246
angiogenesis, 138, 209
angiography, 163, 210
Anselmino, M., 238

antagonistic pleiotropy theory of aging
    (Williams), 179, 185, 210
anthrax, 98
antidiuretic hormone (ADH), 37, 209
antiemetics, 198–199, 210, 247
antihypertensive medications, 48
anti-inflammatory drugs, 190
antioxidants, 188
anxiety disorders, 44
Aparicio, A., 236
apolipoprotien E protein, 173
apoptosis (cell death), 145, 181, 202, 210
APP gene mutations, 170, 172, 210
aquaporins (water channels), 32, 210
Ariga, M., 232
arrhythmias, 67–68, 210
atherosclerosis, 48, 190, 210, 234
Atkins, P., 225, 250
ATP (adenosine triphosphate), 20, 35, 39, 82, 143,
    210
atrial septal defect, 27, 210
attention deficit hyperactivity disorder (ADHD),
    112
Atwal, J. K., 243
Atwood, M. (author), 187, 245
Avendano, M., 243
axon hillock, 42, 44, 215
axons, 44, 210

B

Bailey, S., 233
Baker, D. J., 246
Balaban, R. S., 244
Basso, K., 240
Bates, J. H. T., 248
B cells, 64*f*, 185, 210
BCR-ABL fusion oncogene, 154, 210
Beasley, T. M., 245
Beber, J., 246
Bedell, B. J., 243
behavioral disorders, 166
Berbatis, C. G., 234
Berenbaum M. R., 226
Berg, H. C., 226, 250
Berger, S. L., 240
Bernard, C., 224, 231
Bernard, C. (physiologist), 71, 75–76, 90
beta-amyloidosis, in Alzheimer's disease, 170,
    172, 209, 210
beta blockers (antihypertensive medications), 48
bifurcation, 54, 210
Billen, D., 230
biological complexity, 51–69
    emergent properties of, 59–62
    examples of, 62–66
    fractal geometry and physiology in, 58–59
    in health and disease, 66–69
    interdependent, nonlinear components of, 55–56
    system conditions and states, 52–55

unpredictable behavior in, 56–58
biomarkers
    for cancer early detection, 156
    C-reactive proteins, 128
    definition of, 211
    genetic, 106–107
biophysical determinism, 42
biotechnology, 6
bipolar disorder, 62
Bissell, M. J., 239, 240
Black, A., 241
Black, W. C., 233, 240
Blake, G. J., 246
Blalock, J. E., 245
Bleiler, L., 242
blood-brain barrier, 42, 229
blood doping, 111–112, 211
blood flow, 45, 48
blood perfusion, to organs, 89–90
BMI (body mass index), 117–119, 235
body mass index (BMI), 117–119, 235
Boffey, P. M., 243
Bonawitz, N. D., 245
bone marrow stem cells, 13
bottom-up causation, DNA-directed synthesis
    as, 203
Boutwell, R. K. (scientist), 146, 239
brain, 163–176
    age-associated neurodegenerative diseases of,
        168–176
    cancer in, 130–131
    computational capacity of, 225
    information processing by, 165
    mental states and, 166
    mind and body, 167–168
    modularity and plasticity of, 167
    neural plasticity of, 62, 85, 211
    overview, 163–164
Brain Activity Map initiative, 176
Brave New World (Huxley), 7
breast cancer, 147
Brockman, M., 231
Broeck, D., 226
Brookmeyer, R., 243
Brownian motion, 37, 211
Buklijas, T., 237
Bullock, T. H., 226
Bulsara, M., 234
Buys, S. S., 241

C

CABG (coronary artery bypass graft), 211
cachexia, tumor (wasting disease), 139, 143, 150,
    211
CAD (coronary artery disease), 120, 236
calorie restriction (CR) diets, 184, 244–245
Cambier, J., 244
Campisi, J., 244, 245, 246
cancer, 134–162

aging and, 178*f*
bipolar disorder negatively correlated with, 62
brain, 130–131
complexity of, 16, 98, 141–146
consolidated view of, 150–152
DNA methylation disruption and, 126
drug evaluation for, 233
ductal carcinoma in situ (DCIS), 94, 96, 155
as evolutionary and ecological process, 147–148
false-positive test rates, 100*t*
five-year survival rates, 99*t*
gene mutations and, 63
immune deficiency and, 183
leukemia, 241
lung, 136–137, 148
lymphoma, 241
mortality rates, 136*f*, 137*f*
as multistage process, 146–147
overview, 135–141, 211
pediatric, 235, 239
prevention, 158–162
proliferation barriers to, 202
risk factors, 160*t*
screening, 155–158
self-assembly capacity of, 59–60
skin, 236
as systems biology problem, 148–150
treatment of, 152–154
tumor growth *versus* stromal forces, 49–50
two-species competition model of, 196
World Health Organization's International Agency
    for Research on Cancer (IARC), 130
Cannon, W. B. (physiologist), 76, 90, 224, 231, 250
Cantet, C., 242
capacitance, in cell membranes, 38–39, 42, 211
capillaries, 45–47, 46*f*
carbonic acid-bicarbonate buffer, 81
cardiac power, 48
cardiomyocyte, 119, 211
cardiovascular diseases, 117, 177.
    See also heart disease
cardiovascular system, 47–49
Carnes, B. A., 245
Carroll, L. (author), 25
Carroll, M. D., 235
Cartesian dualism, 167
Cartwright, N. B., 224
Cassell, C., 245
Castellani, B., 247
catheterization, heart, 114, 211
causation, 67, 198, 203, 211, 236.
    See also cigarette smoking, as causal factor
cells
    action at level of, 49–50
    age-related molecular damage to, 180–182
    cell cycle checkpoint machinery, 181
    proliferation *vs.* differentiation, 12–13
central obesity, 116–118
Chaisson, C., 246
Chaisson, E. J., 229, 250

Chandramohan, D., 235
Changeaux, J. P., 224, 228, 232, 242, 250
channels, in neurons, 40–41
chaos
    definition of, 211
    deterministic, 57
    disproportionate response in, 56
    living system resiliency and fragility explained by,
        200
    "noise" *versus*, 58
    stability *versus* adaptability and, 77–78
    unpredictability from, 54
chaos theory, 2–3, 68
chaperone proteins, 34
chemotherapy, 145, 152, 211, 240, 241
Chencharick, J., 246
Cheyne-Stokes respiration, 91, 211
Chin, J., 242, 243
Chlebowski, R. T., 239
cholera, 32–33, 225–226
Chorzempa, A., 237
Chou, R., 231, 241
chronic degenerative diseases, 16, 102–103.
    See also Alzheimer's disease
chronic myelogenous leukemia (CML), 153
Chu, E., 233
cigarette smoking, as causal factor
    in cancer and heart disease, 130, 136, 148, 158
    in complex disease, 128
    mutagenic chemicals in, 236, 239
Clark, C. M., 243
classical laws of physics, 19
Cleeman, J. I., 235
climate system, complexity of, 27, 54
"clinical horizon" of tumors, 134
closed systems, 21–22, 25, 212
CML (chronic myelogenous leukemia), 153
codons, 212, 220
cognitive sciences, 6
coherence, larger-scale, 59
Colditz, G. A., 241
Collins, K. M., 238
Colman, R. J., 244
Colmes, R. H., 246
colorectal cancer, 126
combination therapies, as cancer treatment, 152
comorbidities, 116, 168, 212
complexity paradox, overview of, 1–17
    book overview, 15–17
    chaos theory, 2–3
    complex structure of living systems, 8–9
    definition, 212
    determinate *vs.* indeterminate systems, 1–2
    emergence concept, 5–6
    energy in living systems, 9–11
    fractal anatomy, 3–4
    growth and development in living systems, 12–13
    information retrieval in living systems, 7–8
    life redefined, 13–15
    response to change by living systems, 11–12

complexity paradox, overview of (*Cont.*)
  stability and adaptive capacity, 4–5
  See also biological complexity
computed tomography (CT) scans, 241
concentration gradient
  definition of, 215
  diffusion driven by, 20, 21*f*
  ion pumps for, 34–35
  membrane movement and, 33
  Na⁺ (sodium), 10*f*
  order in living systems from, 9
conditions, system, 52–55, 212
constancy theory (Bernard), 75–76, 90
Cooke, S., 243
Cori cycle, 212
coronary angiogram, 114, 212
coronary artery bypass graft (CABG), 211
coronary artery disease (CAD), 120, 236
CR (calorie restriction) diets, 184, 244–245
C-reactive protein, 128
Crespi, B., 240
Cronin, K. A., 233
Croswell, J. M., 231
CT (computed tomography) scans, 241
Cubbon, R., 235, 236, 237
cultural model of medicine and disease, 110
curative therapy, 95*f*, 103
cybernetics, 76
cytokines, inflammatory, 178*f*, 189–190
cytology, 155, 212
cytolysis, 212

D

Dale, K. M., 246
Dana, T., 231
Daniels, S. R., 235
Dantico, M., 238
Darwin, C. (naturalist), 75–76
Daugherty, J. R., 233
Davies, K. E., 228
Davies, P. (scientist), 22, 224, 225, 229, 230, 250
DCIS (ductal carcinoma in situ), 94, 96, 155, 212
Debasish, S., 226
deficiency diseases, 96
degeneracy of systems, 84, 129, 202–203
de Grey, A. (aging researcher), 186–187, 245
de la Monte, S. M., 243
dementia
  Alzheimer's disease *versus*, 174
  definition of, 212
  example of, 163–164
  mind-body problem in, 168–170
  See also Alzheimer's disease
demyelination of axons, 44
depolarization of membranes, 39–41, 40*f*, 44, 212
depression, 44, 62
DeRubeis, R. J., 228
de Ruyter van Steveninck, R. R., 226

Descartes, R. (mathematician), 5, 167, 223
detection efficiency, 73
determinism
  biophysical, 42
  definition of, 213
  in disease diagnosis, 31
  indeterminate systems *versus*, 1–2
  in laws of life, 30–31
  limits of, in living systems, 28–29
  Newtonian mechanics and, 19
  simple causal relationships in, 27
deterministic chaos, 57, 212
Deutsch, D., 242, 246, 250
DeVita, V. T., 233
diabetes
  brain, 172
  type 1, 70, 235
  type 2, 119–120, 129–130, 213, 235
diagnosis, medical, 95*f*
diet
  antioxidants in, 188
  CR (calorie restriction), 184
  metabolic syndrome and, 131
differentiation of cells, 12–13, 213
diffusion
  Brownian motion for, 37
  concentration gradients driving, 20, 21*f*
  description of, 33
  Fick's law of, 38, 58, 226
  ion pumps for, 34–35
  movement across membranes by, 33–34
  osmosis as, 36
  second law of thermodynamics and, 23
  simple, 35, 35*f*
digital rectal examination (DRE), 157
Discourse on Method (Descartes), 167
disease
  behavioral disorders, 166
  biological complexity in, 66–69
  complexity in, 112–113
  cultural model of medicine and, 110
  definition of, 213
  determinism in diagnosis of, 31
  as deviation from homeostasis, 89–91
  early detection of, 99–107
  evidence-based biomedical model of, 110
  medical treatment variation, 109–111
  organic, 83, 218
  scalability of, 195
  social and cultural definition, 107–109
  as stochastic process, 204
  See also aging; cancer; emergence medicine;
    metabolic syndrome
disposable soma theory of aging (Kirkwood), 180,
  182
dissipative structures
  cancer tumors as, 142–143, 150
  definition of, 213
  far-from-equilibrium conditions for, 54

Prigogine work on, 23
diuretics, 229
DNA (deoxyribonucleic acid)
    bottom-up causation directed by, 203
    cell information stored in, 7–8
    description of, 213
    energy-dependent order built by, 23–24
    methylation disruption in, 126
    mutation increase with age, 180–181
    spontaneous damage to, 230
    telomere shortening in, 180
Dobzhansky, T. (geneticist), 198, 223, 247
Doll, R. (epidemiologist), 148, 159, 238, 241
Dollinger, M., 234
Domann, F. E., 236, 237, 240, 247
Donnenberg, A. D., 240
Donnenberg, V. S., 240
dopamine, 44
Dow, M. W., 242
Dowdy, D., 236
Down syndrome patients, Alzheimer's disease
    and, 170
Drazner, M. H., 235
DRE (digital rectal examination), 157
drugs
    analgesic, 88t, 209
    anti-inflammatory, 190
    cancer, 233
    dose vs. response curves, 104, 104f
    homeostasis perturbations by, 90
    nootropic, 175
    plasma half-life of, 87, 88t, 89f
    thalidomide toxicity, 247
Druker, B. J., 240
dualism doctrine (Descartes), 5
ductal carcinoma in situ (DCIS), 94, 96, 155, 212
Dunlop, D., 234
Dutta, R., 227
dyslipidemia, 120, 129–130, 213

E

Eagleman, D. M., 231
early detection of disease, 99–107
    cancer mortality and, 137
    cancer survival rates based on, 99–100, 99t
    complication versus cure in, 105–107
    diagnostic and screening test value, 100–102
    medical intervention, 102–103
    for successful management, 133
    therapy decisions, 103–105
Eason, E., 246
Ebbeling, C. B., 235
ECF (extracellular fluid), 45, 214, 228
echocardiogram, stress, 234
Ecker, J. R., 230
Eddingon, A. S. (scientist), 22, 225
Edelman, G. M., 232, 247
edema, 47, 213

"edge of chaos," 54, 200
edges, in networks, 63, 213
efficiency, theoretical limits of, 22
Egger, G., 236
Einstein, A. (physicist), 15, 224
electrical charges, 38–44
electrochemical gradients, 38
elementalism, 17, 194, 213
emergence concept
    in aging, 192
    in biological complexity, 59–62
    brain, 165–166
    in cancer, 138–139
    minimal level of complexity in, 29
    overview of, 5–6, 213
emergence medicine
    complex disease management, 203–207
    complexity dimensions in, 196–197
    evolution versus functional dynamics, 197–199
    natural system unpredictability, 199–202
    overview, 193–196
    unified theory of biology, 202–203
Enck, P., 242
ENCODE (Encyclopedia of DNA Elements)
    project, 64–65
Encyclopedia of DNA Elements (ENCODE)
    project, 64–65
endothelium, vascular, 119, 213
energy
    environmental exchanges in open systems, 24
    in living systems, 9–11
    processing of, 20–25
energy flow density, 10–11, 11f, 197, 213,
    224, 246
engines, efficiency of, 22
Enos, W. F., 246
enterotoxin, 32, 213
entropy
    definition of, 213
    movement toward, 15
    in natural systems, 1
    process movement determined by, 22
environmental energy exchanges, 24
environmental factors
    cancer growth promoted by, 138
    disease probability from, 122–124, 123f
    genetic factors versus, 126–131, 127t
environmental signal discrimination, 39
enzymes, 40–41, 62
epidemiology, 124, 159, 213
epigenetics, 123–126, 123f, 149, 203, 213
epithelial cells, 32, 36, 46, 126, 213
Epstein-Barr virus, 139, 183, 227
equilibrium
    death as, 53
    definition of, 214
    far-from-equilibrium conditions, 54
    as steady-state special case, 9
erythropoietin, 94, 111, 211, 214

Ethyol (amifostine, radiation therapy drug),
    245–246
etiology, 96, 113, 123–124, 144, 214
European Union (EU), 161
evidence-based biomedical model, 110
evolution, 5, 15, 199
exchange surfaces, 36
excitable membranes, 39, 214
extracellular fluid (ECF), 45, 214, 228

F

facilitated diffusion, 34, 214
false-negative and -positive medical test rates,
    100–102, 214
Faraday, M. (scientist), 19
far-from-equilibrium conditions, 54
Farias, G., 243
Fearon, E. R., 240
feedback
    classical physics laws *versus,* 26
    life controlled by, 78–81
    negative, 65
    in systems-control engineering, 76
Feinberg, A. P., 237
Feldman, F. A., 235
fetal environmental factors, 124
FFAs (free fatty acids), 119–120
fibroblast, 119–120, 180, 214
Fick's law of diffusion, 38, 58, 226
Fidler, I. J., 239
Finkel, T., 244
first law of thermodynamics, 20
Fisch, A., 226
Flegal, K. M., 235
Fleming, M. T., 231
"flight-or-fight" response, 71–72, 180, 246
florbetapir (Amyvid) tracer for Alzheimer's
    disease, 174
fluid dynamics, 25
fluoxetine (Prozac), 44
fMRI (functional magnetic resonance imaging),
    166, 166f
forces of nature, 32–50
    cardiovascular system, 47–49
    at cellular level, 49–50
    diffusion, 33–37
    electrical charges, 38–44
    movement, 45–47
Ford, E. (geneticist), 148
formalism, 1
Foulds, L., 239
Fournier, J. C., 228
fractal anatomy, 3–4
fractal geometry and physiology, 58–59, 214
fragility in living systems, 85
Frank, S. A., 239, 240
Frankenstein (Shelley), 14
Frayling, T. M., 235

free fatty acids (FFAs), 119–120
free radicals, 189, 214
Frisoni, G. B., 243
FTO (fat mass and obesity-associated) gene, 118,
    214
functional dynamics, 197–199, 214
functional magnetic resonance imaging(fMRI),
    166, 166f
Furukawa, K., 237
Futscher, B. E., 236, 237, 240, 247

G

GABA (gamma-aminobutyric acid), 44
Gale, E. A. M., 235
Gally, J. A., 232, 247
gamma-aminobutyric acid (GABA), 44
Gatenby, R. A., 247
Gazzaniga, M. S., 223, 232
Gell-Mann, M. (physicist), 55, 230
gender, as disease risk factor, 121
generalized inflammatory response, 47
gene silencing, 125, 214
genetic and environmental factors in disease,
    126–131, 127t
genetic biomarkers, 106–107
genetic code, 84, 214
genetic diseases, 96
genetic drift, 147, 214
genetic mutations. *See* mutations
genotoxic agents, 159, 215
genotype-phenotype dynamic, 123f, 203, 219
Gerich, J. E., 237
Gerlinger, M., 240
gerontology, 186, 215
Gerwirtz, P., 243
gestaltism. *See* emergence concept; emergence
    medicine
Giaccia, A. J., 246
Gibson, D. G., 223
Gillies, R. J., 247
Gillik, M. R., 234
Glass, L., 230, 232
Gleevec drug treatment for CML, 153
Gleick, J., 230, 246, 247, 249
glioblastoma (brain tumor), 139f, 215
gliomas (brain tumors), 131, 238
Global Burden of Disease Study 2010, 247–248
Gluckman, P. D., 237
Go, A. S., 234
Godtfredsen, N. S., 239, 241
Gohlke, H., 238
Goldberger, A. L., 230–231
Goldman equation, 38–39, 215, 227
Gompertzian growth model, 244
Gould, S. J., 238
gradient. *See* concentration gradient
Gray, S., 243
Greaves, M., 239

Grinnell, A., 226
Groopman, J. E., 225, 234
Gross, C. G., 247
Grotmaker, S. L., 235
growth and development in living systems, 12–13
Grubbs, R., 237
Grundy, S. M., 235
Guarente, L., 244, 245
Guerrero-Bosagna, C., 236
Gupta, S., 240

H
Hadley, E. C., 242, 245
Hafferty, F. W., 247
half-life, 86–89, 88*t*, 89*f*, 215
Hall, E. J., 246
Hall, K. D., 235
Hampel, H., 243
Hanahan, D., 238, 239
Hansen, E., 242
Hanson, M. A., 237
Hardy, J., 243
Hare, R. D., 242
Harris, S., 242
Harvard University, 76
Harvey, W. (scientist), 5, 167
Hauser, W., 242
Hawking, S. (physicist), 225
Hayflick, L. (microbiologist), 180, 244
"Hayflick limit," 180, 215
hCG (human chorionic gonadotropin), 198, 215
HDL-cholesterol, 114–115, 130, 215
heart disease
  aging and, 178*f*
  anti-inflammatory drugs to reduce risk of, 190
  complexity of, 98
  in metabolic syndrome, 120
  mortality rates, 13*f*, 103, 136*f*
heart pacemaker, oscillatory behavior of, 67–68, 82–83, 83*f*
heart rate, irregularity in, 56–57, 57*f*
Heavner, J. E., 227
Hegi, M. E., 238
Heisenberg uncertainty principle, 230
Heller, C., 226
Heller, G., 231
hemodynamics, 25, 215
Henderson, L. J., 231
Hill, A. B. (epidemiologist), 148
Hillis, D. M., 226
Hippocrates, 76
His-Purkinje network, 3–4
histamine, 47
HIV (human immunodeficiency virus), 121, 183, 215
HMG-CoA, 215
Hollon, S. D., 228
homeostasis

complexity description of, 68–69
  definition of, 215
  description of, 224
  disease as deviation from, 16, 89–91
  environmental response and, 12
  feedback control for, 78
  milieu interieur described by, 76
  physiologic adjustments to maintain, 9
  as stability in living systems, 73
homocysteine, 128, 215
hormone replacement therapy (HRT), 147
Horvath, C., 226
host factors, 95, 113, 127, 215
Houghton, P. J., 245
HRT (hormone replacement therapy), 147
Huang, S., 245
human chorionic gonadotropin (hCG), 198, 215
Human Genome Project, 65, 106, 176, 203
human immunodeficiency virus
  (HIV), 121, 183
Huxley, A. F. (author), 7, 227
hydatidiform mole, 198, 215
hydrostatic pressure, 45–47, 46*f*
hyperlipidemia, 190, 216
hyperpolarization of membranes, 39, 216
hypertension
  causal factors not well understood, 103
  definition of, 216
  scalability of, 98
  screening for, 109*f*
  unpredictability of, 224
hypotension, 110, 216
hypothalamus, 37, 80
hypoxia, 202, 216

I
iatrogenic effect, 216
Ichiro Kawachi, I., 243
IGF1 pathway mutations, 186
immune system failure, in aging, 182–183, 183*f*, 216
Inch, R. S., 234
indeterminate *vs.* determinate systems, 1–2
Industrial Revolution, 22
infectious disease management, 239
inflammatory processes
  in aging and chronic diseases, 178*f*, 189–190
  definition of, 216
  self-assembly capacity in, 59–60
information retrieval in living systems, 7–8
information technology, 6
Institute of Medicine, 237
insulin. *See* diabetes
Insulin Resistance Syndrome.
  See metabolic syndrome
insulin signaling, 129
interleukins, in inflammatory response, 178, 216
internal energy, 22, 24, 216

International Statistical Classification of Diseases and Related Health Problems (ICD, World Health Organization), 96, 233
interstitial fluid, 45–47, 81, 216
intrauterine growth restriction, 124–125
ion channels, 38, 216
ionizing radiation, 159–160
ion pumps, 34–35, 40
irreversibility, in natural systems, 1
ischemia, 202, 216, 246
isothermal processes, 23, 216

J

J. Craig Venter Institute, 7, 13
Jemal, A., 238
Jenkins, G. W., 229
Jessell, T. M., 227
Jobs, S. (Apple, Inc., founder), 187, 245
Johnson, C. L., 235
Jonsson, T., 243
"junk DNA," 65

K

Kahn, M., 235
Kandel, E. R., 227
Kanwal, R., 240
Kapadia, S. R., 234, 237
Kaptoge, S., 235
Karim, M., 226
Karns, C. M., 242
Kauffman, S., 229, 231, 240, 249–250
Kawas, C., 243
Kearney, M. T., 235
Kelly, K., 247
Kemnitz, C. P., 229
Kenny, P. A., 239, 240
kidneys, osmoregulation by, 37, 227
Kiehl, K. A., 242
Kirkwood, T. (biologist), 180, 243, 244
Kleinsmith, L. J., 230, 239, 240, 244, 247
Knight, J. R., 234
Koch, R. (microbiologist), 97–98
Koch's postulates, 233
Koeppen, B. M., 231
Kraemer, K. H., 236
Krogsboll, L., 247
Kubrick, S. (film maker), 6

L

Lachish, U., 226
Lacroix, R., 246
Lakatta, E. G., 242, 245
Lambert, J. C., 243
Laplace, P.-S. (mathematician), 1, 57, 223
larger-scale coherence, 59
Lasley, E. N., 231
Laughlin, S. B., 226
Lawrence, T. S., 233
laws of life, 18–31

deterministic, 30–31
energy processing, 20–25
life laws *versus*, 18–20
physics and reductionism, 28–30
prediction accuracy of, 25–28
laws of thermodynamics, 225. *See also* second law of thermodynamics
LDL cholesterol, 114–115, 121, 129–130, 216
lesions. *See* cancer
leukemia, 241
Levin, R., 247
Levy, D., 235
Lewin, R., 249
Lewis, G., 234
Liang, G., 236
Libby, P., 246
life, free and independent, 70–91
acid-base buffers, 81
feedback control, 78–81
homeostasis for, 89–91
random processes in, 86–89
reliable systems for, 83–86
rhythms, 82–83
stability, 71–78
life laws, laws of life *versus*, 18–20
life spans, 185–187, 187f
Lilly, L. S., 246
Lim, S. S., 248
linear dynamics, 1
linear nonthreshold (LNT) function, in cancer risk factors, 160–161
lipogenesis, 120, 216
Lipsitz, L. A., 231
living systems
complex structure of, 8–9
energy in, 9–11
growth and development in, 12–13
information retrieval in, 7–8
redefined, 13–15
response to change by, 11–12
stability and adaptive capacity in, 4–5
Lloyd-Jones, D. M., 234
LNT (linear nonthreshold) function, in cancer risk factors, 160–161, 2161
Loeb, L. A., 238
Lonn, S., 237
Lopaschuk, G. D., 236
Lorenz, E., 230
Loustaunau, M. O., 234
Lozano, R., 248
lumen of small intestine, 32, 36, 48, 97, 217
lung cancer, 136–137, 148
lungs, 36, 58–59, 59f
Lydon, N. B., 240
lymphatic system, 47, 217
lymphomas, 183, 241

M

Maccioni, R. B., 243
Mackey, M. C., 230, 232

MacKinnon, R., 227
Macklem, P., 248
macrophage, 190, 217
Maley, C. C., 239
mammography screening, 102, 102*f*
Mandelblatt, J. S., 233, 241
Manikkam, M., 236
Maravec, N., 225
Marsh, G. N., 234
Martin, M., 229
Martinson, M. L., 243
Mascie-Taylor, C. G. N., 234
Mason, W. P., 238
Mathewkutty, S., 235
Mattison, J. A., 244–245
Maxwell, J. C. (scientist), 19, 226
Mazoteras, M. V., 242
McCabe, S. E., 234
McCall, R. P., 229
McEwen, B. (physiologist), 77, 231
McGregor, J. L., 245
McGuire, D. K., 235
McKane, A. J., 225
McQuaid, J., 232
MDR (multiple drug resistance) transport
     proteins, 150
Medawar, P. B. (biologist), 179, 244
medical treatment, variation in, 109–111
medicine. *See* emergence medicine
Medvedev, Z. A., 243
Mehlman, M. J., 234
meiosis, 224
Mellbin, L., 238
Melzack, R., 246
membrane resting potential, 38–39, 165, 217, 227
membranes
     acid-base buffers and, 81
     concentration gradients for movement across, 33
     conductance of, 217
     electrical charge movement across, 38
     excitable, 39
     nerve, 40
     permeability of, 34, 35*f*
     water transport across, 36
memory loss, 176
mental states, 166
Merlo, L. M. F., 239, 240
messenger RNA (ribonucleic acid), 7, 217
metabolic syndrome, 114–133
     causes and risks, 120–126
     definition of, 217
     diabetes, 119–120
     genetic and environmental factors, 126–131
     heart disease, 120
     obesity, 117–119
     overview, 114–117
     preventive measures for, 131–133
metabolism, 9–11, 183–185
metastable states, 94, 141, 153, 217
metastasis, 138, 146, 217. *See also* cancer

milieu interieur (Bernard), 75, 90
Mister, S. J., 229
Mitchell, M., 246, 247, 250
Mitchell, S. D., 224, 237, 240, 250
mitogen, 152, 180, 217
mitosis, for cell proliferation, 12, 217
mobile phones, radiation from, 130–131, 161
modularity of brain, 167, 217
molecular pumps, 9
monoclonal antibody systems, 106
Morales, I., 243
morphology, 73, 180–181, 217
Morris, M. J., 231
Morrison-Bogorad, M., 243, 245
Mossman, K. L., 241, 245, 246, 247
movement, 45–47
Moyer, V. A., 241
mRNA (ribonucleic acid), 7, 217
MS (multiple sclerosis), 44, 227
mTOR longevity gene, 186
Mucke, L., 242
Mukherjee, S., 232, 238, 240, 241
multiple drug resistance (MDR) transport
     proteins, 150
multiple sclerosis (MS), 44, 227
multistage model of tumor growth, 141, 146–147
Mulvihill, S. J., 234
Murray, C. J. L., 248
mutation accumulation theory of aging
     (Medawar), 179
mutations
     age accumulation of, 180–181
     APP gene, 170
     cancer arising from, 63–64, 138, 146
     disease susceptibility from, 122, 123*f*
     genetic, 214
     genetic drift, 147
     in *IGF1* pathway, 186
     in *MYC* subnetwork, 63–64, 64*f*, 66, 148
     in *PSEN1* gene, 173
     MYC subnetwork, 63–64, 64*f*, 66, 148
myelin coating on nerve fibers, 42, 44
myosin, in skeletal muscle contractions, 45, 217,
     228

N

Nagy, J. D., 225, 232
nanotechnology, 6, 217
Na$^+$ (sodium) concentration gradients, 10*f*, 21*f*, 217
National Aeronautical and Space Administration
     (NASA), 19
National Cancer Act of 1971, 136
National Institutes of Health, 170
natural selection, 73, 75, 147–148, 179, 217
NBIC (nanotechnology, biotechnology,
     information technology, cognitive sciences)
     technologies, 6
negative feedback, in life control systems, 78–79,
     79*f*, 217

"negligible senescence" (de Grey), 245
Nemoto, S., 244
neo-Darwinism, 202, 217
neoplasias, 117, 217
nerve cells, excitable membranes in, 39–40
nerve impulse conduction, 23
nervous system, 33, 51
Nesse, R. M., 247
Nessim, S., 234
neural plasticity of brain, 62, 85, 165, 167, 219
neurodegenerative diseases
    age and, 168–176
    definition of, 218
    mind-body problem in, 167–168
    overview, 117
    See also aging; Alzheimer's disease
neuroenhancment, 111–112
neurofibrillary tangles (NFTs), in Alzheimer's
        disease, 187, 218
neurons, anatomy of, 43*f*
neurotransmitters, 44, 165, 227–228
Neville, H. J., 242
Newman, T. J., 225, 232
Newton, I. (scientist), 15, 19
Newton's laws of motion, 26, 228
New York Times, 250
NFTs (neurofibrillary tangles), in Alzheimer's
        disease, 187
Nickerson, C. A., 229
Nicolis, G., 231, 239
Niebly, J. R., 247
nocebo effect, 168, 218
nodes, in networks, 63, 218
nodes of Ranvier, in nerves, 42–43, 218
"noise," 58, 72
nonlinear dynamics, 2, 26
nootropic drugs, 175, 218
normal-tissue tolerance, 105
normative standards, for health, 108
normotensive range, for blood pressure, 29, 218
Nowak, K. J., 228
Nowell, P. C. (scientist), 147, 239

O
Obama, B. (U.S. president), 176
obesity, in metabolic syndrome, 116*f*, 117–119
O'Brien, J. T., 243
obsessive-compulsive disorder, 44
occlusion, 115, 218
Ockham's razor, 3
Ogden, C. L., 235
Ohm's law, 25, 38, 48
Oken, B. S., 242
Olshansky, S. J., 245
oncogenes, 154, 218, 230
open systems, 24, 197, 218
organ blood perfusion, 89–90
organic disease, 83, 218
Orkand, R., 226

Oryx and Crake (Atwood), 187
oscillating membrane potentials, 165
oscillatory behavior
    in biological systems, 65
    of bodily fluid concentrations, 77
    disease as changes in, 91
    heart pacemaker, 67–68, 82–83, 83*f*
Osler, M., 239
Osler, W. (physician), 206
osmoregulation, 37
osmosis
    cholera impact on, 32–33
    definition of, 218
    hydrostatic pressure and, 45–47, 46*f*
    second law of thermodynamics and, 23
    water transported by, 36
osmotic pressure, 229
Ott, C. M., 229
oxidative phosphorylation, 195, 218

P
Page, R. E., 240
palliative therapy, 95*f*, 103, 218
parasympathetic nervous system, 76, 218
Parkinson's disease, 44, 117, 139
paroxetine (Paxil), 44
Partridge, A. H., 241
Partridge, E., 241
pathogenesis, 125, 218
pathogenic diseases, 96, 218
pathophysiology, 69, 113, 153, 170, 218
Patterson, K. D., 233
Pavlopoulos, E., 243
Paxil (paroxetine), 44
Payer, L., 234
Pearce, M. S., 241
Penrose, R., 242, 250
Pepper, J. W., 239
perfusion, organ blood, 89–90, 219
peripheral excess body fat, 118
permeability of membranes, 34, 219
personality disorders, 44
personalized medicine, 106
Peto, J., 244, 247
Peto, R. (epidemiologist), 159, 238, 241
PET (positron emission tomography) imaging,
        166, 174, 219
p53 tumor suppression gene, 145, 181
pH control, 81
phenotype. *See* genotype-phenotype dynamic
physics, laws of, 19, 28–30
physiological diseases, 96–97
Picard, F., 244, 245
Pilkey, O. H., 247
Pilkey-Jarvis, L., 247
Pinney, S. E., 236
Piraino, S., 229
pituitary gland, posterior, 37
placebo effect, 167–168, 219

planetary motion, 15
plasma half-life of drugs, 87, 88t, 89f
plasticity. *See* brain
pleiotropy, 179, 185, 210, 219
Poincaré, H. (mathematician), 2, 57, 199, 223, 232, 247
Poiseuille's law, 48
polarity of membranes, 41, 219. *See also* membranes
polymorphism, 173, 219
pores, in neurons, 41
positive feedback, in life control systems, 80–81, 219
positive predictive value (PPV), in screening, 156f, 219, 240
positron emission tomography (PET) imaging, 166, 174, 219
potential energy, 21, 219
Poznansky, A., 225
PPV (positive predictive value), in screening, 156f, 219, 240
Prescott, E., 239
presenilin, 173, 219
pressure gradients, in heart function, 45
Preston, D. L., 237
prevention of cancer, 158–162
Prigogine, I. (scientist), 23, 224, 229, 231, 239, 240, 250
Prince, M., 242
proliferation of cells, 12–13
promotion stage, in tumor growth, 146, 181, 202
prophylaxis, 95f, 103, 131, 219
prostate specific antigen (PSA), 68, 101, 157, 220, 231
proteins
    aging effects on, 188–189
    apolipoprotien E, 173
    channel, carrier, and pump, 34
    C-reactive, 128
    MDR (multiple drug resistance) transport, 150
    messenger RNA (ribonucleic acid) regulation of, 7
    in neurons, 40
    RbAp48, memory loss and, 176
    in skeletal muscle contractions, 45
    tau, 171–175
proteomics, 68, 220
proto-oncogenes, 64f, 146, 148, 220, 230
proximal causation, 198
Prozac (fluoxetine), 44
PSA (prostate specific antigen), 68, 101, 157, 220, 231
PSEN1 gene mutations, 173
pseudodisease, 73, 94, 149, 155, 205, 220
public health policy, 204, 241. *See also* emergence medicine
Pyle, G. F., 233

Q

quiescent cells, 181, 220

R

radiation therapy, 106, 145, 152, 220
radiofrequency electromagnetic radiation, from mobile phones, 130–131
Ravusin, E., 235
Ray, W. A., 233
RbAp48 protein, memory loss and, 176
RB tumor suppression gene, 181
Reasner, C. A., 238
Reaven, G. M. (endocrinologist), 116, 235
receptors, 40–41, 44
recovery kinetics, 74–75
reductionism, 28–30, 30f, 220
redundancy of systems, 83–84, 129, 220
Reichman, N. E., 243
Reid, B. J., 239
reliable systems for life, 83–86
replication, biological complexity and, 15
reserve capacity, for reliability, 84–85, 85t, 232
response to change by living systems, 11–12
resting membrane potential, 38–39, 165, 220
rhythms of life, 82–83
Ridker, P. M., 246
Ringman, J. M., 243
risk factors. *See* aging; cancer; disease
Ritz, P., 227
Roberson, E. D., 242
robustness of systems, 83–84, 129, 220
Roger, V. L., 234
Rombo, L., 226
Rose, S., 232
Rosenbaum, E. H., 234
Rosenberg, S. A., 233
Roth, G. S., 245
Ryden, L., 238
Rzhetsky, A., 230

S

Sacks, G., 235
Sadava, D., 226
safety margins, 85
Sagan, D., 225, 229, 245, 250
Saif, M. W., 233
Salle, A., 227
saltatory conduction, in nerves, 42, 220
Sari, I., 235
saturation effects, 51
Saunders, J., 235
Schiffman, S. S., 246
schizophrenia, 62
Schleifstein, M., 232
Schneider, E. D., 225, 229, 245, 250
Schneider, J. A., 243
Schrödinger, E. (physicist), 13, 18, 23, 93, 201, 224, 225, 230, 250
Schrödinger's cat paradox, 93–95
Schwartz, J. H., 227
scientific determinism, 1

screening
  benefits of, 205
  cancer, 155–158, 156*f*
  medical, 95*f*
  sensitivity, specificity, and predictive value,
    240–241
Secemsky, E. A., 236
second law of thermodynamics
  importance of, 15
  in living systems, 20–25, 184
  osmosis consistent with, 36
  waste returned to environment, 197
"seed and soil" hypothesis, in cancer, 146, 153
selective serotonin reuptake inhibitor (SSRI)
    drugs, 44
self-assembly capacity, emergence as, 59–60
self-renewal capacity, for reliability, 84–85
senescence (cell aging)
  in cancer modeling, 202
  definition of, 220
  immunosenecence, 183*f*
  "negligible," 245
  to stop division of damaged cells, 244
  telomere shortening as, 180–182
  tumor cells constrained by, 192
sensitivity of detection, 73, 220, 240
sensory systems
  age-related losses in, 190–191
  environmental response and, 11–12
  resting membrane potential in, 39
  spontaneous nerve oscillation in, 83
  tracking in, 50
serotonin, 44
sertraline (Zoloft), 44
Seshsasai, S. R. K., 235
Shay, J. W., 244
Shearer, N. B. C., 238
Shelley, M. (author), 14
Shermer, M., 242
Sica, D. A., 237
Siegal, R., 238
signal discrimination, 72, 83
signal processing, 51
signs of disease, 31–32, 50, 220
silent information regulator *(SIR)* genes, 245
Silver, N., 223
Simard, G., 227
Simmons, R. A., 236
simple diffusion, 35, 35*f*
simple domain, 1
SIR (silent information regulator) genes, 245
skeletal muscle contraction and relaxation, 228
skin cancer, 236
Skinner, M. A., 236
Skloot, R., 240
Slor, H., 236
Smale, S., 246
small intestine, 36
Smith, A. M., 242

Smith, D. S., 234
Smith, E. M., 245
Smith, H. (scientist), 7
Snow, C. P. (author), 22, 225
Sobo, E. J., 234
sodium (Na⁺) concentration gradients, 10*f*, 21*f*
sodium-potassium pump, 38
solar ultraviolet (UV) light, 236
solute gradients, 35, 220
solvents, 34, 221
Soto, C., 243, 245
Soydinc, S., 235
species competition models, 246
specificity, 106, 130, 155–156, 221, 240
SSRI (selective serotonin reuptake inhibitors)
    drugs, 44, 221
stability in living systems, 71–78
  adaptability *versus*, 77–78
  allostasis, 77
  "flight-or-fight" response, 71–72
  homeostasis as, 73–74
  internal control for, 75–76
  overview, 4–5
  recovery kinetics, 74–75
  signal discrimination, 72–73
Stämpfli, R., 227
Starfield, B., 232
states, system, 92–113
  disease complexity, 112–113
  early disease detection, 99–107
  malfunctions in, 95–99
  medical treatment variation, 109–111
  neuroenhancment, 111–112
  overview, 52–55
  Schrödinger's cat paradox, 93–95
  social and cultural disease definition, 107–109
statin therapy, for hyperlipidemia, 190, 221
steady-state processes, 9, 10*f*, 65, 221
Stefanini, M. O., 225, 232
Stein, C. M., 233
Stein, Z., 237
Steinberg, S., 243
stem cells, 13, 94, 188, 221
Stewart, P. (US Supreme Court justice), 177
Stipp, D., 245
stochastic processes, 86–89, 204, 221
Stontop, B. A., 231
stress echocardiogram, 234
stress response, 72*f*
stroma, 49, 221
structural elements, in neurons, 40
Stupp, R., 238
suicide, 44
Summers, K., 240
Sunday Times of London, 247
Sunderland, V. B., 234
superposition, in quantum theory, 94, 221
supportive therapy, 103
surgery, as cancer treatment, 152

Swain, J. F., 235
Swinburn, B. A., 235
Sylven, C., 246
sympathetic nervous system, 76, 221
symptoms, 31–32, 50, 89, 95–97, 220.
    See also disease
synaptic membrane potentials, 165
Syndrome X. *See* metabolic syndrome
synergy, 153, 221
systems biology
    aging as problem of, 180
    cancer as problem in, 148–150
    definition of, 221
    holistic approach of, 65–66
    threshold level of complexity, 60
    See also biological complexity
Sznol, M., 233

T

tamoxifen breast cancer therapy, 147, 221
targeted therapies, 106, 153
taste stimulus-response function, 51–52, 53*f*
tau protein, 171–175, 221
Tchaikovsky, P. I. (composer), 32
Teitler, J. O., 243
telomere shortening, in DNA, 180, 222
Temparo, M., 234
temporal asymmetry, 51
tests, diagnostic. *See* screening
Teter, C. J., 234
thalidomide drug toxicity, 247
T helper cells (immune cells), 183
therapy-enhancement dynamic, 112, 222
thermodynamics, laws of, 20, 225.
    See also second law of thermodynamics
Thies, W., 242
Thompson, A., 235
threshold level of complexity, 60
thrombus, 117, 195, 222
Through the Looking Glass (Carroll), 25
Timpson, N. J., 235
Tirosh-Samuelson, H., 245
Tisdale, M. J., 238
tissue repair, senescence for, 181
tissue swelling, 47, 105
tobacco control, 130.
    See also cigarette smoking, as causal factor
tonicity, 226–227
top-down causation, epigenetics as, 203
Totora, G. J., 229
Trans Alaska Pipeline System, 48
transcription regulatory network, 63, 63*f*
transplant medicine, 56, 183
Trapp, B. D., 227
Tsang, C. K., 245
Tseng, Z. H., 236
tumor cachexia (wasting disease), 139, 143, 150, 211, 222

tumor suppression, 181, 222
turgor pressure, 37, 222
Tutar, E., 234, 237
Tuzcu, E. M., 234, 237
two-species competition model, 196
2001: A Space Odyssey (film), 6

U

ultimate causation, 198
uncertainty, 1
unified theory of biology, 202–203
Uniform Definition of Death Act of 1980, 224
United States Preventative Task Force,
    156–157, 241

V

Van't Hoff's law, 226
vascular endothelium, 119, 213, 222
vasoconstriction, 48, 222
vasodilation, 48, 222
vasopressin (ADH), 37
Venter, J. C. (scientist), 7
villi, in small intestine, 36, 222
Vioxx (NSAID), 105, 233
Virchow, R. (pathologist), 158
viruses, 224
vitalism, 75, 222
vitamin D, 227
vitamin E, 188
Vogelstein, B., 237, 240
voltage across membranes, 38
voltage-gating, 40–41, 222

W

Wallace, R. B., 234
Wands, J. R., 243
Ward, E., 238
waste energy, 16, 22–25, 222, 229, 244
wasting disease, from tumor cachexia, 139, 143, 150
water, osmosis to transport, 36
water channels (aquaporins), 32
Wechsler, H., 234
Weedom, M. N., 235
Weibel, E. R., 230
Weibull failure model, 182, 244
Weinberg, A., 232
Weinberg, R. A., 238, 239
Welch, H. G., 231, 233, 240
wellness model of healthcare management, 234
West, B. J., 230
What Is Life? (Schrödinger), 13, 23, 201, 224, 225
Whewell, J. B., 234
Wiener, N. (mathematician), 76, 225, 231
Willett, W. C., 237, 247
William of Ockham, 3
Williams, G. C. (biologist), 179, 185, 244, 245, 247
Wilmoth, J. R., 245

Wimo, A., 242
Winer, E. P., 241
Wisdom of the Body (Cannon), 76
Wolfram, S., 247
World Health Organization, 130, 233
Wright, W. E., 244

X
xeroderma pigmentosum, 236

Xu, J., 238

Y
Young, J. L., 246

Z
Zimmet, P. Z., 235
Zoloft (sertraline), 44
Zuckerman, J., 226